Advances in
PARASITOLOGY

VOLUME 75

Chagas Disease, Part A

Advances in PARASITOLOGY

VOLUME **75**

Chagas Disease, Part A

Edited by

LOUIS M. WEISS
Departments of Pathology and Medicine,
Albert Einstein College of Medicine, Bronx
New York, USA

HERBERT B. TANOWITZ
Departments of Pathology and Medicine,
Albert Einstein College of Medicine, Bronx
New York, USA

LOUIS V. KIRCHHOFF
Departments of Internal Medicine and Epidemiology,
Department of Veterans Affairs Medical Center,
University of Iowa, Iowa, USA

ELSEVIER

AMSTERDAM • BOSTON • HEIDELBERG • LONDON
NEW YORK • OXFORD • PARIS • SAN DIEGO
SAN FRANCISCO • SINGAPORE • SYDNEY • TOKYO
Academic Press is an imprint of Elsevier

Academic Press is an imprint of Elsevier

32 Jamestown Road, London, NW1 7BY, UK
525 B Street, Suite 1900, San Diego, CA 92101-4495, USA
225 Wyman Street, Waltham, MA 02451, USA
Radarweg 29, PO Box 211, 1000 AE Amsterdam, The Netherlands

First edition 2011

ISBN: 978-0-12-385863-4
ISSN: 0065-308X

For information on all Academic Press publications
visit our website at www.elsevierdirect.com

Printed and bound by CPI Group (UK) Ltd, Croydon, CR0 4YY

Transferred to Digital Print 2012

CONTENTS OF VOLUME 75

CONTENTS OF VOLUME 76

CONTRIBUTORS OF VOLUME 75

Andrea Rodrigues Ávila
Instituto Carlos Chagas, ICC—Fiocruz-PR, Rua Prof. Algacyr Munhoz Mader, Curitiba, PR, Brazil

Patrícia R. Araújo
Departamento de Bioquímica e Imunologia, Universidade Federal de Minas Gerais, Belo Horizone, MG, Brazil

Caryn Bern
Parasitic Diseases Branch, Division of Parasitic Diseases and Malaria, Centers for Disease Control and Prevention, Atlanta, Georgia, USA

John Blangero
Department of Genetics, Texas Biomedical Research Institute, San Antonio, Texas, USA

Frederick S. Buckner
Department of Medicine, University of Washington, Seattle, Washington, USA

Antonio C. Campos de Carvalho
Carlos Chagas Filho Institute of Biophysics, Federal University of Rio de Janeiro and National Cardiology Institute, Rio de Janeiro, RJ, Brazil

Adriana B. Carvalho
Carlos Chagas Filho Institute of Biophysics, Federal University of Rio de Janeiro and National Cardiology Institute, Rio de Janeiro, RJ, Brazil

Rodrigo Corrêa-Oliveira
Centro de Pesquisas Rene Rachou, FIOCRUZ; and Instituto Nacional de Ciencia e Tecnologia em Doenças Tropicais—INCTDT, BeloHorizonte, MinasGerais, Brazil

Roberto Docampo
Department of Cellular Biology and Center for Tropical and Global Emerging Diseases, University of Georgia, Athens, Georgia, USA

Patricia L. Dorn
Department of Biological Sciences, Loyola University of New Orleans, New Orleans, Los Angeles, USA

Najib M. El-Sayed
Department of Cell Biology and Molecular Genetics, Center for Bioinformatics and Computational Biology, University of Maryland, College Park, Maryland, USA

Nisha Jain Garg
Department of Microbiology and Immunology; Department of Pathology; Member of the Institute for Human Infections and Immunity, University of Texas Medical Branch, Galveston, Texas, USA

Robert H. Gilman
Johns Hopkins University Bloomberg School of Public Health, Baltimore, Maryland, USA

Regina C.S. Goldenberg
Carlos Chagas Filho Institute of Biophysics, Federal University of Rio de Janeiro and National Cardiology Institute, Rio de Janeiro, RJ, Brazil

Samuel Goldenberg
Instituto Carlos Chagas, ICC—Fiocruz-PR, Rua Prof. Algacyr Munhoz Mader, Curitiba, PR, Brazil

Shivali Gupta
Department of Microbiology and Immunology, University of Texas Medical Branch, Galveston, Texas, USA

Huan Huang
Department of Pathology, Albert Einstein College of Medicine, Bronx, New York, USA

Linda A. Jelicks
Department of Physiology and Biophysics, Albert Einstein College of Medicine, Bronx, New York, USA

Veronica Jimenez
Department of Cellular Biology and Center for Tropical and Global Emerging Diseases, University of Georgia, Athens, Georgia, USA

John M. Kelly
Department of Pathogen Molecular Biology, London School of Hygiene and Tropical Medicine, London, United Kingdom

Sharon King-Keller
Department of Cellular Biology and Center for Tropical and Global Emerging Diseases, University of Georgia, Athens, Georgia, USA

Louis V. Kirchhoff
Departments of Internal Medicine and Epidemiology; and Department of Veterans Affairs Medical Center, University of Iowa, Iowa City, Iowa, USA

John H. Klotz
Department of Entomology, University of California Riverside, Riverside, California, USA

Stephen A. Klotz
Section of Infectious Diseases, University of Arizona, Tucson, Arizona, USA

Galina I. Lepesheva
Department of Biochemistry School of Medicine, Vanderbilt University, Nashville, Tennessee, USA

Zhu-hong Li
Department of Cellular Biology and Center for Tropical and Global Emerging Diseases, University of Georgia, Athens, Georgia, USA

David Lucero
Department of Biology, University of Vermont, Burlington, Vermont, USA

Diana L. Martin
Parasitic Diseases Branch, Division of Parasitic Diseases and Malaria, Centers for Disease Control and Prevention, Atlanta, Georgia, USA

Silvia N.J. Moreno
Department of Cellular Biology and Center for Tropical and Global Emerging Diseases, University of Georgia, Athens, Georgia, USA

Sheila C. Nardelli
Departamento de Microbiologia, Imunologia e Parasitologia, Universidade Federal de São Paulo, São Paulo, Brazil

Bruno dos Santos Pascoalino
Departamento de Microbiologia, Imunologia e Parasitologia, Universidade Federal de São Paulo, São Paulo, Brazil

Sergio Schenkman
Departamento de Microbiologia, Imunologia e Parasitologia, Universidade Federal de São Paulo, São Paulo, Brazil; and Center for Tropical and Emerging Diseases, University of Georgia, Athens, Georgia, USA

Justin O. Schmidt
Southwestern Biological Institute, Tucson, Arizona, USA

Lori Stevens
Department of Biology, University of Vermont, Burlington, Vermont, USA

Herbert B. Tanowitz
Departments of Pathology; and Department of Medicine, Albert Einstein College of Medicine, Bronx, New York, USA

Martin C. Taylor
Department of Pathogen Molecular Biology, London School of Hygiene and Tropical Medicine, London, United Kingdom

Santuza M. Teixeira
Departamento de Bioquímica e Imunologia, Universidade Federal de Minas Gerais, Belo Horizone, MG, Brazil

Juan C. Vázquez-Chagoyán
Centro de Investigación y Estudios Avanzados en Salud Animal, Facultad de Medicina Veterinaria y Zootecnia, Universidad Autónoma de Estado de México, Toluca, Mexico

John L. VandeBerg
Department of Genetics, Texas Biomedical Research Institute; and Southwest National Primate Research Center, San Antonio, Texas, USA

Fernando Villalta
Department of Microbiology and Immunology, Meharry Medical College, Nashville, Tennessee, USA

Michael R. Waterman
Department of Biochemistry School of Medicine, Vanderbilt University, Nashville, Tennessee, USA

Sarah Williams-Blangero
Department of Genetics, Texas Biomedical Research Institute, San Antonio, Texas, USA

Louis M. Weiss
Departments of Pathology and Medicine, Albert Einstein College of Medicine, Bronx, NY, USA

PREFACE

Chagas disease or American trypanosomiasis is caused by the hemoflagellate *Trypanosoma cruzi* which was first described by Carlos Chagas shortly after the turn of the twentieth century. Chagas disease has been designated a neglected tropical disease designated by the World Health Organization and the National Institutes of Health. Interestingly, palaeoparasitological studies have shown that *T. cruzi* was present in tissues obtained from mummies in northern Chile and southern Peru from the period 4000 BC to AD 1400, obviously long before it was discovered by Carlos Chagas in 1909 (Aufderheide et al., 2004).

Carlos Justiniano Ribeiro das Chagas (Fig. 1A and B) was born in the state of Minas Gerais, Brazil, on 9 July 1879, and after his basic education and a brief brush with engineering in the city of Ouro Preto, he began his studies of medicine in Rio de Janeiro where he trained under the guidance of Dr. Oswaldo Cruz. After graduation from medical school, while working in 1909 as a malaria control officer in Lassance, Minas Gerias, Chagas observed microscopic flagellated organisms in the blood of a febrile child named Berenice. When the fever abated, there were no longer any organisms in her blood. Chagas named the organism *T. cruzi* in honour of his mentor. In a period of several months, working for the most part by himself, he described the pathogen, its vector and the clinical features of the disease that bears his name an accomplishment unique in the history of medicine (Chagas, 1909; Lewinsohn, 2003). Although his achievements ultimately gained widespread recognition, he was never awarded a Nobel Prize for this important work. Carlos Chagas died in 1935. In the 1960s, Berenice was located and was found to be seropositive for Chagas disease reflecting the typical lifelong infection with this parasite. She was, however, free of clinical manifestations of her chronic infection and died due to unrelated "natural causes" in 1973. In 2009 the scientific world celebrated the centenary of Chagas' achievements in numerous symposia and review articles on the clinical and research aspects of *T. cruzi* and of Chagas disease (Apt, 2010; Biolo et al., 2010; Buckner and Navabi, 2010; Casadei, 2010; Epting et al., 2010; Junqueira et al., 2010; Rassi et al., 2010; Villalta et al., 2009).

Since Chagas's original observations were published, an enormous amount of information has accumulated on the biology, pathology, pathogenesis, epidemiology and clinical manifestations of the disease. The completion of the genome of the CL Brener strain and the anticipated completion of the genomes of other strains will continue to add to our knowledge of this complex human parasite and provide fertile ground for researchers of this neglected tropical disease. Moreover, use of the modern tools of molecular biology, biochemistry, cell biology and immunology has greatly expanded our knowledge of the complex biology of this organism and the host responses to this infection. The advances made through the application of the methods of these disciplines have raised hopes for the development of sorely needed new therapeutic and prophylactic agents for the management of *T. cruzi* infection.

This volume in *Advances in Parasitology* is not meant to be a comprehensive "novel" on Chagas disease but rather a collection of "short stories" in which experts in the field have highlighted historical perspectives and detailed descriptions of innovative experimental work based on cutting-edge methodologies applied to the challenges of Chagas disease. Our hope is that by bringing together in one place reviews of some of the best current work in Chagas disease research, readers will be informed and perhaps even stimulated to become involved in combating the illness

A

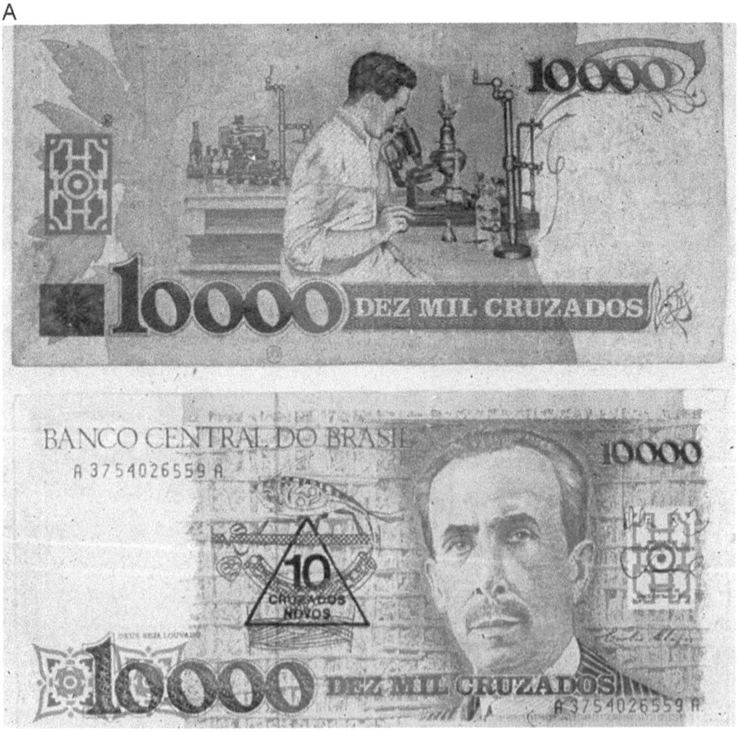

B

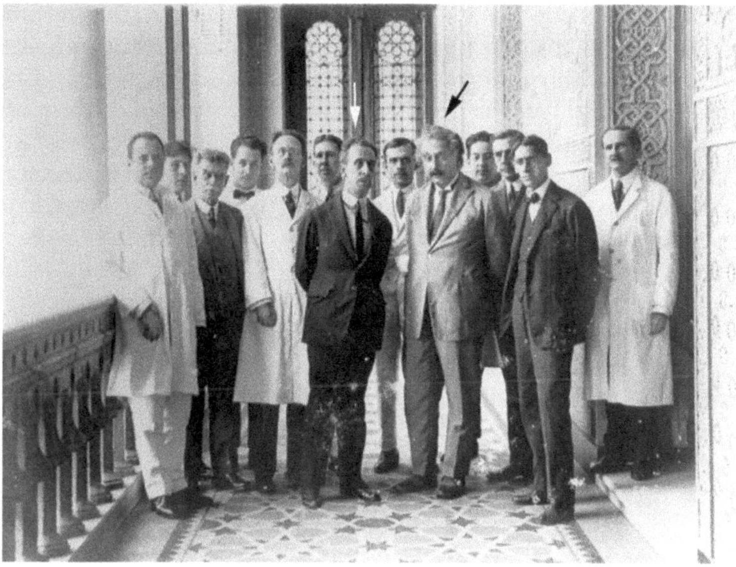

FIGURE 1 (A) Carlos Chagas on the 10,000 Cruzados Banknote from Brazil. (B) A photograph of Carlos Chagas (white arrow) and Albert Einstein (black arrow) taken during Einstein's visit to the Oswaldo Cruz Institute in 1925 (Lewinsohn, 2003). With permission of Casa de Oswaldo Cruz-Fiocruz, Arquivo e Documentação, Rio de Janeiro, Brazil.

that, despite over 100 years of research, still is the most important parasitic disease in the Americas.

Chagas disease is present in the countries of Latin America with the exception of the Caribbean. Vector-borne transmission of the *T. cruzi* parasite usually occurs in individuals living in primitive houses in areas where the sylvatic cycle is active. The parasite has a complex life cycle which is detailed in the epidemiology chapter. One of the important recent changes in the epidemiology of Chagas diseases has been the increased immigration of infected, usually asymptomatic, individuals from endemic areas to non-endemic areas such as North America, Europe, Japan and Australia. Thus, Chagas disease is being recognized with increasing frequency worldwide. This immigration into non-endemic areas of potentially chronically infected individuals has led to screening of blood donors to identify people who are asymptomatic but have the potential to transmit the infection via blood transfusion and organ transplantation. Interestingly, as a result of the immigration of populations into non-endemic areas, congenital Chagas disease has now been diagnosed in Europe among immigrants from Latin America.

The exacerbation of Chagas disease in the setting of immune suppression has been documented among individuals with HIV/AIDS and among those who receive immunosuppressive therapy in the setting of treatment for other immune disorders or organ transplantation. Acute Chagas disease and congenital Chagas disease are well described in the chapters in this volume. These are areas that have not received intensive investigation in recent years. The description of chronic Chagas disease has been dealt with in several excellent recent reviews, and the reader is referred to these for discussion of these topics (Carod-Artal et al., 2011; Lima-Costa et al., 2010; Rassi et al., 2010; Tanowitz et al., 2009).

Diagnostic testing is not covered in a separate chapter, as this is in a state of flux; however, there have been a number of reviews on this topic (Britto, 2009; Shah et al., 2010). At the present time, the diagnosis of acute *T. cruzi* infection is usually made by the detection of parasites in wet mounts of blood or cerebrospinal fluid and in Giemsa-stained slides. Testing for anti-*T. cruzi* IgM antibodies is not useful. Polymerase chain reaction (PCR) tests can detect the parasite and are useful in diagnosis. In acute or congenital Chagas disease, PCR is thought to be the most sensitive method for detecting infection; however, it is not widely available. The diagnosis of chronic Chagas disease is usually based on detecting specific antibodies. Several serologic assays are employed such as the indirect immunofluorescence (IFA) and enzyme-linked immunosorbent assay (ELISA). Serologic assays are used widely for clinical diagnosis and for screening of donated blood, as well as in epidemiologic studies. A radio immunoprecipitation assay (RIPA) based on iodinated *T. cruzi* proteins is specific and sensitive and is being used as the confirmatory assay to test all donor samples that are positive in the screening test (Shah et al., 2010). The utility of various diagnostic modalities have been published and has generated controversy, and the reader is referred to the following for a discussion of these issues (Otani et al., 2009; Shah et al., 2010). A critical unmet need is for tests that deal with the issue of parasitological cure; currently, no test can accurately predict that cure has been achieved following drug treatment.

Other chapters in this *Advances in Parasitology* volume (Parts A and B) deal with advances in the therapy of Chagas disease such as cell-based therapy for chronic Chagas cardiomyopathy which could obviate the need for heart transplantation. There are important chapters which focus on advances in chemotherapy as well as the current state of vaccine development. One of the intriguing questions of this disease is what role human genetic variability contributes to susceptibility to infection and the final clinical outcome of infection with *T. cruzi*. Chapters on molecular biology, cell biology, host cell invasion, stage differentiation and parasite signalling follow. For example, there is a comprehensive review of the current state of knowledge of the unique organelle, the acidocalcisome, an organelle which the author of this chapter, was instrumental in describing in several protozoa. The last several chapters are diverse and deal with topics in pathogenesis including those on eicosanoids, oxidative stress, vascular pathophysiology, and myocardial inflammation. One of the chapters deals with the question of autoimmunity. This has intrigued investigators for decades and the controversy continues as to what role, if any, does autoimmunity play in the pathogenesis of Chagas disease. The work on parasite-derived neurotropic factors is reviewed, and there is a review on myocardial inflammation and Chagas disease. As there have been excellent recent reviews on immunology in Chagas disease, the editors decided to concentrate on myocardial inflammation rather than the entire gamut of immunology which could be a topic of an entire volume. In recent years, there has been an increase in obesity and diabetes in Chagas endemic areas which has alarmed many and has resulted in an increase in the investigation as to the role of adipose tissue and diabetes in infections caused by parasites. To this end, we have included a review which explores this relationship demonstrating the complex interaction that is resulting from the intersection of the obesity epidemic with this endemic tropical disease.

The editors wish to thank their families, friends, laboratory members and colleagues who have made it possible to achieve all that we have done. In addition, they acknowledge the efforts of the entire Chagas disease research community who have contributed their talents to unravel the complex interactions of *T. cruzi* and humans.

Only a life lived for others is a life worthwhile.

We can't solve problems by using the same kind of thinking we used when we created them

Albert Einstein

Louis M. Weiss
Herbert B. Tanowitz
April 2011

REFERENCES

Apt, W., 2010. Current and developing therapeutic agents in the treatment of Chagas disease. Drug Des. Devel. Ther. 4, 243–253.

Aufderheide, A.C., Salo, W., Madden, M., Streitz, J., Buikstra, J., Guhl, F., et al., 2004. A 9,000-year record of Chagas' disease. Proc. Natl. Acad. Sci. USA. 101, 2034–2039.

Biolo, A., Ribeiro, A.L., Clausell, N., 2010. Chagas cardiomyopathy—where do we stand after a hundred years? Prog. Cardiovasc. Dis. 52, 300–316.

Britto, C.C., 2009. Usefulness of PCR-based assays to assess drug efficacy in Chagas disease chemotherapy: value and limitations. Mem. Inst. Oswaldo Cruz 104 (Suppl. 1), 122–135.

Buckner, F.S., Navabi, N., 2010. Advances in Chagas disease drug development: 2009–2010. Curr. Opin. Infect. Dis. 23, 609–616.

Carod-Artal, F.J., Vargas, A.P., Falcao, T., 2011. Stroke in asymptomatic *Trypanosoma cruzi*-infected patients. Cerebrovasc. Dis. 31, 24–28.

Casadei, D., 2010. Chagas' disease and solid organ transplantation. Transplant. Proc. 42, 3354–3359.

Chagas, C., 1909. Nova tripanozomiase humana: Estudos sobre a morfolojia e o ciclo evolutivo do schizotrypanum cruzi n. Gen., n. Sp., ajente etiolojico de nova entidade morbida do homem. (New human trypanosomiasis. Studies about the morphology and life-cycle of Schizotripanum cruzi, etiological agent of a new morbid entity of man). Med. Inst. Oswaldo Cruz 1, 159–218.

Epting, C.L., Coates, B.M., Engman, D.M., 2010. Molecular mechanisms of host cell invasion by *Trypanosoma cruzi*. Exp. Parasitol. 126, 283–291.

Junqueira, C., Caetano, B., Bartholomeu, D.C., Melo, M.B., Ropert, C., Rodrigues, M.M., et al., 2010. The endless race between *Trypanosoma cruzi* and host immunity: lessons for and beyond Chagas disease. Expert Rev. Mol. Med. 12, e29.

Lewinsohn, R., 2003. Prophet in his own country: Carlos Chagas and the Nobel Prize. Perspect. Biol. Med. 46, 532–549.

Lima-Costa, M.F., Matos, D.L., Ribeiro, A.L., 2010. Chagas disease predicts 10-year stroke mortality in community-dwelling elderly: the Bambui cohort study of aging. Stroke 41, 2477–2482.

Otani, M.M., Vinelli, E., Kirchhoff, L.V., del Pozo, A., Sands, A., Vercauteren, G., et al., 2009. WHO comparative evaluation of serologic assays for Chagas disease. Transfusion 49, 1076–1082.

Rassi, A., Jr., Rassi, A., Marin-Neto, J.A., 2010. Chagas disease. Lancet 375, 1388–1402.

Shah, D.O., Chang, C.D., Cheng, K.Y., Salbilla, V.A., Adya, N., Marchlewicz, B.A., et al., 2010. Comparison of the analytic sensitivities of a recombinant immunoblot assay and the radioimmune precipitation assay for the detection of antibodies to *Trypanosoma cruzi* in patients with Chagas disease. Diagn. Microbiol. Infect. Dis. 67, 402–405.

Tanowitz, H.B., Machado, F.S., Jelicks, L.A., Shirani, J., de Carvalho, A.C., Spray, D.C., et al., 2009. Perspectives on *Trypanosoma cruzi*-induced heart disease (Chagas disease). Prog. Cardiovasc. Dis. 51, 524–539.

Villalta, F., Scharfstein, J., Ashton, A.W., Tyler, K.M., Guan, F., Mukherjee, S., et al., 2009. Perspectives on the *Trypanosoma cruzi*-host cell receptor interactions. Parasitol. Res. 104, 1251–1260.

CHAPTER 1

Epidemiology of American Trypanosomiasis (Chagas Disease)

Louis V. Kirchhoff*,†

Contents

* Departments of Internal Medicine and Epidemiology, University of Iowa, Iowa City, Iowa, USA
† Department of Veterans Affairs Medical Center, University of Iowa, Iowa City, Iowa, USA

Advances in Parasitology, Volume 75
ISSN 0065-308X, DOI: 10.1016/B978-0-12-385863-4.00001-0

Abstract

Trypanosoma cruzi, the cause of American trypanosomiasis, or Chagas disease, is a protozoan parasite that is enzootic and endemic in much of the Americas, where it infects a wide variety of wild and domestic mammals as well as many species of triatomine vectors, in addition to humans. Historically, vector-borne transmission of *T. cruzi* has been the most important mechanism through which humans have become infected with the parasite, but transmission by blood transfusion and congenital transmission also have been important. In many of the endemic countries transmission of *T. cruzi* has improved markedly in recent years as vector control and donor screening programs have been implemented on a widespread basis.

In the United States autochthonous transmission of *T. cruzi* appears to be extremely rare. Five persons are known to have become infected with *T. cruzi* through organ transplants here, and prior to the implementation of blood donor screening in 2007 five instances of transmission by transfusion had been reported. Current estimates put the total number of *T. cruzi*-infected persons living in the United States at 300,000, essentially all of whom are immigrants from the endemic countries. The obstacles that stand in the way of the total elimination of *T. cruzi* transmission throughout the endemic range are economic and political, and no major technological advances are needed to accomplish this goal.

1.1. HISTORICAL BACKGROUND

Trypanosoma cruzi, the cause of American trypanosomiasis, or Chagas disease, is a protozoan parasite that is enzootic and endemic in much of the Americas, where it infects a wide variety of wild and domestic mammals as well as many species of triatomine vectors, in addition to humans. The only other members of the genus *Trypanosoma* that cause disease in humans are two subspecies of African trypanosomes, *Trypanosoma brucei gambiense* and *T.b. rhodesiense*. These organisms cause West African and East African trypanosomiases, or sleeping sickness, respectively. The enzootic and endemic ranges of the American and African trypanosomes do not overlap. The distinct geographic distribution of *T. cruzi* and *T. brucei* is not new, as comparative phylogenetic analyses suggest that their two lineages separated around 100 million years ago (Stevens et al., 1999).

1.2. MECHANISMS OF TRANSMISSION OF *TRYPANOSOMA CRUZI*

1.2.1. Sylvatic transmission of *Trypanosoma cruzi*

Triatomine insects (cone-nosed or kissing bugs) are exclusively haematophagous and become infected with *T. cruzi* when they take blood meals from mammals that contain free-swimming, non-dividing bloodstream trypomastigotes. This is the only route through which they can become infected, as transovarial transmission does not occur. Once inside the gut of an insect, the latter transform into epimastigotes, which are a replicative form that has a different morphology. As the epimastigotes multiply to large numbers, some are carried down to the hindgut of the insects, where they transform into metacyclic trypomastigotes, which is a form of *T. cruzi* that is capable of infecting mammals. When infected insects defecate during subsequent blood meals they often deposit parasite-laden faeces that can result in transmission by coming into contact with vulnerable surfaces such as the conjunctivas, nasal and oral mucosas, or the bug bite itself. The metacyclic trypomastigotes penetrate local cells and transform into amastigotes, which have yet another distinct morphologic form, that in turn multiply intracellularly. After many rounds of multiplication, amastigotes transform to bloodstream trypomastigotes and are released as the host cells rupture. These parasites can then infect adjacent cells or be swept into the lymphatics or bloodstream, ultimately infecting host cells in a wide variety of distant tissues. The cycle of transmission is completed when circulating trypomastigotes are taken up in blood meals by vectors (Fig. 1.1).

There are several other mechanisms of transmission of *T. cruzi* in sylvatic cycles in addition to the contaminative scenario described above. Many of the mammalian species that are reservoirs for *T. cruzi* are omnivorous and may become infected when they ingest and chew *T. cruzi*-infected vectors, thus exposing their oral and gastrointestinal mucosas to infective metacyclic trypomastigotes. It has been demonstrated experimentally that deposition of extremely small numbers of infective parasites on the oral mucosa of mice can result in infection (Kirchhoff and Hoft, 1990), and it has also been shown that when omnivorous mammals are fed *T. cruzi*-infected vectors they in turn become infected.

T. cruzi transmission also can occur when carnivores kill and eat other mammals that are infected with the parasite. An example of this would be wild canids (e.g. coyotes) or domestic dogs (e.g. coonhounds) that kill and eat raccoons, opossums, armadillos, and other small mammals that often are infected (Barr et al., 1995; Bradley et al., 2000). In the case of *T. cruzi*-infected coonhounds living in enzootic areas, there is simply no way to determine how they become infected, as they are known to eat potentially

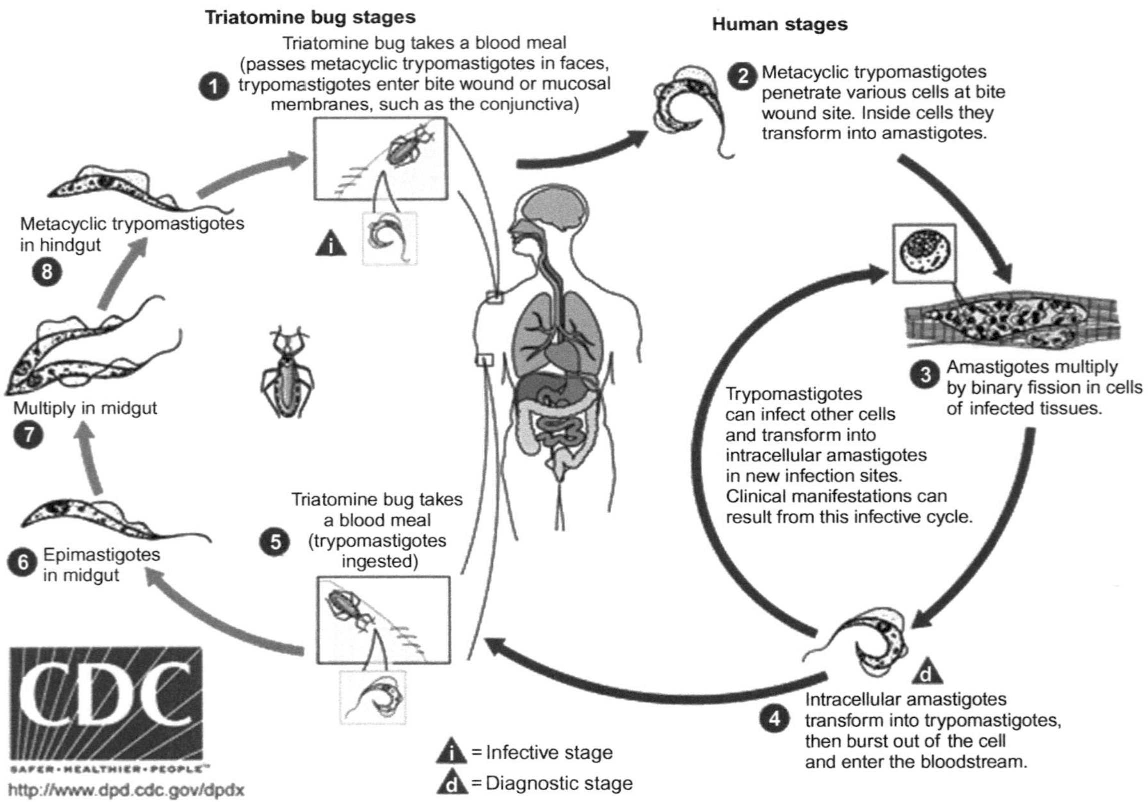

FIGURE 1.1 Life cycle of *Trypansoma cruzi*. Figure from the Centers for Disease Control (http://www.cdc.gov/parasites/chagas/biology.html).

infected mammalian reservoirs and also typically are housed outside, where they would be exposed to vectors.

Congenital transmission may play an important role of the maintenance of *T. cruzi* infection in mammalian reservoirs, and such transmission has been documented in domestic dogs in at least one instance (Barr et al., 1995). The relative importance in sylvatic cycles of *T. cruzi* transmission by these various routes is not known.

1.2.2. Mechanisms of *Trypanosoma cruzi* transmission to humans

The life cycle of *T. cruzi* is essentially the same as that described above, independent of whether the mammalian reservoirs are non-human or human. As with the other mammalian hosts, *T. cruzi* infection in humans is not a dead end, since chronically infected persons have persistent parasitaemias and act as a source of infection for the vectors that take blood meals from them.

Historically, vector-borne transmission of *T. cruzi* has been the most important mechanism through which humans have become infected with the parasite. This occurs when people live in structures in which vectors have become domiciliary and are bitten by the insects while sleeping. Although the vectors can penetrate intact skin, they apparently most often take blood meals from the oral or nasal mucosa or the conjunctivas. This behaviour probably is the result of the insects' being attracted to the face because of its relative warmth or the CO_2 being exhaled, or because penetration of the mucosas is easier for feeding. In any event, feeding around the face favours transmission of *T. cruzi*, since the probability of parasite-laden faeces being accidentally smeared on surfaces through which transmission can take place is much higher there than elsewhere on the body. This is critical in the cycle of transmission since the parasites cannot penetrate intact skin.

Transmission of *T. cruzi* can also occur through transfusion of whole blood or derivative products obtained from donors who are chronically infected with the parasite (Kirchhoff et al., 2006; Schmunis and Cruz, 2005; Wendel, 2010). Platelets from infected donors appear to carry the highest risk of transmission, followed by whole blood. The high risk associated with platelets results from the fact that trypomastigotes end up in the platelet fraction during centrifugation. Transmission can also occur through transplantation of organs obtained from *T. cruzi*-infected persons (Centers for Disease Control and Prevention, 2006). Presumably, this occurs because some host cells in the donor organs contain intracellular amastigote forms of *T. cruzi*, which after organ transplantation ultimately transform into trypomastigotes that infect adjacent tissues and cells at distant sites after rupture of the host cells, thus establishing systemic infection.

The occurrence of congenital transmission of *T. cruzi* has been well characterized by investigators in the endemic countries (Altcheh et al., 2005; Freilij and Altcheh, 1995; Gurtler et al., 2003; Jercic et al., 2010; Sanchez Negrette et al., 2005). Transmission of the parasite is transplacental and in a number of studies 1–10% of infants born to mothers with chronic *T. cruzi* infections were found to be infected. In two studies, higher levels of circulating parasites in infected mothers have been shown to increase the likelihood of congenital transmission (Bern et al., 2009; Brutus et al., 2010), but beyond this the factors that affect the probability of congenital transmission are not known.

Two other mechanisms of transmission of *T. cruzi* to people merit comment. The first is oral transmission resulting from the ingestion of food or drink that is infected with parasites. The fact that oral transmission occurs in this manner is not surprising in view of data demonstrating the ease with which oral transmission can be achieved in experimental animals (Kirchhoff and Hoft, 1990). More importantly, this type of transmission would be expected when one considers that an unknown but presumably substantial proportion of vector-borne transmission occurs through contamination of the oral mucosa with parasites. The second mechanism is transmission through laboratory accidents, which would be expected given the ease with which infected forms of *T. cruzi* can be produced in the laboratory (Herwaldt, 2006). Finally, transmission of *T. cruzi* from chronically infected mothers to their nursing infants has not been definitively documented and thus *T. cruzi* infection in mothers is not viewed as a contraindication to breast feeding. Experts do raise caution, however, if bleeding of the nipples is present (Ferreira et al., 2001). Sexual transmission of *T. cruzi* is not known to occur.

Ingestion of *T. cruzi*-infected insects is not known to be a mechanism through which *T. cruzi* is transmitted to humans, even though some people in endemic regions are known to eat insects. Obviously transmission of *T. cruzi* could only occur if infected vectors were not processed in a manner that would kill any parasites they might contain. Similarly, acquisition of *T. cruzi* through ingestion of meat or blood from infected mammals has not been reported. It merits mention, however, that in some enzootic areas small mammals that typically harbour *T. cruzi* (e.g. armadillos) are often consumed, but in my experience in Brazil they were always thoroughly cooked, so it is unlikely that ingestion of this food item would lead to transmission of infection. Although transmission of *T. cruzi* via these two mechanisms may seem to unlikely, in a biologic sense there are really no barriers to its occurrence, and occasional cases of acute Chagas disease resulting from such events likely would never be recognized and reported.

1.3. EPIZOOTIOLOGY OF *TRYPANOSOMA CRUZI*

T. cruzi, which as noted above is present only in the Americas, is found mostly in wild and domestic mammals and triatomine insect vectors (Bradley et al., 2000; Houk et al., 2010; Lent and Wygodzinsky, 1979; Sarkar et al., 2010; Villegas-Garcia and Santillan-Alarcon, 2004). The many species of vectors that transmit the parasite are found in spotty distributions from the southern third of the United States to central Argentina and Chile. Burrows, hollow trees, palm trees, and other enclosures in which mammals seek shelter are typical places where transmission takes place among mammalian reservoirs and vectors. Moreover, large numbers of vectors often can be found in piles of old vegetation and other debris around houses as well as in stacks of roof tiles and boards, and these can play a major role in the establishment of a domiciliary cycle of transmission of the parasite that in turn can involve domestic animals, primarily dogs, as well as the people who live in the houses (Cohen and Gurtler, 2001; Enger et al., 2004; Starr et al., 1991).

T. cruzi has been isolated from more than 100 species of wild and domestic mammals (Barbabosa-Pliego et al., 2011; Barr et al., 1995; Campos et al., 2010; Maloney et al., 2010; Wisnivesky-Colli et al., 1992; Yaeger, 1988). Racoons, wood rats, opossums, non-human primates (Monteiro et al., 2010), and dogs are typical mammalian reservoirs. Moreover, non-typical hosts can become infected when held in captivity (Jaime-Andrade et al., 1997; Lisboa et al., 2004; Williams et al., 2009). *T. cruzi* infection is not a problem livestock. The wide variety of mammalian hosts that *T. cruzi* can infect and the fact that chronically infected animals have persistent parasitaemias result in an enormous sylvatic and domestic reservoir in enzootic regions, and this in turn drives the establishment of the domiciliary cycle of transmission of the parasite in human dwellings.

1.4. EPIDEMIOLOGY OF HUMAN *TRYPANOSOMA CRUZI* INFECTION IN THE ENDEMIC COUNTRIES

T. cruzi is only found in the Americas, and since humans have been here only for about 13,000 years, this parasite is a relatively recent pathogen of humans. Current thinking is that *T. cruzi* infection in humans is as old as their presence in enzootic regions of our hemisphere (Araujo et al., 2009a, b). The new arrivals inadvertently joined the many other mammalian species that served as reservoirs of *T. cruzi*, and this could occur because of the parasite's lack of host specificity, which contrasts sharply with that of other parasites such as *Plasmodium falciparum*. PCR-based studies of mummies found in the Atacama Desert of northern Chile and southern Peru that were dated to 9000 years before present indicated clearly that *T. cruzi* infection was present (Araujo et al., 2009a,b; Aufderheide et al., 2004). The process that likely resulted in infections in members of such prehistoric communities has continued into modern times, as people have continued to live in areas of active enzootic transmission of *T. cruzi* and become infected through contact with vectors. This typically occurs in rural settings in which subsistence farmers and ranchers live in primitive structures to which vectors and mammalian reservoirs have free access. Thus historically, Chagas disease has been a problem among poor people who live in the countryside, but with the advent of blood transfusion and migration of large numbers of people to cities the *T. cruzi* infection has been urbanized.

Early reports suggested that most vector-borne cases of acute *T. cruzi* infection occurred in children, since most acutely infected persons that came to medical attention were young (Laranja et al., 1956). Prevalence data support this perspective, but since most acute cases of *T. cruzi* infection are mild and are not diagnosed specifically, few geographic and aged-specific incidence data have been published.

The endemic range of Chagas disease includes all the countries of Central and South America as well as Mexico. The World Health Organization currently estimates that 10 million persons are chronically infected with *T. cruzi* and that about 10,000 deaths each can be attributed to Chagas disease (WHO, 2010). Both of these estimates are substantially less than they were in earlier years (Santo, 2009). The highest prevalence rates are found in Bolivia (6.75%), and several other countries also have substantial rates, such as Argentina (4.13%), El Salvador (3.37%), Honduras (3.05%), and Paraguay (2.54%) (Bern and Montgomery, 2009). Importantly, Brazil and Mexico both have prevalence rates around 1%, and because of their large populations about one-third of all *T. cruzi*-infected persons live in these two countries. There is no Chagas disease in any of the Caribbean islands.

In 2000, the aggregate cost of the morbidity and mortality associated with chronic Chagas disease was estimated to be more than US $8 billion (Schmunis, 2000). Despite this substantial burden of infection and its consequences, however, in recent years the epidemiologic situation of Chagas disease has improved strikingly in many of the endemic countries as vector control and donor screening programs have been implemented on a widespread basis. In many areas, successful efforts to break the cycle of vector-borne transmission have resulted in substantial reduction of *T. cruzi* prevalence rates among children and blood donors (Borges et al., 2006; Segura et al., 2000). Much of the progress in controlling vector transmission has occurred in the framework of the Southern Cone Initiative (SCI), which began in 1991 with the support of the World Health

Organization, PAHO, and the national health ministries of the participating countries, which include Argentina, Bolivia, Brazil, Chile, Paraguay, and Uruguay. This program is based on the low-technology approaches of improving housing conditions, spraying of residual insecticides, and educating persons at-risk for *T. cruzi* infection. Uruguay, Chile, and Brazil were certified free of transmission of *T. cruzi* in 1997, 1999, and 2006, respectively, and marked reduction of transmission of the parasite also has been achieved in the other SCI countries (Coura and Dias, 2009; Moncayo and Silveira, 2009; Rassi et al., 2003; Schofield et al., 2006). The accomplishments of the SCI are a tribute to the thousands of persons who have worked on the design and implementation of the SCI, which has served as a model for the development of control programs in the other endemic regions. Vector control programs have been in operation for some years in the Andean nations (Salvatella, 2007) and also in the countries of Central America (Anonymous, 1998). In Mexico, a growing awareness of Chagas disease as a public health problem is reflected in an expansion of vector control and blood screening programs (Cruz-Reyes and Pickering-Lopez, 2006; Guzman-Bracho, 2001; Ramos-Ligonio et al., 2010; Secretaría de Salud, 2002). Moreover, throughout the endemic range, with the notable exception of Mexico, effective national blood donor screening programs for Chagas disease have been implemented, based on the commercial availability of a variety of sensitive and specific serodiagnostic assays (Chang et al., 2006; Ortho-Clinical Diagnostics, Inc., 2006; Otani et al., 2009). With the exception of some limited situations in which all donated blood is not screened, it is fair to say that the risk of transfusion transmission of *T. cruzi* in the endemic countries is extremely low (Schmunis and Cruz, 2005).

In the context of the widespread successful efforts to control *T. cruzi* transmission, nonetheless, in the endemic countries an estimated 41,200 instances of vector-borne transmission occurred in 2005, and about 14,000 infants were born with congenital disease (Salvatella, 2006). Although these numbers of new cases of *T. cruzi* infection are far fewer that those that occurred in the years prior to the initiation of the control programs, they do indicate that the programs still need to be extended and maintained.

There are, however, other aspects of *T. cruzi* transmission for which acceptable solutions are not available. By far the most important of these is congenital transmission, the incidence of which is simply a function of the prevalence of chronic *T. cruzi* infection among women of child-bearing age and the birth rate. At present, there are no options available for treating *T. cruzi*-infected pregnant women with the goal of reducing the likelihood of congenital transmission. Moreover, no data are available from controlled trials that support the concept that treating women of child-bearing age prior to pregnancy with benznidazole or nifurtimox, which generally are not parasitologically curative in adults, significantly reduces the probability of congenital transmission. Even if such reduction could be achieved by treatment, moreover, the logistical challenges and costs involved in serologically identifying women in the endemic countries with chronic *T. cruzi* infection and treating them prior to pregnancy would be a major barrier to making substantial progress in reducing the overall number of congenital cases. What is available to deal with this problem, however, is highly effective treatment for babies with congenital Chagas disease, who if treated within the first year of life are highly likely to be cured parasitologically. Nonetheless, the logistics and expense of implementing widespread programs for screening at-risk pregnant women serologically for *T. cruzi* infection and then testing their babies parasitologically at birth and/or serologically months later for *T. cruzi* infection would be daunting.

A second question relating to the transmission of *T. cruzi* is how best to eliminate outbreaks of food-borne transmission of *T. cruzi*, of which fortunately only a handful have been reported since the first description appeared more than 40 years ago (Alarcon de Noya et al., 2010; Bastos et al., 2010; Beltrao et al., 2009; Benchimol-Barbosa, 2010; Dias et al., 2008; Guimaraes et al., 1968). In essence, the occurrence of these outbreaks reflects general problems with food safety, rather than Chagas disease-specific issues. The outbreaks reported to date appear to have resulted from the contamination of food or drink with parasites from sylvatic cycles and since elimination of the latter is not a feasible goal, the avoidance of such outbreaks must depend on increased focus on general food safety.

1.5. EPIDEMIOLOGY OF *TRYPANOSOMA CRUZI* INFECTION IN THE UNITED STATES

1.5.1. Incidence

In terms of the incidence of vector-borne *T. cruzi* infection in the United States, even though as noted mammalian reservoirs of *T. cruzi* and triatomine vectors that transmit the parasite among these animals are spread widely across the southern and southwestern states, autochthonous transmission of *T. cruzi* here appears to be extremely rare. To date, only six such cases have been reported. The lower overall density of infected vectors and our higher housing standards, in comparison to areas of active transmission to humans in the endemic countries, are thought to be the factors that account for the rarity of transmission of the parasite to people here.

Prior to 2007, the large number of immigrants from Chagas-endemic countries who reside in the United States (see below) posed a risk of transmission of *T. cruzi* by transfusion. Several large studies of U.S.

blood donors showed clearly that *T. cruzi*-infected persons occasionally donated blood (Leiby et al., 2002, 2008), and not surprisingly five cases of transfusion-related transmission of *T. cruzi* in the United States had been reported, in addition to two in Canada. In all these instances, acute *T. cruzi* infection was diagnosed in the recipients only because they were immunocompromised and as a consequence had fulminant courses of acute Chagas disease. Since acute *T. cruzi* infection transmitted by any means would be expected to follow a relatively mild course in immunocompetent recipients, it was widely assumed that far more cases than the small number reported had occurred but went undiagnosed.

In January 2007, serological screening of U.S. blood donors for Chagas disease began and since then the risk of transfusion transmission of *T. cruzi* in the United States presumably has been negligible. To date, over 1400 *T. cruzi*-infected donors have been identified and permanently deferred from donation, reflecting an overall prevalence in the donor population of about 1:28,000. Retrospective studies done many years ago in the endemic countries indicated that the overall rate of transmission by transfusion was 13-26%, and a recent study in Mexico found that four of nine recipients (44%) of blood products from infected donors were infected with *T. cruzi*, two of whom had received platelets and two had been given whole blood (Kirchhoff et al., 2006). The implementation of donor screening here in 2007 has provided the opportunity to do trace-back studies to estimate the transmission rate in our context. Interestingly, in these studies only 2 of 271 (0.7%) recipients who had been transfused with a blood product prior to 2007 from a *T. cruzi*-infected donor who was identified as such after screening began here were found to be infected. Several factors may underlie the wide discrepancy between the historical and our pre-2007 rate of transmission, such as the length of storage of the blood products prior to transfusion and the use of leukocyte filters.

The implementation of donor screening for Chagas disease in the United States also provided a context to look for evidence of autochthonous transmission of *T. cruzi* here. Almost all the *T. cruzi*-infected donors identified through screening and deferred from further donation have had geographic risk for Chagas disease, that is, they were born in or had spent substantial periods of time in the endemic countries. There have been a small number of donors, however, identified among the tens of millions of persons screened serologically since the initiation of serologic screening, who do not have geographic risk and are not children of mothers with such risk and thus appear to have acquired *T. cruzi* infection autochthonously (Cantey et al., 2010). The vagaries of serologic and parasitological testing for *T. cruzi* infection make determination of the exact number of such donors difficult. Nonetheless, the data do support the concept that autochthonous transmission of *T. cruzi* to humans does occur in the United States, albeit extremely rarely.

1.5.2. Incidence of congenital transmission in the United States

Current estimates put the total number of *T. cruzi*-infected persons living in the United States at 300,000 (Bern and Montgomery, 2009). If we assume that the birth rate in this group is that of Mexico (19.39 births/ 1000 population per year), since the majority are Mexican immigrants, and that the rate of congenital transmission is 1-10%, we would expect the number of babies born in the United States each year with congenital Chagas disease to be between 58 and 582 (Yadon and Schmunis, 2009). Curiously, only one infant born in the United States with congenital disease has been reported (Baram et al., 2011). The fact that there is little knowledge about congenital Chagas disease among caregivers who deal with pregnant women at-risk for chronic *T. cruzi* infection and their infants (Verani et al., 2010) likely is the primary factor underlying this lack of diagnosed cases. The fact that infected infants typically have few or no symptoms also likely plays a role. Infants born to at-risk mothers have been diagnosed with congenital Chagas disease in Switzerland and Spain (Jackson et al., 2010; Martinez de Tejada et al., 2009; Piron et al., 2008), where in clinics that serve immigrant populations the awareness of Chagas disease is greater, pregnant at-risk women are often screened, and infants born to serologically positive women are tested specifically for *T. cruzi* infection.

1.5.3. Transmission of *Trypanosoma cruzi* in the United States associated with organ transplantation

As noted, *T. cruzi* can be transmitted through transplantation of organs obtained from chronically infected donors. Given the sizable numbers of infected persons living in the United States it is not surprising that several such incidents have occurred. Some years ago three persons received organs from a *T. cruzi*-infected immigrant and subsequently developed acute Chagas disease (Centers for Disease Control and Prevention, 2002) and one of the recipients died of the infection. More recently, two recipients of hearts obtained from *T. cruzi*-infected donors became infected (Centers for Disease Control and Prevention, 2006). In all these cases, the infection status of the donors was not known at the time the transplants were performed and came to light only after acute infection developed in the recipients.

1.5.4. Laboratory accidents involving transmission of *Trypanosoma cruzi*

Many incidents of transmission of *T. cruzi* transmission in research laboratories in the endemic countries were reported years ago and several occurred in the United States as well. Given the understandable reluctance for reporting such incidents, it is a safe assumption that the number reported was substantially fewer than the number that actually occurred. In recent years, further reports of this type have not appeared, and this likely reflects the widespread adoption of more effective biosafety standards in research laboratories.

1.5.5. Prevalence of *Trypanosoma cruzi* infection in the United States

It was estimated recently that 300,000 persons with chronic *T. cruzi* infections live in the United States (Bern and Montgomery, 2009). This number was obtained by multiplying country-specific *T. cruzi* prevalence rates by U.S. country-specific immigrant population estimates. Census data indicate that about 23 million immigrants from the Chagas-endemic countries currently live in the United States and that 17 million of these persons are Mexican nationals. Thus, the overall prevalence in the at-risk population would be about 1.3%. Screening of all persons living in the United States who are at-risk for *T. cruzi* infection has been recommended for many years (Kirchhoff and Neva, 1985; Kirchhoff et al., 1985). Importantly, the millions of Cubans, Dominicans, Hatians, and Puerto Ricans, all of whom are Latin Americans, do not need to be screened because as indicated there is no Chagas disease in the Caribbean. Identification of *T. cruzi*-infected persons is important so that long-term cardiac monitoring (i.e. EKGs) can be carried out, parasite-specific treatment can be offered, and infants born to infected mothers can be tested for congenital Chagas disease (Bern et al., 2007). Unfortunately only a small proportion of immigrants at-risk for Chagas disease have been screened here, largely because of the lack of awareness of Chagas disease in the U.S. medical community.

1.6. *TRYPANOSOMA CRUZI* INFECTION IN NON-ENDEMIC COUNTRIES OTHER THAN THE UNITED STATES

Substantial numbers of persons have emigrated from Chagas-endemic countries to countries other than the United States. Canada, Australia, Japan, France, Switzerland, and England are on this list, but by far the largest population of immigrants from Chagas-endemic countries lives in Spain (Piron et al., 2008). Importantly, a high proportion of the immigrants in Spain are Bolivians, who as indicated above have the highest national *T. cruzi* prevalence of all the endemic countries. The challenges presented in Spain by the presence of these at-risk immigrants are similar to those faced by caregivers in the United States.

1.7. PERSPECTIVES ON THE CONTROL OF CHAGAS DISEASE

The obstacles that stand in the way of the total elimination of *T. cruzi* transmission to humans are economic and political, and no major technological advances are needed to accomplish this goal. It appears unlikely that the detailed understanding of the molecular aspects of *T. cruzi* biology, the intricacies of human immune responses to infection with the parasite, and the mechanisms of pathogenesis will contribute in a substantial way to the overall control of Chagas disease. Rather, the low-technology approaches that are the backbone of the SCI clearly constitute appropriate, affordable, and implementable methods for elimination of transmission and can serve as a paradigm for the development of other infectious disease control programs. Several challenges, however, do remain. Far and away, the most important of these is the development of a new drug with fewer side effects than benznidazole and nifurtimox that has a high rate of parasitological cure when given over a short period of time. The impact of such a drug would not be as much in terms of reducing vector-borne transmission, given the inevitable persistence of the sylvatic cycle throughout the enzootic range, but rather in reducing pathogenesis and clinical manifestations in the estimated 10 million persons already infected. Importantly, however, widespread curative treatment of infected persons would inevitably include large numbers of infected girls and women and thus would eliminate the possibility of congenital transmission of the parasite to the children they would have subsequent to treatment. Finally, an accurate, rapid, simple, and inexpensive tool for diagnosing congenital Chagas disease is sorely needed, as current methods for the parasitological diagnosis of infected newborns are tedious and difficult to implement on a widespread basis. Although having such a tool obviously would not reduce the rate of congenital transmission, as parasitological cure generally can be achieved in infected infants even with the currently available drugs, it would reduce the number of persons who have chronic *T. cruzi* infections as a consequence congenital transmission.

REFERENCES

Alarcon de Noya, B., Diaz-Bello, Z., Colmenares, C., Ruiz-Guevara, R., Mauriello, L., Zavala-Jaspe, R., et al., 2010. Large urban outbreak of orally acquired acute Chagas disease at a school in Caracas, Venezuela. J. Infect. Dis. 201 (9), 1308–1315.

Altcheh, J., Biancardi, M., Lapena, A., Ballering, G., Freilij, H., 2005. Congenital Chagas disease: experience in the Hospital de Ninos, Ricardo Gutierrez, Buenos Aires, Argentina. Rev. Soc. Bras. Med. Trop. 45 (Suppl. 2), 41–45.

Anonymous, 1998. Chagas disease: Central American initiative launched. TDR News 55, 6.

Araujo, A., Jansen, A.M., Reinhard, K., Ferreira, L.F., 2009a. Paleoparasitology of Chagas disease—a review. Mem. Inst. Oswaldo Cruz 104 (Suppl. 1), 9–16.

Araujo, C.A., Waniek, P.J., Jansen, A.M., 2009b. An overview of Chagas disease and the role of triatomines on its distribution in Brazil. Vector Borne Zoonotic Dis. 9 (3), 227–234.

Aufderheide, A.C., Salo, W., Madden, M., Streitz, J., Buikstra, J., Guhl, F., et al., 2004. A 9,000-year record of Chagas' disease. Proc. Natl. Acad. Sci. USA 101 (7), 2034–2039.

Baram, M., Nassif, D.S., Lazarte, R.A., Litman-Mazo, F.R., Moore, A.C., Kamat, R., et al., 2011. Congenital Chagas disease (American trypanosomiasis) in the United States. (submitted).

Barbabosa-Pliego, A., Gil, P.C., Hernandez, D.O., Aparicio-Burgos, J.E., de Oca-jimenez, R.M., Martinez-Castaneda, J.S., et al., 2011. Prevalence of Trypanosoma cruzi in dogs (Canis familiaris) and triatomines during 2008 in a sanitary region of the State of Mexico, Mexico. Vector Borne Zoonotic Dis. 11 (2), 151–156.

Barr, S.C., Van Beek, O., Carlisle-Nowak, M.S., Lopez, J.W., Kirchhoff, L.V., Zajac, A., et al., 1995. *Trypanosoma cruzi* infection in Walker hounds in Virginia. Am. J. Vet. Res. 56, 1937–1944.

Bastos, C.J., Aras, R., Mota, G., Reis, F., Dias, J.P., de Jesus, R.S., et al., 2010. Clinical outcomes of thirteen patients with acute chagas disease acquired through oral transmission from two urban outbreaks in northeastern Brazil. PLoS Negl. Trop. Dis. 4 (6), e711.

Beltrao, H.B., Cerroni, M.P., Freitas, D.R., Pinto, A.Y., Valente, V.C., Valente, S.A., et al., 2009. Investigation of two outbreaks of suspected oral transmission of acute Chagas disease in the Amazon region, Para State, Brazil, in 2007. Trop. Doct. 39 (4), 231–232.

Benchimol-Barbosa, P.R., 2010. Trends on acute Chagas' disease transmitted by oral route in Brazil: steady increase in new cases and a concealed residual fluctuation. Int. J. Cardiol. 145 (3), 494–496.

Bern, C., Montgomery, S.P., 2009. An estimate of the burden of Chagas disease in the United States. Clin. Infect. Dis. 49 (5), e52–e54.

Bern, C., Montgomery, S.P., Herwaldt, B.L., Rassi, A., Jr., Marin-Neto, J.A., Dantas, R.O., et al., 2007. Evaluation and treatment of Chagas disease in the United States: A Systematic Review. JAMA. 298, 2171–2181.

Bern, C., Verastegui, M., Gilman, R.H., Lafuente, C., Galdos-Cardenas, G., Calderon, M., et al., 2009. Congenital Trypanosoma cruzi transmission in Santa Cruz, Bolivia. Clin. Infect. Dis. 49 (11), 1667–1674.

Borges, J.D., Assis, G.F., Gomes, L.V., Dias, J.C., Pinto, I.D., Martins-Filho, O.A., et al., 2006. Seroprevalence of Chagas disease in schoolchildren from two municipalities of Jequitinhonha Valley, Minas Gerais, Brazil; six years following the onset of epidemiological surveillance. Rev. Inst. Med. Trop. Sao Paulo 48 (2), 81–86.

Bradley, K.K., Bergman, D.K., Woods, J.P., Crutcher, J.M., Kirchhoff, L.V., 2000. Prevalence of American trypanosomiasis (Chagas disease) among dogs in Oklahoma. J. Am. Vet. Med. Assoc. 217 (12), 1853–1857.

Brutus, L., Castillo, H., Bernal, C., Salas, N.A., Schneider, D., Santalla, J.A., et al., 2010. Detectable Trypanosoma cruzi parasitemia during pregnancy and delivery as a risk factor for congenital Chagas disease. Am. J. Trop. Med. Hyg. 83 (5), 1044–1047.

Campos, R., Botto-Mahan, C., Ortiz, S., Coronado, X., Solari, A., 2010. Temporal fluctuation of infection with different Trypanosoma cruzi genotypes in the wild rodent Octodon degus. Am. J. Trop. Med. Hyg. 83 (2), 380–381.

Cantey, P.T., Stramer, S.L., Kamel, H., Currier, M., Townsend, R.L., Winton, C., et al., 2010. The U.S. Trypanosoma Cruzi Infection Study: evidence for autochthonous Trypanosoma Cruzi transmission among United States Blood Donors (Abstract S70-030F). Transfusion 50 (Suppl.), 32A.

Centers for Disease Control and Prevention, 2002. Chagas disease after organ transplantation—United States, 2001. MMWR 51 (10), 210–212.

Centers for Disease Control and Prevention, 2006. Chagas disease after organ transplantation—Los Angeles, California, 2006. MMWR 55 (29), 798–800.

Chang, C.D., Cheng, K.Y., Jiang, L., Salbilla, V.A., Haller, A.S., Yem, A.W., et al., 2006. Evaluation of a prototype Trypanosoma cruzi antibody assay with recombinant antigens on a fully automated chemiluminescence analyzer for blood donor screening. Transfusion 46 (10), 1737–1744.

Cohen, J.E., Gurtler, R.E., 2001. Modeling household transmission of American trypanosomiasis. Science 293 (5530), 694–698.

Coura, J.R., Dias, J.C., 2009. Epidemiology, control and surveillance of Chagas disease: 100 years after its discovery. Mem. Inst. Oswaldo Cruz 104 (Suppl. 1), 31–40.

Cruz-Reyes, A., Pickering-Lopez, J.M., 2006. Chagas disease in Mexico: an analysis of geographical distribution during the past 76 years—a review. Mem. Inst. Oswaldo Cruz 101 (4), 345–354.

Dias, J.P., Bastos, C., Araujo, E., Mascarenhas, A.V., Martins, N.E., Grassi, F., et al., 2008. Acute Chagas disease outbreak associated with oral transmission. Rev. Soc. Bras. Med. Trop. 41 (3), 296–300.

Enger, K.S., Ordonez, R., Wilson, M.L., Ramsey, J.M., 2004. Evaluation of risk factors for rural infestation by Triatoma pallidipennis (Hemiptera: Triatominae), a Mexican vector of Chagas disease. J. Med. Entomol. 41 (4), 760–767.

Ferreira, C.S., Martinho, P.C., Amato, N.V., Cruz, R.R., 2001. Pasteurization of human milk to prevent transmission of Chagas disease. Rev. Inst. Med. Trop. Sao Paulo 43, 161–162.

Freilij, H., Altcheh, J., 1995. Congenital Chagas' disease: diagnostic and clinical aspects. Clin. Infect. Dis. 21 (3), 551–555.

Guimaraes, F.N., Da Silva, N.N., Clausell, D.T., De Mello, A.L., Rapone, T., Snell, T., et al., 1968. [Epidemic outbreak of Chagas' disease in Teutonia (Estrela-Rio Grande do Sul) probably due to gastrointestinal infection]. Hospital (Rio J.) 73 (6), 1767–1804.

Gurtler, R.E., Segura, E.L., Cohen, J.E., 2003. Congenital transmission of Trypanosoma cruzi infection in Argentina. Emerg. Infect. Dis. 9 (1), 29–32.

Guzman-Bracho, C., 2001. Epidemiology of Chagas disease in Mexico: an update. Trends Parasitol. 17 (8), 372–376.

Herwaldt, B.L., 2006. Protozoa and helminths. In: Fleming, D.O., Hunt, D.L. (Eds.), Biological Safety: Principles and Practice. fourth ed. American Society for Microbiology, Washington, DC, pp. 115–161.

Houk, A.E., Goodwin, D.G., Zajac, A.M., Barr, S.C., Dubey, J.P., Lindsay, D.S., 2010. Prevalence of antibodies to Trypanosoma cruzi, Toxoplasma gondii, Encephalitozoon cuniculi, Sarcocystis neurona, Besnoitia darlingi, and Neospora caninum in North American opossums, Didelphis virginiana, from southern Louisiana. J. Parasitol. 96 (6), 1119–1122.

Jackson, Y., Getaz, L., Wolff, H., Holst, M., Mauris, A., Tardin, A., et al., 2010. Prevalence, clinical staging and risk for blood-borne transmission of Chagas disease among Latin American migrants in Geneva, Switzerland. PLoS Negl. Trop. Dis. 4 (2), e592.

Jaime-Andrade, G.J., Avila-Figueroa, D., Lozano-Kasten, F.J., Hernandez-Gutierrez, R.J., Magallon-Gastelum, E., Kasten-Monges, M.J., et al., 1997. Acute Chagas' cardiopathy in a polar bear (*Ursus maritimus*) in Guadalajara, Mexico. Rev. Soc. Bras. Med. Trop. 30 (4), 337–340.

Jercic, M.I., Mercado, R., Villarroel, R., 2010. Congenital Trypanosoma cruzi infection in neonates and infants from two regions of Chile where Chagas' disease is endemic. J. Clin. Microbiol. 48 (10), 3824–3826.

Kirchhoff, L.V., Hoft, D.F., 1990. Immunization and challenge of mice with insect-derived metacyclic trypomastigotes of *Trypanosoma cruzi*. Parasite Immunol. 12, 65–74.

Kirchhoff, L.V., Neva, F.A., 1985. Chagas' disease in Latin American immigrants. JAMA 254, 3058–3060.

Kirchhoff, L.V., Gam, A.A., Gilliam, F.C., 1985. Chagas' disease (American trypanosomiasis) among Central American immigrants. Clin. Res. 33, 407A Ref Type: Abstract.

Kirchhoff, L.V., Paredes, P., Lomeli-Guerrero, A., Paredes-Espinoza, M., Ron-Guerrero, C., Delgado-Mejia, M., et al., 2006. Transfusion-associated Chagas' disease (American trypanosomiasis) in Mexico: implications for transfusion medicine in the United States. Transfusion 46 (2), 298–304.

Laranja, F.S., Dias, E., Nobrega, G., Miranda, A., 1956. Chagas' disease: a clinical, epidemiologic, and pathologic study. Circulation 14, 1035–1060.

Leiby, D.A., Herron, R.M., Jr., Read, E.J., Lenes, B.A., Stumpf, R.J., 2002. Trypanosoma cruzi in Los Angeles and Miami blood donors: impact of evolving donor demographics on seroprevalence and implications for transfusion transmission. Transfusion 42 (5), 549–555.

Leiby, D.A., Herron, R.M., Jr., Garratty, G., Herwaldt, B.L., 2008. Trypanosoma cruzi parasitemia in US blood donors with serologic evidence of infection. J. Infect. Dis. 198 (4), 609–613.

Lent, H., Wygodzinsky, P., 1979. Revision of the Triatominae (Hemiptera, Reduviidae), and their significance as vectors of Chagas' disease. Bull. Am. Mus. Nat. Hist. 163, 123–520.

Lisboa, C.V., Mangia, R.H., Rubiao, E., de Lima, N.R., das Chagas Xavier, S.C., Picinatti, A., et al., 2004. Trypanosoma cruzi transmission in a captive primate unit, Rio de Janeiro, Brazil. Acta Trop. 90 (1), 97–106.

Maloney, J., Newsome, A., Huang, J., Kirby, J., Kranz, M., Wateska, A., et al., 2010. Seroprevalence of Trypanosoma cruzi in raccoons from Tennessee. J. Parasitol. 96 (2), 353–358.

Martinez de Tejada, B., Jackson, Y., Paccolat, C., Irion, O., 2009. Congenital Chagas disease in Geneva: diagnostic and clinical aspects [French]. Rev. Med. Suisse 5 (222), 2091–2092.

Moncayo, A., Silveira, A.C., 2009. Current epidemiological trends for Chagas disease in Latin America and future challenges in epidemiology, surveillance and health policy. Mem. Inst. Oswaldo Cruz 104 (Suppl. 1), 17–30.

Monteiro, R.V., Dietz, J.M., Jansen, A.M., 2010. The impact of concomitant infections by Trypanosoma cruzi and intestinal helminths on the health of wild golden and golden-headed lion tamarins. Res. Vet. Sci. 89, 27–35.

Ortho-Clinical Diagnostics, Inc., 2006. *Trypanosoma cruzi (T. cruzi)*, Whole Cell Lysate Antigen, *ORTHO®* *T. cruzi* ELISA Test System (Package insert). Ref Type: Pamphlet.

Otani, M.M., Vinelli, E., Kirchhoff, L.V., del Pozo, A., Sands, A., Vercauteren, G., et al., 2009. WHO comparative evaluation of serologic assays for Chagas disease. Transfusion 49, 1076–1082.

Piron, M., Verges, M., Munoz, J., Casamitjana, N., Sanz, S., Maymo, R.M., et al., 2008. Seroprevalence of Trypanosoma cruzi infection in at-risk blood donors in Catalonia (Spain). Transfusion 48 (9), 1862–1868.

Ramos-Ligonio, A., Lopez-Monteon, A., Guzman-Gomez, D., Rosales-Encina, J.L., Limon-Flores, Y., Dumonteil, E., 2010. Identification of a hyperendemic area for Trypanosoma cruzi infection in central Veracruz, Mexico. Am. J. Trop. Med. Hyg. 83 (1), 164–170.

Rassi, A., Luquetti, A.O., Ornelas, J.F., Ervilha, J.F., Rassi, G.G., Rassi Junior, A., et al., 2003. The impact of the extensive chemical control of Triatoma infestans on the incidence of acute cases and the prevalence of human Chagas disease. The example of Montalvania, Minas Gerais State. [Portuguese]. Rev. Soc. Bras. Med. Trop. 36 (6), 719–727.

Salvatella, R., 2006. Current Status of Chagas Disease. Pan American Health Association, Washington, DC Ref Type: Pamphlet.

Salvatella, R., 2007. Andean subregional Chagas disease area and the Andean initiative of Chagas disease. Mem. Inst. Oswaldo Cruz 102 (Suppl. 1), 39–40. Epub;%2007 Nov 5.

Sanchez Negrette, O., Mora, M.C., Basombrio, M.A., 2005. High prevalence of congenital Trypanosoma cruzi infection and family clustering in Salta, Argentina. Pediatrics 115 (6), e668–e672.
Santo, A.H., 2009. Chagas disease-related mortality trends, state of Sao Paulo, Brazil, 1985 to 2006: a study using multiple causes of death. Rev. Panam. Salud Publica 26 (4), 299–309.
Sarkar, S., Strutz, S.E., Frank, D.M., Rivaldi, C.L., Sissel, B., Sanchez-Cordero, V., 2010. Chagas disease risk in Texas. PLoS Negl. Trop. Dis. 4 (10), e836.
Schmunis, G.A., 2000. Portuguese. In: Brener, Z., Andrade, Z.A., Barral-Netto, M. (Eds.), *Trypanosoma cruzi* e Doença de Chagas. second ed. Guanabara Koogan, Rio de Janeiro, pp. 1–20.
Schmunis, G.A., Cruz, J.R., 2005. Safety of the blood supply in Latin America. Clin. Microbiol. Rev. 18 (1), 12–29.
Schofield, C.J., Jannin, J., Salvatella, R., 2006. The future of Chagas disease control. Trends Parasitol. 22, 583–588.
Secretaría de Salud, 2002. Norma Oficial Mexicana NOM-032-SSA2-202, para la Vigilancia Epidemiológica, Prevención y Control de Enfermedades Transmitidas por Vector. http://www.mex.ops-oms.org/documentos/chagas/NOM%20032%20SSA2%202002.pdf Estados Unidos Mexicanos. Ref Type: Electronic Citation.
Segura, E.L., Cura, E.N., Estani, S.A., Andrade, J., Lansetti, J.C., de Rissio, A.M., et al., 2000. Long-term effects of a nationwide control program on the seropositivity for Trypanosoma cruzi infection in young men from Argentina. Am. J. Trop. Med. Hyg. 62 (3), 353–362.
Starr, M.D., Rojas, J.C., Zeledon, R., Hird, D.W., Carpenter, T.E., 1991. Chagas' disease: risk factors for house infestation by *Triatoma dimidiata*, the major vector of Trypanosoma cruzi in Costa Rica. Am. J. Epidemiol. 133, 740–747.
Stevens, J.R., Noyes, H.A., Dover, G.A., Gibson, W.C., 1999. The ancient and divergent origins of the human pathogenic trypanosomes, *Trypanosoma brucei* and *T. cruzi*. Parasitology 1, 107–116.
Verani, J.R., Montgomery, S.P., Schulkin, J., Anderson, B., Jones, J.L., 2010. Survey of obstetrician-gynecologists in the United States about Chagas disease. Am. J. Trop. Med. Hyg. 83 (4), 891–895.
Villegas-Garcia, J.C., Santillan-Alarcon, S., 2004. American trypanosomiasis in central Mexico: *Trypanosoma cruzi* infection in triatomine bugs and mammals from the municipality of Jiutepec in the state of Morelos. Ann. Trop. Med. Parasitol. 98 (5), 529–532.
Wendel, S., 2010. Transfusion transmitted Chagas disease: is it really under control? Acta Trop. 115 (1–2), 28–34.
WHO, 2010. Chagas disease (American trypanosomiasis) fact sheet (revised in June 2010). Wkly. Epidemiol. Rec. 85 (34), 334–336.
Williams, J.T., Dick, E.J., Jr., Vandeberg, J.L., Hubbard, G.B., 2009. Natural Chagas disease in four baboons. J. Med. Primatol. 38 (2), 107–113.
Wisnivesky-Colli, C., Schweigmann, N.J., Alberti, A., Pietrokovsky, S.M., Conti, O., Montoya, S., et al., 1992. Sylvatic American trypanosomiasis in Argentina. Trypanosoma cruzi infection in mammals from the Chaco forest in Santiago del Estero. Trans. R. Soc. Trop. Med. Hyg. 86, 38–41.
Yadon, Z.E., Schmunis, G.A., 2009. Congenital Chagas disease: estimating the potential risk in the United States. Am. J. Trop. Med. Hyg. 81 (6), 927–933.
Yaeger, R.G., 1988. The prevalence of *Trypanosoma cruzi* infection in armadillos collected at a site near New Orleans, Louisiana. Am. J. Trop. Med. Hyg. 38, 323–326.

CHAPTER 2

Acute and Congenital Chagas Disease

Caryn Bern,* **Diana L. Martin,*** and **Robert H. Gilman**†

Contents

* Parasitic Diseases Branch, Division of Parasitic Diseases and Malaria, Centers for Disease Control and Prevention, Atlanta, Georgia, USA
† Johns Hopkins University Bloomberg School of Public Health, Baltimore, Maryland, USA

Advances in Parasitology, Volume 75
ISSN 0065-308X, DOI: 10.1016/B978-0-12-385863-4.00002-2

Abstract The acute phase of Chagas disease lasts 4–8 weeks and is characterized by microscopically detectable parasitaemia. Symptoms are usually mild with severe acute disease occurring in less than 1% of patients. Orally transmitted *Trypanosoma cruzi* outbreaks can have more severe acute morbidity and higher mortality than vector-borne infection. Congenital *T. cruzi* infection occurs in 1–10% of infants of infected mothers. Most congenital infections are asymptomatic or cause non-specific signs, requiring laboratory screening for detection. A small proportion of congenital infections cause severe morbidity with hepatosplenomegaly, anaemia, meningoencephalitis and/or respiratory insufficiency, with an associated high mortality. Infected infants are presumed to carry the same 20–30% lifetime risk of cardiac or gastrointestinal disease as other infected individuals. Most control programs in Latin America employ prenatal serological screening followed by microscopic examination of cord blood from infants of seropositive mothers. Recent data confirm that polymerase chain reaction (PCR) is more sensitive and detects congenital infections earlier than conventional techniques. For infants not diagnosed at birth, conventional serology is recommended at at 6 to 9 months of age. In programs that have been evaluated, less than 20% of at risk infants completed all steps of the screening algorithm. A sensitive, specific and practical screening test for newborns is needed to enable Chagas disease to be added to newborn screening programs.

2.1. INTRODUCTION

Chagas disease, caused by the protozoan parasite *Trypanosoma cruzi*, leads to more morbidity and mortality in the Americas than any other parasitic disease (Rassi et al., 2010). In 2004 estimates for the American region, Chagas disease accounted for nearly five times as many disability adjusted life years lost as malaria (World Health Organization, 2008). An estimated 8 million people are currently infected; 20–30% of these will develop symptomatic, potentially life-threatening Chagas disease (Organización Panamericana de la Salud, 2006). *T. cruzi* is carried in the gut of haematophagous triatomine bugs, and transmission occurs when infected bug faeces contaminate the bite site or intact mucous membranes. *T. cruzi* can also be transmitted through transfusion, transplant and congenitally (Maguire, 2004; Rassi et al., 2010). Since 1991, several subregional initiatives have made major advances in control of domiciliated Chagas disease vectors and *T. cruzi* screening of the blood supply (Dias et al., 2002; Schmunis and Cruz, 2005). Uruguay, Chile and Brazil, as well as many areas of Argentina and Paraguay, have been certified free of Chagas transmission by the domestic vectors *Triatoma infestans* and *Panstrongylus megistus*. Nevertheless, *T. cruzi* seroprevalence remains high in adults in many countries of Latin America (Moncayo, 2003; Rassi et al., 2010). Because *T. cruzi* infection is life-long, women infected in childhood will remain at risk for transmission to their infants for a generation to come, even if vector-borne transmission were interrupted today (Carlier and Torrico, 2003). Congenitally infected women can also transmit to their children, sustaining the cycle across generations in the absence of the vector (Schenone et al., 1987).

2.2. ACUTE PHASE

2.2.1. Clinical manifestations

The incubation period following vector-borne *T. cruzi* exposure is 1–2 weeks, after which the acute phase of Chagas disease begins (Rassi et al., 2010). The acute phase lasts 4–8 weeks and is characterized by circulating trypomastigotes detectable by microscopy of fresh blood or buffy coat smears. Most patients have only mild, non-specific symptoms such as fever or are asymptomatic, so do not come to clinical attention during the acute phase. In a minority of patients, acute infection may be associated with inflammation and swelling at the site of inoculation, known as a chagoma. Chagomas typically occur on the face or extremities; in some cases, parasites can be demonstrated in the lesion. Inoculation via the conjunctiva may lead to characteristic unilateral swelling of the upper and lower eyelid known as Romaña's sign. Severe acute disease occurs in less than 1% of patients. Manifestations may include acute myocarditis, pericardial effusion and/or meningoencephalitis (Acquatella, 2007; Maguire, 2004). Severe acute Chagas disease carries a substantial risk of mortality.

In the setting of transfusion- and transplant-associated infections, the incubation period may be as long as 4 months, and immunosuppression may lead to more severe acute manifestations (Centers for Disease Control and Prevention, 2002; Kun et al., 2009). In published reports, all seven patients known to have been infected through blood component transfusion in the United States (five) or Canada (two) had underlying malignancies and received chemotherapy; platelet units were implicated in several cases (Centers for Disease Control and Prevention, 2007; Cimo et al., 1993; Grant et al., 1989; Leiby et al., 1999; Nickerson et al., 1989; Young et al., 2007). Four of the five infected patients with available clinical data presented with severe manifestations of Chagas disease, including acute myocarditis, acute atrioventricular block, severe congestive heart failure, pericarditis with *T. cruzi* in the pericardial fluid and possible meningoencephalitis (Cimo et al., 1993; Grant et al., 1989; Nickerson et al., 1989; Young et al., 2007). The recipient of platelets detected as infected during a research study had *T. cruzi* infection detects by PCR and serology during prospective monitoring, but never developed symptoms (Leiby et al., 1999).

In the setting of organ derived transmission, symptoms of acute *T. cruzi* infection can include fever, malaise, anorexia, hepatosplenomegaly, skin lesions, acute myocarditis and decreased cardiac function. Several clusters of organ transplant transmission of *T. cruzi* have been described in the United States since 2001 (Centers for Disease Control and Prevention, 2002; Kun et al., 2009). Of the five infected recipients with published clinical data, one died from acute Chagas myocarditis despite a full course of nifurtimox treatment. Three others presented with febrile illnesses, received antitrypanosomal therapy and died from causes not directly related to Chagas disease (Centers for Disease Control and Prevention, 2002; Kun et al., 2009). One recipient was asymptomatic and was tested because she received an organ from the same donor as the first recipient described above; she was treated with nifurtimox and had a good clinical outcome (Centers for Disease Control and Prevention, 2002).

Recently, increasing attention has focused on the oral route of *T. cruzi* transmission; common source outbreaks from contaminated fruit or sugar cane juice have been reported from Brazil and Venezuela (Beltrao et al., 2009; de Noya et al., 2010; Nobrega et al., 2009). Most outbreaks are small, often affecting family groups in the Amazon region, where the palm fruit açaí is a dietary staple that appears to be particularly vulnerable to contamination, perhaps from infected triatomine vectors living in the trees themselves (Coura et al., 2002; Nobrega et al., 2009). The largest reported outbreak to date led to more than 100 infections among students and staff at a school in Caracas; locally prepared guava juice was implicated (de Noya et al., 2010). Orally transmitted *T. cruzi* infection appears to be associated with more severe acute morbidity and higher mortality than vector-borne infection (Beltrao et al., 2009; Secretaria de Vigilancia em Saude de Brasil, 2007). For example, 75% of 103 infected individuals in the Caracas outbreak were symptomatic, 59% had electrocardiogram (ECG) abnormalities, 20% were hospitalized and there was one death from acute myocarditis (de Noya et al., 2010). Among 13 patients infected in two outbreaks associated with infected sugar cane juice in northeastern Brazil, 92% had ECG abnormalities, 27% had ejection fractions below 55%

and two individuals died of acute Chagas disease (Bastos et al., 2010). Among survivors, nearly all cardiac abnormalities resolved after treatment with benznidazole. Recent laboratory data suggest that parasite contact with host gastric acid may render trypomastigotes more invasive through changes in parasite surface glycoproteins, and that this interaction may underlie the increased clinical severity seen in orally acquired Chagas disease (Covarrubias et al., 2007; Yoshida, 2008).

2.2.2. Diagnosis

In the acute phase, the level of parasitaemia is high, and motile trypomastigotes can often be detected by microscopy of fresh preparations of anticoagulated blood or buffy coat (WHO Expert Committee, 2002). The level of parasitaemia decreases within 90 days of infection, even without treatment, and is undetectable by microscopy in the chronic phase (Wegner and Rohwedder, 1972; WHO Expert Committee, 2002). PCR is a sensitive diagnostic tool in the acute phase of Chagas disease. It may also be used to monitor for acute *T. cruzi* infection in the recipient of an infected organ or after accidental exposure (Herwaldt, 2001; Herwaldt et al., 2000; Kun et al., 2009). When *T. cruzi*-infected organ donors are detected before or soon after the transplant, microscopy and PCR of serial blood specimens are recommended to monitor for infection in the recipient (Chin-Hong et al., 2011; Riarte et al., 1999). A frequently recommended monitoring schedule consists of weekly specimens for 2 months post-transplant, every 2 weeks for the 3rd month and then monthly afterwards depending on the clinical status of the patient (Chin-Hong et al., 2011; Riarte et al., 1999). Patients with infections detected in this way can be treated immediately and have favourable outcomes in the majority of cases (Chin-Hong et al., 2011; Riarte et al., 1999). PCR assays generally demonstrate positive results days to weeks before circulating trypomastigotes are detectable by microscopy (Schijman et al., 2000).

2.2.3. The immunology of acute *Trypanosoma cruzi* infection

Experimental models of acute *T. cruzi* infection have demonstrated a critical role for type 1 immunity in control of infection, via toll-like receptor (TLR)-mediated and TLR-independent cytokine production (Bafica et al., 2006; Koga et al., 2006; Monteiro et al., 2006). While early data suggested a degree of immunosuppression caused by *T. cruzi* infection, the development of tools to directly monitor antigen-specific lymphocytes have shown a robust anti-parasite response during acute experimental infection (Martin et al., 2006; Tzelepis et al., 2006, 2008). The limited data in acute human *T. cruzi* infection also indicate a bias towards type 1 immunity. Two acutely infected schoolchildren in Paraguay (parasitaemic with the Romaña sign) displayed cytokine mRNA profiles from peripheral blood mononuclear cells (PBMCs) biased towards interferon (IFN)-γ, interleukin (IL)-2 and IL-10, with low levels of IL-4 (Samudio et al., 1998). In the same study, the 23 children with asymptomatic chronic *T. cruzi* infection had upregulated IL-4 mRNA, suggesting that following type 1 immune-mediated clearance of parasitaemia, a balance of type 1 and type 2 responses combine to suppress parasite load, with the type 2 cytokines theoretically protecting against immunopathology (Samudio et al., 1998). Serum specimens from children with acute infection in a study in northern Argentina showed higher serum levels of tumour necrosis factor (TNF)-α, sIL2R, sCD8, sCD4 and IL-6, but no change in IL-2, IL-12 and IL-8, compared to healthy controls or children with asymptomatic chronic *T. cruzi* infection (Moretti et al., 2002). Benznidazole treatment and decreased parasitaemia levels were associated with a decrease in the previously elevated serum cytokine levels.

2.3. CLINICAL AND DIAGNOSTIC ASPECTS OF CONGENITAL *TRYPANOSOMA CRUZI* INFECTION

2.3.1. Clinical aspects

Congenital *T. cruzi* infection causes a spectrum of clinical manifestations. Disease severity may be related in part to the period of pregnancy during which transmission occurs. Although data are sparse, transmission early in pregnancy appears to increase risk of spontaneous abortion, while infection after 22 weeks of gestation is thought to be more likely to lead to a late stillbirth or infected live-born infant (Azogue et al., 1985; Bittencourt and Barbosa, 1972; Bittencourt et al., 1974). Infected live-born infants fall into three clinical categories: (1) severe disease at birth with high risk of neonatal death, (2) apparently well at birth with progression to symptoms in the first weeks to months and (3) asymptomatic throughout infancy, but with the risk of chronic cardiac or gastrointestinal Chagas disease decades later. Most infected newborns are asymptomatic or have subtle findings, and fall into categories (2) or (3) (Bern et al., 2009; Torrico et al., 2004).

The manifestations of symptomatic congenital Chagas disease can include low birth weight, prematurity, low Apgar scores, hepatosplenomegaly, anaemia and thrombocytopenia (Bittencourt et al., 1975, 1981; Maguire, 2004; Torrico et al., 2004). Severely affected neonates may have meningoencephalitis, gastrointestinal megasyndromes, anasarca, pneumonitis and/or respiratory distress (Bittencourt et al., 1975, 1981, 1984; Torrico et al., 2004). Mortality among infected infants is significantly higher than in uninfected infants, ranging from <5% to 20% in published studies (Bittencourt, 1992; Torrico et al., 2004). However, even severe congenital Chagas disease may not be recognized because signs are often non-specific, or the diagnosis is not considered (Torrico et al., 2004).

2.3.2. Diagnosis of congenital *Trypanosoma cruzi* infection

2.3.2.1. Diagnosis in the first 6–9 months of life

Direct parasitologic methods based on microscopic visualization of parasites have the advantage of very high specificity when performed by an experienced laboratory. Concentration methods yield better sensitivity than direct examination of fresh blood. The microhaematocrit method or "micromethod" is the most widely used technique in Latin American health facilities, and consists of centrifugation of fresh cord or neonatal blood sealed in four to six heparinized microhaematocrit tubes followed by light microscopic examination of the buffy coat layer (Azogue et al., 1985; Freilij et al., 1983; La Fuente et al., 1984). The micromethod uses a small volume of blood and requires less processing than the classic Strout concentration method (Strout, 1962). The major limitation of the micromethod is suboptimal sensitivity. In published studies, testing a single specimen (e.g., cord blood) misses 40–100% of infected infants (Azogue and Darras, 1991; Bern et al., 2009; Mora et al., 2005). Repeated sampling increases the sensitivity. In part, this may reflect the finding that parasitaemia levels in infected infants increase in the weeks after birth, peaking around 30–60 days of life (Bern et al., 2009; Bittencourt, 1976). In a study of neonatal diagnostic testing in Santa Cruz, Bolivia, a total of four specimens were examined in the first 2 weeks of life: all infected infants had circulating parasites found on at least one examination, but all four examinations were necessary to diagnose all of the infants (cumulative detection on day 0: 61%, day 4: 67%, day 7: 83%, day 15: 100%) (Azogue and Darras, 1991). In a subsequent study in the same city, none of the 10 infected infants had positive microhaematocrit results in cord blood, but parasites were detected in subsequent neonatal specimens from four (40%) infants (Bern et al., 2009). However, repeated neonatal blood sampling is often unacceptable to parents and impractical for large-scale screening.

Molecular techniques have substantially higher sensitivity and detect congenital infections earlier in life compared to the micromethod (Bern et al., 2009; Duffy et al., 2009; Russomando et al., 1998). However, transient detection of parasite DNA has occasionally been reported in infants who subsequently are found to be uninfected (Bern et al., 2009; Oliveira et al., 2010). For this reason, positive PCR on two separate samples may be used as a criterion for confirmation of congenital infection (Bern et al., 2009). Parasite DNA can be detected in umbilical cord tissue; the sensitivity of PCR in this specimen type appears to be higher than in cord blood specimens (Bern et al.,

2009). Although not yet widely implemented in the context of screening programs, PCR is increasingly used for the early diagnosis of congenital Chagas disease in Latin America and is the method of choice in industrialized countries (Carlier and Torrico, 2003; Jackson et al., 2009; Muñoz et al., 2007; Russomando et al., 1998; Schijman, 2006). The sensitivity of *T. cruzi* PCR techniques reported in the literature varies widely, depending on the specific extraction methods, primers, population tested and investigator experience (Britto et al., 1993, 1995; Moser et al., 1989; Souto and Zingales, 1993; Virreira et al., 2003; Wincker et al., 1994a,b). Nonetheless, PCR applied in a single infant specimen can achieve sensitivity equivalent to or higher than that achieved by testing multiple specimens by conventional parasitologic techniques (Virreira et al., 2003). Several primer sets targeting kinetoplast DNA minicircles (S35/S36, 121/122) or nuclear DNA satellite repeats (Tcz1/Tcz2) are widely used for *T. cruzi* detection in blood or tissue (Vago et al., 1996; Virreira et al., 2003; Wincker et al., 1994b). The kinetoplast minicircle primers have been used with success to screen infants of infected mothers for congenital infection and to monitor congenitally infected infants for response to treatment (Bern et al., 2009; Mora et al., 2005; Russomando et al., 1998; Schijman et al., 2003).

Classic indirect parasitologic techniques, xenodiagnosis, haemoculture and suckling mouse inoculation, can have high specificity in expert hands (Freilij et al., 1983). However, sensitivity is more variable and each of these techniques has stringent requirements and requires substantial resources and expertise (laboratory-reared triatomine colonies for xenodiagnosis, labour-intensive techniques and a contamination-free environment for haemoculture, and animal facilities for mouse inoculation), making them impractical for routine diagnosis or large-scale screening. Moreover, results from these assays are not available for 30–60 days. Histologic examination of the placenta has moderately high sensitivity, but low positive predictive value. Only a portion of pregnancies with positive placental histopathology result in infected infants (Torrico et al., 2004). In addition, placental examination requires substantial resources and expertise.

Several serological tests have been proposed for use to diagnose congenital or acute infection, but these tests are currently available only in a few research settings and current data are insufficient to recommend their wide application. A test with high reported sensitivity and specificity was developed using *T. cruzi* trypomastigote excretion–secretion antigens (TESA) as antigens in IgG and IgM immunoblot assays. Sera from patients with chronic infection show a broad band at 150–160 kDa on the IgG immunoblot, while those from acute and congenital Chagas disease patients demonstrate a characteristic ladder-like set of bands at 130–200 kDa on the IgM immunoblot (Umezawa et al., 1996). The ladder-like bands appear to correspond to shed acute phase antigens

(SAPA) that occur in acute and congenital Chagas disease (Breniere et al., 1997). In published data in specimens from acutely infected patients, including just four congenitally infected infants, TESA (SAPA)-IgM sensitivity is reported to be high (Umezawa et al., 1996, 2001). However, in a subsequent cohort study, only 56% of congenitally infected infants were detected by TESA (SAPA)-IgM (Bern et al., 2009). In the same study, TESA (SAPA)-IgM specificity was 100% in 92 cord blood specimens and 207 follow-up specimens from uninfected infants. An IgG ELISA based on recombinant SAPA antigen has been employed in one recent study; 50% of mothers had positive SAPA-ELISA, so the diagnosis of infection in the infant depended on subtracting the maternal ELISA absorbance value from the absorbance value in the infant specimen (Mallimaci et al., 2010). Based on this technique, all three infected infants in the study were identified within the first 30 days of life. Anti-*T. cruzi* lysate IgM assays have proved neither highly sensitive nor highly specific, possibly due in part to suppression of foetal IgM production by circulating maternal IgG antibodies (Reyes et al., 1990).

2.3.2.2. Diagnosis in later infancy or childhood

For infants not diagnosed at birth, conventional IgG serology is recommended after 6–9 months of age, when transferred maternal antibody has disappeared and the congenital infection has passed into the chronic phase (Carlier and Torrico, 2003; Carlier and Truyens, 2010). Diagnosis of chronic infection relies on detection of serum IgG antibodies to *T. cruzi*, principally by ELISA using whole parasite lysates or recombinant antigens, and immunofluorescent antibody (IFA) test. No single serological assay has sufficiently high sensitivity and specificity to be relied on alone; serum specimens are therefore tested by at least two assays based on different antigens or principles (WHO Expert Committee, 2002). The age at which maternal antibodies disappear has been reported as ranging from 6 to 9 months, and depends on the sensitivity of the test; the more sensitive the test used, the longer transferred maternal antibodies will be detectable. A less sensitive test such as the indirect haemagglutination assay is likely to show negative results in most or all infants at 6 months of age. However, when a highly sensitive commercial ELISA was employed, 78% of infants had positive serology at 6 months and 2.5% at 9 months of age (Bern et al., 2009).

2.4. ANTITRYPANOSOMAL DRUG TREATMENT

Nifurtimox and benznidazole are the only licensed drugs with proven efficacy against Chagas disease (Coura and de Castro, 2002; Maguire, 2004). In acute and early congenital Chagas disease both drugs reduce the severity of symptoms, shorten the clinical course and reduce the duration of detectable parasitaemia (Cancado and Brener, 1979; Wegner and Rohwedder, 1972). In the acute phase parasitological cure is thought to occur in 60–85% of patients treated (Cancado and Brener, 1979; Wegner and Rohwedder, 1972). Currently, treatment of an infant requires benznidazole or nifurtimox tablets to be crushed and prepared as a syrup or slurry in a compounding pharmacy, but a paediatric liquid formulation of benznidazole is under development (Drugs for Neglected Disease Initiative, 2010). Although longitudinal data are lacking, successful treatment of congenital infection is assumed to decrease or eliminate risk of later complications (Freilij and Altcheh, 1995; Schijman, 2006). Early diagnosis and treatment is therefore a high priority in control programs.

2.4.1. Nifurtimox

Nifurtimox (Lampit, Bayer 2502) is a nitrofuran active against trypomastigotes and amastigotes. The drug interferes with *T. cruzi* carbohydrate metabolism by inhibiting pyruvic acid synthesis. Side effects include tremors, irritability, insomnia, anorexia and weight loss. The more serious adverse effects, peripheral neuropathy, psychosis, and haemolytic anaemia associated with G6PD deficiency, are dose-dependent, appear towards the end of treatment and usually resolve when treatment is stopped. The standard dosage regimen varies by age: 10–15 mg/kg/day for children 10 years or younger; 12.5–15 mg/kg/day for 11–16 years and 8–10 mg/kg/day for those 17 years or older. For all regimens, the drug is administered orally in 3 or 4 divided doses for 90 days. Higher doses are often used in infants than in older children, and tolerance is better in children than adults. In one case series of congenitally infected children, adverse effects from nifurtimox were common, but most were mild (24% poor feeding, 14.5% irritability and 6.5% vomiting; Freilij and Altcheh, 1995). Three (4.8%) of 62 children had reversible leukopenia and thrombocytopenia (Freilij and Altcheh, 1995).

2.4.2. Benznidazole

Benznidazole (Rochagon, Roche 7-1051) is a nitroimidazole derivative, considered more trypanocidal than nifurtimox. Side effects fall into three categories, hypersensitivity (light-sensitive rashes that can progress to exfoliative dermatitis), bone marrow suppression (thrombocytopenia, neutroenia, agranulocytosis) and neurologic (peripheral neuropathy). The standard benznidazole dosage regimens are 10 mg/kg/day for children younger than 12 years and 5–7 mg/kg/day for those 12 years or older. The drug is administered orally in two divided doses for 60 days. Benznidazole was well tolerated in two placebo-controlled trials in children (12% rash and <5% with gastrointestinal symptoms in one study; <10% moderate reversible side effects in the other study) (Andrade et al., 1996; Sosa-Estani and Segura, 1999).

2.4.3. Clinical trial data

The earliest trials of antitrypanosomal drugs were conducted in patients with acute Chagas disease in the 1960s and 1970s using nifurtimox (Cancado and Brener, 1979; Wegner and Rohwedder, 1972). Early in life, congenital Chagas disease is an acute phase infection with patent parasitaemia, and was included in the earliest treatment recommendations (Cancado and Brener, 1979). Although trial data for benznidazole are not available, 210 infants were included in the clinical trial for nifurtimox in acute Chagas disease conducted by Bayer (Wegner and Rohwedder, 1972). Infants and young children had significantly lower rates of side effects. For example, anorexia was seen in 25% of children compared to >70% of adults, and neuropathy was reported in 0% of children compared to 23% of adults (Wegner and Rohwedder, 1972). Serological cure was documented at the 12-month follow-up in 81% of those treated in the acute phase (Wegner and Rohwedder, 1972). Observational studies confirm that treatment with either nifurtimox or benznidazole is tolerated better in infants than in older children or adults, and yields high cure rates (Freilij and Altcheh, 1995; Russomando et al., 1998).

Until recently, only the acute phase, including early congenital infection, was thought to be responsive to etiological therapy. However, in the 1990s, two placebo-controlled trials of benznidazole treatment in children with chronic *T. cruzi* infection demonstrated approximately 60% cure as measured by conversion to negative serology 3–4 years after the end of treatment (Andrade et al., 1996; Sosa-Estani et al., 1998). Several follow-up studies suggest that the earlier in life the children are treated, the higher the rate of reversion to negative serology (Andrade et al., 2004; Streiger et al., 2004). Together with growing clinical experience across Latin America, these studies revolutionized management of children with Chagas disease, making early diagnosis and antitrypanosomal drug therapy the standard of care throughout the region (Maguire, 2004; WHO Expert Committee, 2002). There is currently a growing movement to offer treatment to adult patients, including those with early cardiomyopathy (Bern et al., 2007; Viotti et al., 2006; WHO Expert Committee, 2002). This change in standards of practice is based in part on non-randomized, non-blinded longitudinal studies that demonstrate decreased progression of Chagas cardiomyopathy and decreased mortality in adult patients treated with benznidazole (Viotti et al., 1994, 2006). A multi-centre, randomized, placebo-controlled, double-blinded trial of benznidazole for patients with mild to moderate Chagas cardiomyopathy is currently underway and may help to clarify treatment efficacy for this group (http://clinicaltrials.gov/show/NCT00123916).

2.5. EPIDEMIOLOGY OF CONGENITAL CHAGAS DISEASE

2.5.1. Cohort studies of congenital Chagas disease: Transmission rates

Most *T. cruzi*-infected women are asymptomatic and most congenital infections cannot be detected based on clinical findings. Therefore, a prospective birth cohort, in which maternal infection is detected by serologic assays and the infants of infected mothers are tested for congenital *T. cruzi* infection, provides the only study design that can determine vertical transmission rates and the full spectrum of congenital disease. A total of 20 such cohort studies have been described in the published literature since 1980 (Table 2.1) (Arcavi et al., 1993; Azogue and Darras, 1991; Azogue et al., 1985; Bern et al., 2009; Bittencourt et al., 1985; Blanco et al., 2000; Brutus et al., 2008; De Rissio et al., 2009, 2010; Mallimaci et al., 2010; Mora et al., 2005; Nisida et al., 1999; Olivera Mar et al., 2006; Russomando et al., 1998; Salas et al., 2007; Streiger et al., 1995; Tello et al., 1982; Torrico et al., 2004). The *T. cruzi* infection prevalence among pregnant women in these studies varied from <1% to 54%. Even in studies conducted after 2005, seroprevalence among women in some rural areas of Bolivia remains as high as 42% and the prevalence in a public hospital in the largest city in Bolivia was 29% in 2006–2007 (Bern et al., 2009; Brutus et al., 2008; Salas et al., 2007). Prevalence rose with increasing maternal age, reflecting progress in control of vectorial transmission, but infected women younger than 20 years old remain, implying that congenital transmission will continue to pose a risk for the next 25–30 years (Bern et al., 2009; Brutus et al., 2008).

The sensitivity of available diagnostic testing varies, with the highest sensitivity achieved when multiple specimens are tested and serological screening in late infancy is included. For this reason, the completeness of ascertainment in these studies is likely to be heterogeneous. Of the 20 studies, 11 tested only at birth or during the first 30 days of life; 16 of 20 used the micromethod as the only neonatal diagnostic technique. Molecular techniques were used in four studies, but only two of these tested a sufficient number of infants and presented sufficiently complete data to allow transmission rates to be calculated (6.5% in Santa Cruz Bolivia and 9.6% in Salta, Argentina) (Bern et al., 2009; Mora et al., 2005). Direct comparisons of PCR and conventional methods suggest that the use of molecular tools could improve neonatal diagnosis of congenital infection (Bern et al., 2009; Mora et al., 2005). Only 6 of 20 studies tested infants after

TABLE 2.1 Cohort studies of congenital Chagas disease in Latin America published since 1980

Location	Setting	Years	Maternal seroprevalence	Length of infant follow-up	Day of specimen collection	Infant laboratory testing	Infected infants / infants of infected mothers (%)	Reference
Argentina	Endemic province	1975–1991	895/6123 (14.6)	Birth only	0 days	Direct microscopy and/or xenodiagnosis	9/231 (3.9) (664 infants not tested?)	Streiger et al. (1995)
Argentina	Non-endemic area	1990–1991	62/729 (8.5)	Birth	0 days	Micromethod	2/38 (5.1)	Arcavi et al. (1993)
Argentina	Endemic province	1992–1994	927/16,842 (5.5)	12 months (high loss to follow-up)	0, 30 days, 6, 12 months	Micromethod, serology	21/315 (5.7)	Blanco et al. (2000)
Argentina	Non-endemic urban referral centre	1994–2004	Non-representative	12 months (56% loss to follow-up)	0 and 30 days, 6 and 12 months	Micromethod, serology at 12 months	267/4355 (6.1)	De Rissio et al. (2010)
Argentina	Endemic province	1997–2001	Not reported	12 months (30% loss to follow-up)	0 days, 6 and 12 months	Micromethod, PCR, serology	29/302 (9.6)	Mora et al. (2005)
Argentina	Non-endemic urban referral centre	2004–2006	Non-representative	10–18 months	0 and 30 days, 6 and 12+ months	Micromethod, serology at 12 months	29/267 (10.9)	de Rissio et al. (2009)
Argentina	Setting not well described	Not specified	Not reported	9 months	0 days, 9 months, plus specimens at variable times	Micromethod, conventional serology, SAPA-ELISA	3/68 (4.4)	Mallimaci et al. (2010)
Bolivia	Largest city in endemic department	1979–1980	161/317 (50.8)	Birth only	0 days	Strout, placental pathology	18/161 (11.1) + 7 positive only in placenta	Azogue et al. (1985)
Bolivia	Largest city in endemic department	1988–1989	410/760 (53.9)	30 days	0, 4, 7, 15, 20 days	Micromethod, placental pathology	70/410 (17.1) + 8 positive only in placenta	Azogue and Darras (1991)

(*continued*)

TABLE 2.1 *(continued)*

Location	Setting	Years	Maternal seroprevalence	Length of infant follow-up	Day of specimen collection	Infant laboratory testing	Infected infants / infants of infected mothers (%)	Reference
Bolivia	Urban hospital in endemic department	1992–1994	444/1606 (27.6)	Birth and in some cases 30 days	0 and in some cases 30 days	Micromethod and/or haemoculture	22/444 (4.9)	Torrico et al. (2004)
Bolivia	Urban hospital in endemic department	1999–2001	809/3879 (20.8) or 17.3%?	Birth and in some cases 30 days	0 and in some cases 30 days	Micromethod and/or haemoculture	49/811 (6.0)	Torrico et al. (2004)
Bolivia	Hospital in non-endemic area	2002–2004	172/508 (33.9)	Birth	0 days	Micromethod	8/153 (5.2)	Brutus et al. (2008)
Bolivia	Hospital in endemic district	2003–2004	1144/2711 (42.2)	Birth only	0 days	Micromethod	58/1156 (5.0)	Salas et al. (2007)
Bolivia	Largest city in endemic department	2006–2007	154/530 (29.1)	9–12 months	0, 15, 21, 20 days, 3, 6, 9 months	Micromethod, PCR, serology, TESA-blot	10/154 (6.5)	Bern et al. (2009)
Brazil	Urban referral centre	1981–1982	226/2651 (8.5)	Birth only	0 days	Direct microscopy and xenodiagnosis	3/186 (1.6) infants with birth weight >2000 g	Bittencourt et al. (1985)
Brazil	High-risk obstetric services	Not specified	Not reported	Birth	0 days	Micromethod, Quantitative buffy coat (QBC), indirect xenodiagnosis, placental pathology	3/58 (5.2)	Nisida et al. (1999)
Chile	Non-endemic urban referral hospital	1981–1982	27/1000 (2.7)	Birth	0 days	Direct microscopy, xenodiagnosis	3/27 (11.1)	Tello et al. (1982)

Mexico	Regional hospitals in two endemic states	Not specified	3/85 (3.5%) Veracruz, 3/60 (5%) Palenque	Birth	0 days	Serology, haemoculture and PCR	0/6 (0%)	Olivera Mar et al. (2006)
Paraguay	Urban referral centre; rural regional hospital	1991–1992	65/840 (7.7) urban, 107/1022 (10.5) rural	Variable with low completion	Variable	Micromethod and PCR	Unable to determine denominator	Russomando et al. (1998)
Peru	Urban and rural hospitals and health centres	2001–2002	20/3000 (0.73%)	Not reported	Not reported	Micromethod and xenodiagnosis	0/20 (0%)	Mendoza Ticona et al. (2005)

6 months of age with serological techniques, and the reported loss to follow-up for the late infancy specimen was 42–80% (Bern et al., 2009; Blanco et al., 2000; De Rissio et al., 2010). Bearing these limitations in mind, the percentage of infants of infected mothers with congenital *T. cruzi* infection ranged from 0% to 17.1%. However, the two studies which reported no congenital infections lacked sufficient statistical power to estimate the transmission rates, because of the small number of infected women in their study populations (6 and 20 infected women in Mexico and Peru, respectively; Mendoza Ticona et al., 2005; Olivera Mar et al., 2006). One study lacked sufficient data to determine the appropriate denominator for calculating the transmission rate (Russomando et al., 1998). Excluding these three studies, the median transmission rate from infected mothers was 5.7%; for the six studies that included late infancy serological testing, the median was 6.4%. There was no apparent trend in transmission rates over time; the only publication which directly compared cohorts of infants in the same hospital found no difference in the transmission rates in 1992–1994 versus 1999–2001 (Torrico et al., 2004).

2.5.2. Congenital Chagas disease outside of Latin America

In recent years, congenital Chagas disease has been reported in the newborns of Latin American immigrants living in Spain and Switzerland (Jackson et al., 2009; Muñoz et al., 2007). Only one congenital *T. cruzi* infection has been recognized in the United States (CDC, unpublished data, 2010), but estimates of the number of babies with congenital Chagas disease born each year in this country range from 60 to more than 600 (Bern and Montgomery, 2009; Buekens et al., 2008; Yadon and Schmunis, 2009).

2.5.3. Severity spectrum of congenital Chagas disease in epidemiological studies

Early reports of congenital *T. cruzi* infection describe a severe, often lethal clinical picture, ranging from spontaneous abortions and stillbirths to congenital megaesophagus, hydrops fetalis and severe pneumonitis (Bittencourt and Barbosa, 1972; Bittencourt et al., 1972, 1981, 1984). Prematurity and low birth weight were commonly reported (Azogue et al., 1985). However, few studies give a comprehensive description of the clinical spectrum of congenital Chagas disease. One of the seminal studies of congenital Chagas disease was conducted in Cochabamba, Bolivia and compared cohorts of infants born in 1992–1994 and 1999–2001 (Torrico et al., 2004). Half of infected infants were asymptomatic, while half had manifestations attributable to congenital *T. cruzi* infection. A more restrictive analysis, defining "symptomatic" as having at least two severe signs (low birth weight, Apgar <7 at 1 min, respiratory distress syndrome, anasarca), demonstrated significant differences between infected and uninfected infants, as well as a significant decrease in prevalence of symptomatic congenital Chagas disease from the 1992–1994 cohort (50% of infected infants) to the 1999–2001 cohort (18%). The mortality rate also fell from 20% in the earlier cohort to 4% in the later one. Deaths were attributed to respiratory distress syndrome, anaemia, hydrops fetalis and sudden death. Better birth outcomes in the later cohort were considered to be the result of improved prenatal and neonatal health care, and possibly of a decrease in maternal reinfection rates and parasite load due to better vector control. Despite a fall in maternal seroprevalence from 28% in 1992–1994 to 17% in 1999–2001, the congenital transmission rate remained stable at 5–6% of births to infected mothers. A later analysis of the same data suggested that women living in areas with higher vector density were more likely to have positive haemocultures (indicating higher circulating parasite load) than those living in districts with lower vector density (Torrico et al., 2006). Severe disease in the infants also showed a significant association with higher vector density. The authors hypothesized that repeated *T. cruzi* reinfections in women living in infested houses may in turn lead to repeated transplacental transmission, and higher parasite burdens and more severe disease in their infants. Recent cohort data support the notion that the severity of congenital Chagas disease has decreased in the last 20 years, though the role of improved detection in identifying asymptomatically infected infants cannot be ruled out (Bern et al., 2009; Brutus et al., 2008). The majority of congenital infections detected in recent studies are in infants who have normal examinations or only minimal findings (Bern et al., 2009; Brutus et al., 2008).

2.5.4. Epidemiological determinants of congenital transmission

The maternal parasitaemia level is a major biological determinant of transmission risk: the higher the circulating parasite load in the mother at the time of birth, whether measured by haemoculture or quantitative molecular methods, the greater the infection risk for the infant (Bern et al., 2009; Hermann et al., 2004). Younger maternal age, presumed to reflect more recent infection, has been reported to increase transmission risk in some reports but not others (Bern et al., 2009; Bittencourt, 1992; Brutus et al., 2008; Torrico et al., 2004). Limited data suggest that the rate of congenital transmission is higher for HIV-infected women than for immunocompetent mothers (Sartori et al., 2007; Scapellato et al., 2009). This finding may reflect the fact that HIV–*T. cruzi* coinfected individuals have higher parastaemia levels than other persons with chronic *T. cruzi* infection, even in the absence of overt reactivation (Sartori et al., 2002). Infants coinfected with HIV and

T. cruzi may also be more likely to have symptoms, especially neurologic abnormalities (Freilij and Altcheh, 1995; Freilij et al., 1995). Women with one congenitally infected child were found to be more likely to have transmited the parasite to the child's siblings (Sanchez Negrette et al., 2005).

Geographical location (and by extension, parasite strain) has often been cited as a likely risk factor based on the wide variation in reported transmission rates (Bittencourt, 1992). However, at least some of the variation seen among cohort studies is likely attributable to differences in the sensitivity of diagnostic techniques and completeness of follow-up. In an animal model, parasite strain was reported to be an important determinant of transmission risk (Andrade, 1982). Using current tools, no differences have been detected between strained from women who transmitted to their infants and strains from those that did not, but little variation was seen in the *T. cruzi* strains infecting the women under study, all of whom lived in Bolivia or Argentina (Burgos et al., 2007; Corrales et al., 2009; Virreira et al., 2007). Indeed almost none of the available congenital Chagas disease cohort data come from countries outside of the Southern Cone, where *T. cruzi* II, V and VI (formerly IIb, IId and IIe) are predominant (Miles et al., 2009; Zingales et al., 2009). The only cohort studies from areas where *T. cruzi* I is the likely predominant genotype were from Peru and Mexico, and both these studies included such small numbers of infected women that transmission risk could not be quantified (Mendoza Ticona et al., 2005; Olivera Mar et al., 2006).

2.5.5. Immunological responses in the mother and infant

Weak immune responses in the mother have been associated with increased risk of congenital transmission in several studies. Mothers of *T. cruzi*-infected children had lower circulating levels of the pro-inflammatory cytokine tumor necrosis factor alpha (TNFα) and soluble TNF receptor I (TNFRI) (Cardoni et al., 2004; Garcia et al., 2008), and lower production of antigen-stimulated IFNγ and a less activated T cell phenotype than infected mothers of uninfected children (Hermann et al., 2004). The apparent high *T. cruzi* transmission risk for infants of HIV-coinfected women may be related to the higher parasitaemias seen in coinfected individuals, the immunosuppressed state of the HIV-infected mother, or both (Sartori et al., 2002, 2007; Scapellato et al., 2009).

Studies in rats suggest that maternal IFNγ may cross the placenta and provide some protection from congenital *T. cruzi* transmission (Didoli et al., 2000). In a study in southern Bolivia, pregnant women with microscopically detectable parasitaemia had higher serum concentrations of IFNγ, slightly elevated levels of TNFα and decreased levels of transforming growth factor (TGF)β compared to women with undetectable parasitaemia (Cuna et al., 2009). However, no congenital infections were ascertained in this study, probably due to the small sample size, and no direct conclusions can be drawn with respect to congenital transmission risk (Cuna et al., 2009).

In infants with congenital *T. cruzi* infection, cord blood natural killer cell activity was decreased and cord blood CD8+ T cells displayed increased spontaneous T cell apoptosis, oligoclonal expansion of CD8+ T cells with an activated phenotype and parasite-induced IFNγ production (Hermann et al., 2002, 2006). Maternal *T. cruzi* infection has also been shown to modulate the innate immune responses of their uninfected infants. For example, the monocyte-derived cytokines TNFα, IL1β and IL-6 were secreted by cord blood cells from uninfected neonates of infected mothers (Vekemans et al., 2000). Vaccine-induced immune responses also differ in *T. cruzi*-infected versus uninfected infants. IFNγ responses to antigens from hepatitis B virus, diphtheria, or tetanus vaccines were elevated in infants with congenital Chagas disease compared to uninfected infants of either infected or uninfected mothers (Dauby et al., 2009). In contrast, IFNγ responses to *Mycobacterium tuberculosis* purified protein derivative following *Bacillus Calmette-Guerin* (BCG) vaccine were higher in uninfected infants of *T. cruzi*-infected mothers than in either uninfected infants of uninfected mothers or infants with congenital Chagas disease (Dauby et al., 2009). The differential responses may be due to the nature of the vaccines (live attenuated virus in the case of BCG vs. acellular vaccines for the others), the timing of vaccine delivery, or the anti-parasitic treatment given to infants with congenital infection. The altered vaccine-induced response in uninfected infants of *T. cruzi*-infected mothers is indicative of prenatal immune activation due to maternal infection, possibly through soluble parasite antigens or maternal cytokines crossing the placenta. Neonatal immune activation may also confer partial protection from congenital infection, but delineating the relative importance of maternal parasite load, maternal immune responses and neonatal immune activation remains challenging.

2.6. APPROACHES TO THE CONTROL OF CONGENITAL CHAGAS DISEASE

2.6.1. Public health approaches

Conceptually, there are three potential approaches to the control of congenital Chagas disease: primary, secondary and tertiary prevention. Primary prevention depends on prevention of maternal infection, which is already being addressed as a long-term strategy through vector control initiatives (Dias et al., 2002). Antitrypanosomal drug treatment is estimated to cure approximately 60% of children younger than 15 years; the efficacy is thought to be inversely proportional to the time since initial infection (Andrade et al., 1996, 2004; Sosa-Estani et al., 1998). Although data are sparse, girls and women treated before pregnancy are thought to be less likely to transmit to their offspring (Sosa-Estani et al., 2009). Screening and treatment of children with *T. cruzi* infection may therefore help to decrease the congenital transmission risk in the future. Without broad program coverage, however, potentially infectious women will be present in the population for the next generation.

Secondary prevention, antenatal screening to identify seropositive women followed by maternal antitrypanosomal treatment or *in utero* treatment of the foetus, will not be feasible without safer, more effective drugs. No human data are available on teratogenicity and toxicity during pregnancy of benznidazole and nifurtimox, but both drugs have been associated with increased detection of chromosomal aberrations in children being treated for Chagas disease (Gorla et al., 1988, 1989). Both drugs are contraindicated in pregnancy. One attempt to treat a severely affected foetus with hydrops secondary to Chagas disease with exchange transfusions *in utero* was unsuccessful (Okumura et al., 2004).

The approach that carries the most current promise is tertiary prevention: the detection and treatment of infected neonates. Appropriate treatment of newborns has a high cure rate (Carlier and Torrico, 2003; Russomando et al., 1998). Diagnostic testing could be incorporated into existing newborn screening programs (Neto et al., 2004) and may be the impetus to establish screening for metabolic and other disorders in countries such as Bolivia which do not yet have programs (Carlier and Torrico, 2003). The lack of a sensitive, specific and practical *T. cruzi* screening test for newborns represents a major obstacle to this approach.

2.6.2. Current congenital Chagas disease detection programs

The current approach to screening relies on the identification of seropositive pregnant women followed by direct parasitologic testing of infants using the micromethod in cord blood and/or neonatal specimens and for infants not diagnosed parasitologically, conventional IgG serology on specimens after 9 months of age (Blanco et al., 2000; Carlier and Torrico, 2003; Programa Nacional de Control de Chagas, 2007). A central problem in this schema is that the sensitivity of the micromethod is inadequate and may be decreasing over time; the apparent decrease in sensitivity is hypothesized to be related to decreasing maternal and infant parasite loads in areas under vector control (Torrico et al., 2006). In data from the 1980s, the sensitivity of a single micromethod examination in cord blood was ~60% (Azogue and Darras, 1991), but in more recent data, only 40% of infected infants were detected by micromethod in multiple specimens over the first 30 days of life (Bern et al., 2009). New rapid antibody-detection tests could help streamline the maternal step in the screening process and can be applied in cord blood (Luquetti et al., 2003; Ponce et al., 2005; Sosa-Estani et al., 2008). However, when these tests are applied in diverse field sites, their sensitivities have been lower than in the original laboratory analyses and show substantial geographic variation (Roddy et al., 2008; Sosa-Estani et al., 2008; Verani et al., 2009).

Follow-up rates in a pilot screening program in Argentina were low: screening reached 69% of pregnant women, but only 39% of babies of seropositive mothers at birth, and 53% of babies requiring further screening were lost to follow-up in the first year of life (Blanco et al., 2000). In total, only 17% of babies of seropositive mothers completed the required testing algorithm. In practice, these obstacles have been difficult to surmount and few endemic countries currently have effective systematic screening even in highly endemic localities. Prenatal screening is particularly challenging in low prevalence settings such as the United States and will require the development of innovative approaches.

2.7. CONCLUSIONS

As control of vector- and blood-borne *T. cruzi* infection has improved, congenital transmission and outbreaks of orally transmitted acute Chagas disease have become more prominent. Congenital infections are now estimated to represent more than one-quarter of annual new *T. cruzi* infections in Latin America (Organización Panamericana de la Salud, 2006). Adequately powered cohort studies of congenital Chagas disease, preferably with *T. cruzi* genotyping, are needed to assess transmission in geographic areas outside the Southern Cone. Better diagnostic tests with high sensitivity and specificity in cord blood are needed to enable congenital Chagas disease screening programs to improve detection rates and avoid loss to follow-up. Finally, there is still the need to develop safe, efficacious drugs with the ability to cure Chagas disease with shorter, more practical regimens.

REFERENCES

Acquatella, H., 2007. Echocardiography in Chagas heart disease. Circulation 115, 1124–1131.

Andrade, S.G., 1982. The influence of the strain of *Trypanosoma cruzi* in placental infections in mice. Trans. R. Soc. Trop. Med. Hyg. 76, 123–128.

Andrade, A.L., Zicker, F., de Oliveira, R.M., Almeida Silva, S., Luquetti, A., Travassos, L.R., et al., 1996. Randomised trial of efficacy of benznidazole in treatment of early *Trypanosoma cruzi* infection. Lancet 348, 1407–1413.

Andrade, A.L., Martelli, C.M., Oliveira, R.M., Silva, S.A., Aires, A.I., Soussumi, L.M., et al., 2004. Short report: benznidazole efficacy among *Trypanosoma cruzi*-infected adolescents after a six-year follow-up. Am. J. Trop. Med. Hyg. 71, 594–597.
Arcavi, M., Orfus, G., Griemberg, G., 1993. Incidence of Chagas infection in pregnant women and newborn infants in a non-endemic area. Medicina (B Aires) 53, 217–222.
Azogue, E., Darras, C., 1991. Prospective study of Chagas disease in newborn children with placental infection caused by *Trypanosoma cruzi* (Santa Cruz-Bolivia). Rev. Soc. Bras. Med. Trop. 24, 105–109.
Azogue, E., La Fuente, C., Darras, C., 1985. Congenital Chagas' disease in Bolivia: epidemiological aspects and pathological findings. Trans. R. Soc. Trop. Med. Hyg. 79, 176–180.
Bafica, A., Santiago, H.C., Goldszmid, R., Ropert, C., Gazzinelli, R.T., Sher, A., 2006. Cutting edge: TLR9 and TLR2 signaling together account for MyD88-dependent control of parasitemia in *Trypanosoma cruzi* infection. J. Immunol. 177, 3515–3519.
Bastos, C.J., Aras, R., Mota, G., Reis, F., Dias, J.P., de Jesus, R.S., et al., 2010. Clinical outcomes of thirteen patients with acute Chagas disease acquired through oral transmission from two urban outbreaks in northeastern Brazil. PLoS Negl. Trop. Dis. 4, e711.
Beltrao, B., Cerroni, P., Freitas, D.R., Pinto, A.Y., Valente, C., Valente, S.A., et al., 2009. Investigation of two outbreaks of suspected oral transmission of acute Chagas disease in the Amazon region, Para State, Brazil, in 2007. Trop. Doct. 39, 231–232.
Bern, C., Montgomery, S.P., 2009. An estimate of the burden of Chagas disease in the United States. Clin. Infect. Dis. 49, e52–e54.
Bern, C., Montgomery, S.P., Herwaldt, B.L., Rassi, A., Jr., Marin-Neto, J.A., Dantas, R.O., et al., 2007. Evaluation and treatment of Chagas disease in the United States: a systematic review. JAMA 298, 2171–2181.
Bern, C., Verastegui, M., Gilman, R.H., Lafuente, C., Galdos-Cardenas, G., Calderon, M., et al., 2009. Congenital *Trypanosoma cruzi* transmission in Santa Cruz, Bolivia. Clin. Infect. Dis. 49, 1667–1674.
Bittencourt, A.L., 1976. Congenital Chagas disease. Am. J. Dis. Child. 130, 97–103.
Bittencourt, A.L., 1992. Possible risk factors for vertical transmission of Chagas' disease. Rev. Inst. Med. Trop. Sao Paulo 34, 403–408.
Bittencourt, A.L., Barbosa, H.S., 1972. Incidence of congenital transmission of Chagas' disease in abortion. Rev. Inst. Med. Trop. Sao Paulo 14, 257–259.
Bittencourt, A.L., Barbosa, H.S., Rocha, T., Sodre, I., Sodre, A., 1972. Incidence of congenital transmission of Chagas' disease in premature births in the Maternidade Tsylla Balbino (Salvador, Bahia). Rev. Inst. Med. Trop. Sao Paulo 14, 131–134.
Bittencourt, A.L., Barbosa, H.S., Santos, I., Ramos, M.E., 1974. Incidence of congenital transmission of Chagas' disease in full term deliveries. Rev. Inst. Med. Trop. Sao Paulo 16, 197–199.
Bittencourt, A.L., Sadigursky, M., Barbosa, H.S., 1975. Congenital Chagas' disease. Study of 29 cases. Rev. Inst. Med. Trop. Sao Paulo 17, 146–159.
Bittencourt, A.L., Rodrigues de Freitas, L.A., Galvao de Araujo, M.O., Jacomo, K., 1981. Pneumonitis in congenital Chagas' disease. A study of ten cases. Am. J. Trop. Med. Hyg. 30, 38–42.
Bittencourt, A.L., Vieira, G.O., Tavares, H.C., Mota, E., Maguire, J., 1984. Esophageal involvement in congenital Chagas' disease. Report of a case with megaesophagus. Am. J. Trop. Med. Hyg. 33, 30–33.
Bittencourt, A.L., Mota, E., Ribeiro Filho, R., Fernandes, L.G., de Almeida, P.R., Sherlock, I., et al., 1985. Incidence of congenital Chagas' disease in Bahia, Brazil. J. Trop. Pediatr. 31, 242–248.
Blanco, S.B., Segura, E.L., Cura, E.N., Chuit, R., Tulian, L., Flores, I., et al., 2000. Congenital transmission of *Trypanosoma cruzi*: an operational outline for detecting and treating infected infants in north-western Argentina. Trop. Med. Int. Health 5, 293–301.

Breniere, S.F., Yaksic, N., Telleria, J., Bosseno, M.F., Noireau, F., Wincker, P., et al., 1997. Immune response to *Trypanosoma cruzi* shed acute phase antigen in children from an endemic area for Chagas' disease in Bolivia. Mem. Inst. Oswaldo Cruz 92, 503–507.

Britto, C., Cardoso, M.A., Wincker, P., Morel, C.M., 1993. A simple protocol for the physical cleavage of *Trypanosoma cruzi* kinetoplast DNA present in blood samples and its use in polymerase chain reaction (PCR)-based diagnosis of chronic Chagas disease. Mem. Inst. Oswaldo Cruz 88, 171–172.

Britto, C., Cardoso, M.A., Vanni, C.M., Hasslocher-Moreno, A., Xavier, S.S., Oelemann, W., et al., 1995. Polymerase chain reaction detection of *Trypanosoma cruzi* in human blood samples as a tool for diagnosis and treatment evaluation. Parasitology 110 (Pt 3), 241–247.

Brutus, L., Schneider, D., Postigo, J., Romero, M., Santalla, J., Chippaux, J.P., 2008. Congenital Chagas disease: diagnostic and clinical aspects in an area without vectorial transmission, Bermejo, Bolivia. Acta Trop. 106, 195–199.

Buekens, P., Almendares, O., Carlier, Y., Dumonteil, E., Eberhard, M., Gamboa-Leon, R., et al., 2008. Mother-to-child transmission of Chagas' disease in North America: why don't we do more? Matern. Child Health J. 12, 283–286.

Burgos, J.M., Altcheh, J., Bisio, M., Duffy, T., Valadares, H.M., Seidenstein, M.E., et al., 2007. Direct molecular profiling of minicircle signatures and lineages of *Trypanosoma cruzi* bloodstream populations causing congenital Chagas disease. Int. J. Parasitol. 37, 1319–1327.

Cancado, J.R., Brener, Z., 1979. Terapeutica. In: Brener, Z., Andrade, Z. (Eds.), Trypanosoma cruzi e doença de Chagas. Guanabara Koogan, Rio de Janeiro, Brazil, pp. 362–424.

Cardoni, R.L., Garcia, M.M., De Rissio, A.M., 2004. Proinflammatory and anti-inflammatory cytokines in pregnant women chronically infected with *Trypanosoma cruzi*. Acta Trop. 90, 65–72.

Carlier, Y., Torrico, F., 2003. Congenital infection with *Trypanosoma cruzi:* from mechanisms of transmission to strategies for diagnosis and control. Rev. Soc. Bras. Med. Trop. 36, 767–771.

Carlier, Y., Truyens, C., 2010. Maternal-fetal transmission of Trypanosoma cruzi. In: Telleria, J., Tibayrenc, M. (Eds.), American Trypanosomiasis-Chagas Disease: One Hundred Years of Research. Elsevier, New York, NY, pp. 539–581.

Centers for Disease Control and Prevention, 2002. Chagas disease after organ transplantation—United States, 2001. MMWR Morb. Mortal. Wkly Rep. 51, 210–212.

Centers for Disease Control and Prevention, 2007. Blood donor screening for Chagas disease—United States, 2006–2007. MMWR Morb. Mortal. Wkly Rep. 56, 141–143.

Chin-Hong, P.V., Schwartz, B.S., Bern, C., Montgomery, S.P., Kontak, S., Kubak, B., Morris, M.I., Nowicki, M., Wright, C., Ison, M.G., 2011. Screening and Treatment of Chagas Disease in Organ Transplant Recipients in the United States: Recommendations from the Chagas in Transplant Working Group. American Journal of Transplantation. 11, 672–680.

Cimo, P.L., Luper, W.E., Scouros, M.A., 1993. Transfusion-associated Chagas' disease in Texas: report of a case. Tex. Med. 89, 48–50.

Corrales, R.M., Mora, M.C., Negrette, O.S., Diosque, P., Lacunza, D., Virreira, M., et al., 2009. Congenital Chagas disease involves *Trypanosoma cruzi* sub-lineage IId in the northwestern province of Salta, Argentina. Infect. Genet. Evol. 9, 278–282.

Coura, J.R., de Castro, S.L., 2002. A critical review on Chagas disease chemotherapy. Mem. Inst. Oswaldo Cruz 97, 3–24.

Coura, J.R., Junqueira, A.C., Fernandes, O., Valente, S.A., Miles, M.A., 2002. Emerging Chagas disease in Amazonian Brazil. Trends Parasitol. 18, 171–176.

Covarrubias, C., Cortez, M., Ferreira, D., Yoshida, N., 2007. Interaction with host factors exacerbates *Trypanosoma cruzi* cell invasion capacity upon oral infection. Int. J. Parasitol. 37, 1609–1616.

Cuna, W.R., Choque, A.G., Passera, R., Rodriguez, C., 2009. Pro-inflammatory cytokine production in chagasic mothers and their uninfected newborns. J. Parasitol. 95, 891–894.
Dauby, N., Alonso-Vega, C., Suarez, E., Flores, A., Hermann, E., Cordova, M., et al., 2009. Maternal infection with *Trypanosoma cruzi* and congenital Chagas disease induce a trend to a type 1 polarization of infant immune responses to vaccines. PLoS Negl. Trop. Dis. 3, e571.
de Noya, B., Diaz-Bello, Z., Colmenares, C., Ruiz-Guevara, R., Mauriello, L., Zavala-Jaspe, R., et al., 2010. Large urban outbreak of orally acquired acute Chagas disease at a school in Caracas, Venezuela. J. Infect. Dis. 201, 1308–1315.
De Rissio, A.M., Scollo, K., Cardoni, R.L., 2009. Maternal-fetal transmission of *Trypanosoma cruzi* in Argentina. Medicina (B Aires) 69, 529–535.
De Rissio, A.M., Riarte, A.R., Garcia, M.M., Esteva, M.I., Quaglino, M., Ruiz, A.M., 2010. Congenital *Trypanosoma cruzi* infection. Efficacy of its monitoring in an urban reference health center in a non-endemic area of Argentina. Am. J. Trop. Med. Hyg. 82, 838–845.
Dias, J.C., Silveira, A.C., Schofield, C.J., 2002. The impact of Chagas disease control in Latin America: a review. Mem. Inst. Oswaldo Cruz 97, 603–612.
Didoli, G.L., Davila, H.O., Feldman, S., di Masso, R., Revelli, S.S., Bottasso, O.A., 2000. Protected *Trypanosoma cruzi* infection in rats born to mothers receiving interferon-gamma during gestation is associated with a decreased intramacrophage parasite growth and preferential synthesis of specific IgG2b antibodies. Int. J. Immunopharmacol. 22, 45–55.
Drugs for Neglected Disease Initiative, 2010. Chagas disease: DNDi Strategy. http://www.treatchagas.org/rd_dndi_strategy.aspx.
Duffy, T., Bisio, M., Altcheh, J., Burgos, J.M., Diez, M., Levin, M.J., et al., 2009. Accurate real-time PCR strategy for monitoring bloodstream parasitic loads in Chagas disease patients. PLoS Negl. Trop. Dis. 3, e419.
Freilij, H., Altcheh, J., 1995. Congenital Chagas' disease: diagnostic and clinical aspects. Clin. Infect. Dis. 21, 551–555.
Freilij, H., Muller, L., Gonzalez Cappa, S.M., 1983. Direct micromethod for diagnosis of acute and congenital Chagas' disease. J. Clin. Microbiol. 18, 327–330.
Freilij, H., Altcheh, J., Muchinik, G., 1995. Perinatal human immunodeficiency virus infection and congenital Chagas' disease. Pediatr. Infect. Dis. J. 14, 161–162.
Garcia, M.M., De Rissio, A.M., Villalonga, X., Mengoni, E., Cardoni, R.L., 2008. Soluble tumor necrosis factor (TNF) receptors (sTNF-R1 and -R2) in pregnant women chronically infected with *Trypanosoma cruzi* and their children. Am. J. Trop. Med. Hyg. 78, 499–503.
Gorla, N.B., Ledesma, O.S., Barbieri, G.P., Larripa, I.B., 1988. Assessment of cytogenetic damage in chagasic children treated with benznidazole. Mutat. Res. 206, 217–220.
Gorla, N.B., Ledesma, O.S., Barbieri, G.P., Larripa, I.B., 1989. Thirteenfold increase of chromosomal aberrations non-randomly distributed in chagasic children treated with nifurtimox. Mutat. Res. 224, 263–267.
Grant, I.H., Gold, J.W., Wittner, M., Tanowitz, H.B., Nathan, C., Mayer, K., et al., 1989. Transfusion-associated acute Chagas disease acquired in the United States. Ann. Intern. Med. 111, 849–851.
Hermann, E., Truyens, C., Alonso-Vega, C., Even, J., Rodriguez, P., Berthe, A., et al., 2002. Human fetuses are able to mount an adultlike CD8 T-cell response. Blood 100, 2153–2158.
Hermann, E., Truyens, C., Alonso-Vega, C., Rodriguez, P., Berthe, A., Torrico, F., et al., 2004. Congenital transmission of *Trypanosoma cruzi* is associated with maternal enhanced parasitemia and decreased production of interferon-gamma in response to parasite antigens. J. Infect. Dis. 189, 1274–1281.
Hermann, E., Alonso-Vega, C., Berthe, A., Truyens, C., Flores, A., Cordova, M., et al., 2006. Human congenital infection with *Trypanosoma cruzi* induces phenotypic and functional modifications of cord blood NK cells. Pediatr. Res. 60, 38–43.
Herwaldt, B.L., 2001. Laboratory-acquired parasitic infections from accidental exposures. Clin. Microbiol. Rev. 14, 659–688 table of contents.

Herwaldt, B.L., Grijalva, M.J., Newsome, A.L., McGhee, C.R., Powell, M.R., Nemec, D.G., et al., 2000. Use of polymerase chain reaction to diagnose the fifth reported US case of autochthonous transmission of *Trypanosoma cruzi*, in Tennessee, 1998. J. Infect. Dis. 181, 395–399.

Jackson, Y., Myers, C., Diana, A., Marti, H.P., Wolff, H., Chappuis, F., et al., 2009. Congenital transmission of Chagas disease in Latin American immigrants in Switzerland. Emerg. Infect. Dis. 15, 601–603.

Koga, R., Hamano, S., Kuwata, H., Atarashi, K., Ogawa, M., Hisaeda, H., et al., 2006. TLR-dependent induction of IFN-beta mediates host defense against *Trypanosoma cruzi*. J. Immunol. 177, 7059–7066.

Kun, H., Moore, A., Mascola, L., Steurer, F., Lawrence, G., Kubak, B., et al., 2009. Transmission of *Trypanosoma cruzi* by heart transplantation. Clin. Infect. Dis. 48, 1534–1540.

La Fuente, C., Saucedo, E., Urjel, R., 1984. The use of microhaematocrit tubes for the rapid diagnosis of Chagas disease and malaria. Trans. R. Soc. Trop. Med. Hyg. 78, 278–279.

Leiby, D.A., Lenes, B.A., Tibbals, M.A., Tames-Olmedo, M.T., 1999. Prospective evaluation of a patient with *Trypanosoma cruzi* infection transmitted by transfusion. N. Engl. J. Med. 341, 1237–1239.

Luquetti, A.O., Ponce, C., Ponce, E., Esfandiari, J., Schijman, A., Revollo, S., et al., 2003. Chagas' disease diagnosis: a multicentric evaluation of Chagas Stat-Pak, a rapid immunochromatographic assay with recombinant proteins of *Trypanosoma cruzi*. Diagn. Microbiol. Infect. Dis. 46, 265–271.

Maguire, J.H., 2004. Trypanosoma. In: Gorbach, S., Bartlett, J., Blacklow, N. (Eds.), Infectious Diseases. Lippincott, Williams & Wilkins, Philadelphia, pp. 2327–2334.

Mallimaci, M.C., Sosa-Estani, S., Russomando, G., Sanchez, Z., Sijvarger, C., Alvarez, I.M., et al., 2010. Early diagnosis of congenital *Trypanosoma cruzi* infection, using shed acute phase antigen, in Ushuaia, Tierra del Fuego, Argentina. Am. J. Trop. Med. Hyg. 82, 55–59.

Martin, D.L., Weatherly, D.B., Laucella, S.A., Cabinian, M.A., Crim, M.T., Sullivan, S., et al., 2006. CD8+ T-Cell responses to *Trypanosoma cruzi* are highly focused on strain-variant trans-sialidase epitopes. PLoS Pathog. 2, e77.

Mendoza Ticona, C.A., Cordova Benzaquen, E., Ancca Juarez, J., Saldana Diaz, J., Torres Choque, A., Velasquez Talavera, R., et al., 2005. The prevalence of Chagas' disease in puerperal women and congenital transmission in an endemic area of Peru. Rev. Panam. Salud Publica 17, 147–153.

Miles, M.A., Llewellyn, M.S., Lewis, M.D., Yeo, M., Baleela, R., Fitzpatrick, S., et al., 2009. The molecular epidemiology and phylogeography of *Trypanosoma cruzi* and parallel research on Leishmania: looking back and to the future. Parasitology 136, 1509–1528.

Moncayo, A., 2003. Chagas disease: current epidemiological trends after the interruption of vectorial and transfusional transmission in the Southern Cone countries. Mem. Inst. Oswaldo Cruz 98, 577–591.

Monteiro, A.C., Schmitz, V., Svensjo, E., Gazzinelli, R.T., Almeida, I.C., Todorov, A., et al., 2006. Cooperative activation of TLR2 and bradykinin B2 receptor is required for induction of type 1 immunity in a mouse model of subcutaneous infection by *Trypanosoma cruzi*. J. Immunol. 177, 6325–6335.

Mora, M.C., Sanchez Negrette, O., Marco, D., Barrio, A., Ciaccio, M., Segura, M.A., et al., 2005. Early diagnosis of congenital *Trypanosoma cruzi* infection using PCR, hemoculture, and capillary concentration, as compared with delayed serology. J. Parasitol. 91, 1468–1473.

Moretti, E., Basso, B., Cervetta, L., Brigada, A., Barbieri, G., 2002. Patterns of cytokines and soluble cellular receptors in the sera of children with acute Chagas' disease. Clin. Diagn. Lab. Immunol. 9, 1324–1327.

Moser, D.R., Kirchhoff, L.V., Donelson, J.E., 1989. Detection of *Trypanosoma cruzi* by DNA amplification using the polymerase chain reaction. J. Clin. Microbiol. 27, 1477–1482.

Muñoz, J., Portus, M., Corachan, M., Fumado, V., Gascon, J., 2007. Congenital *Trypanosoma cruzi* infection in a non-endemic area. Trans. R. Soc. Trop. Med. Hyg. 101, 1161–1162.

Neto, E.C., Rubin, R., Schulte, J., Giugliani, R., 2004. Newborn screening for congenital infectious diseases. Emerg. Infect. Dis. 10, 1068–1073.

Nickerson, P., Orr, P., Schroeder, M.L., Sekla, L., Johnston, J.B., 1989. Transfusion-associated *Trypanosoma cruzi* infection in a non-endemic area. Ann. Intern. Med. 111, 851–853.

Nisida, I.V., Amato Neto, V., Braz, L.M., Duarte, M.I., Umezawa, E.S., 1999. A survey of congenital Chagas' disease, carried out at three health institutions in Sao Paulo City, Brazil. Rev. Inst. Med. Trop. Sao Paulo 41, 305–311.

Nobrega, A.A., Garcia, M.H., Tatto, E., Obara, M.T., Costa, E., Sobel, J., et al., 2009. Oral transmission of Chagas disease by consumption of acai palm fruit, Brazil. Emerg. Infect. Dis. 15, 653–655.

Okumura, M., Aparecida dos Santos, V., Camargo, M.E., Schultz, R., Zugaib, M., 2004. Prenatal diagnosis of congenital Chagas' disease (American trypanosomiasis). Prenat. Diagn. 24, 179–181.

Oliveira, I., Torrico, F., Munoz, J., Gascon, J., 2010. Congenital transmission of Chagas disease: a clinical approach. Expert Rev. Anti Infect. Ther. 8, 945–956.

Olivera Mar, A., Guillen Ortega, F., Cruz Vidal, S., Hernandez-Becerril, N., Perez Galdamez, E., Cordova Concepcion, G., et al., 2006. Serological and parasitological screening of *Trypanosoma cruzi* infection in mothers and newborns living in two Chagasic areas of Mexico. Arch. Med. Res. 37, 774–777.

Organización Panamericana de la Salud, 2006. Estimación cuantitativa de la enfermedad de Chagas en las Americas. Organización Panamericana de la Salud, Montevideo, Uruguay.

Ponce, C., Ponce, E., Vinelli, E., Montoya, A., de Aguilar, V., Gonzalez, A., et al., 2005. Validation of a rapid and reliable test for diagnosis of Chagas' disease by detection of *Trypanosoma cruzi*-specific antibodies in blood of donors and patients in Central America. J. Clin. Microbiol. 43, 5065–5068.

Programa Nacional de Control de Chagas (Bolivia), 2007. Chagas Congénito: Estrategias de Diagnóstico y Control, p. 1–89, 2nd ed. Digital Dreams, Cochabamba, Bolivia.

Rassi, A., Jr., Rassi, A., Marin-Neto, J.A., 2010. Chagas disease. Lancet 375, 1388–1402.

Reyes, M.B., Lorca, M., Munoz, P., Frasch, A.C., 1990. Fetal IgG specificities against *Trypanosoma cruzi* antigens in infected newborns. Proc. Natl. Acad. Sci. USA 87, 2846–2850.

Riarte, A., Luna, C., Sabatiello, R., Sinagra, A., Schiavelli, R., De Rissio, A., et al., 1999. Chagas' disease in patients with kidney transplants: 7 years of experience 1989-1996. Clin. Infect. Dis. 29, 561–567.

Roddy, P., Goiri, J., Flevaud, L., Palma, P.P., Morote, S., Lima, N., et al., 2008. Field evaluation of a rapid immunochromatographic assay for detection of *Trypanosoma cruzi* infection by use of whole blood. J. Clin. Microbiol. 46, 2022–2027.

Russomando, G., de Tomassone, M.M., de Guillen, I., Acosta, N., Vera, N., Almiron, M., et al., 1998. Treatment of congenital Chagas' disease diagnosed and followed up by the polymerase chain reaction. Am. J. Trop. Med. Hyg. 59, 487–491.

Salas, N.A., Cot, M., Schneider, D., Mendoza, B., Santalla, J.A., Postigo, J., et al., 2007. Risk factors and consequences of congenital Chagas disease in Yacuiba, south Bolivia. Trop. Med. Int. Health 12, 1498–1505.

Samudio, M., Montenegro-James, S., Cabral, M., Martinez, J., Rojas de Arias, A., James, M.A., 1998. Cytokine responses in *Trypanosoma cruzi*-infected children in Paraguay. Am. J. Trop. Med. Hyg. 58, 119–121.

Sanchez Negrette, O., Mora, M.C., Basombrio, M.A., 2005. High prevalence of congenital *Trypanosoma cruzi* infection and family clustering in Salta, Argentina. Pediatrics 115, e668–e672.

Sartori, A.M., Neto, J.E., Nunes, E.V., Braz, L.M., Caiaffa-Filho, H.H., Oliveira Oda, C., Jr., et al., 2002. *Trypanosoma cruzi* parasitemia in chronic Chagas disease: comparison between human immunodeficiency virus (HIV)-positive and HIV-negative patients. J. Infect. Dis. 186, 872–875.

Sartori, A.M., Ibrahim, K.Y., Nunes Westphalen, E.V., Braz, L.M., Oliveira, O.C., Jr., Gakiya, E., et al., 2007. Manifestations of Chagas disease (American trypanosomiasis) in patients with HIV/AIDS. Ann. Trop. Med. Parasitol. 101, 31–50.

Scapellato, P.G., Bottaro, E.G., Rodriguez-Brieschke, M.T., 2009. Mother-child transmission of Chagas disease: could coinfection with human immunodeficiency virus increase the risk? Rev. Soc. Bras. Med. Trop. 42, 107–109.

Schenone, H., Iglesias, J., Schenone, S., Contreras, M.C., 1987. Congenital Chagas' infection of 2d generation. Bol. Chil. Parasitol. 42, 71–73.

Schijman, A.G., 2006. Congenital Chagas disease. In: Mushahwar, I.K. (Ed.), Congenital and Other Related Infectious Diseases of the Newborn. Elsevier, Amsterdam, Netherlands, pp. 223–259.

Schijman, A.G., Vigliano, C., Burgos, J., Favaloro, R., Perrone, S., Laguens, R., et al., 2000. Early diagnosis of recurrence of *Trypanosoma cruzi* infection by polymerase chain reaction after heart transplantation of a chronic Chagas' heart disease patient. J. Heart Lung Transplant. 19, 1114–1117.

Schijman, A.G., Altcheh, J., Burgos, J.M., Biancardi, M., Bisio, M., Levin, M.J., et al., 2003. Aetiological treatment of congenital Chagas' disease diagnosed and monitored by the polymerase chain reaction. J. Antimicrob. Chemother. 52, 441–449.

Schmunis, G.A., Cruz, J.R., 2005. Safety of the blood supply in Latin America. Clin. Microbiol. Rev. 18, 12–29.

Secretaria de Vigilancia em Saude do Brasil, 2007. Doenca de Chagas Aguda. Nota Tecnica, 9 de outubro de 2007. http://portal.saude.gov.br/portal/arquivos/pdf/nota_chagas_091007.pdf.

Sosa-Estani, S., Segura, E.L., 1999. Treatment of *Trypanosoma cruzi* infection in the undetermined phase. Experience and current guidelines of treatment in Argentina. Mem. Inst. Oswaldo Cruz 94 (Suppl. 1), 363–365.

Sosa-Estani, S., Segura, E.L., Ruiz, A.M., Velazquez, E., Porcel, B.M., Yampotis, C., 1998. Efficacy of chemotherapy with benznidazole in children in the indeterminate phase of Chagas' disease. Am. J. Trop. Med. Hyg. 59, 526–529.

Sosa-Estani, S., Gamboa-Leon, M.R., Del Cid-Lemus, J., Althabe, F., Alger, J., Almendares, O., et al., 2008. Use of a rapid test on umbilical cord blood to screen for *Trypanosoma cruzi* infection in pregnant women in Argentina, Bolivia, Honduras, and Mexico. Am. J. Trop. Med. Hyg. 79, 755–759.

Sosa-Estani, S., Cura, E., Velazquez, E., Yampotis, C., Segura, E.L., 2009. Etiological treatment of young women infected with *Trypanosoma cruzi*, and prevention of congenital transmission. Rev. Soc. Bras. Med. Trop. 42, 484–487.

Souto, R.P., Zingales, B., 1993. Sensitive detection and strain classification of *Trypanosoma cruzi* by amplification of a ribosomal RNA sequence. Mol. Biochem. Parasitol. 62, 45–52.

Streiger, M., Fabbro, D., del Barco, M., Beltramino, R., Bovero, N., 1995. Congenital Chagas disease in the city of Santa Fe. Diagnosis and treatment. Medicina (B Aires) 55, 125–132.

Streiger, M.L., del Barco, M.L., Fabbro, D.L., Arias, E.D., Amicone, N.A., 2004. Longitudinal study and specific chemotherapy in children with chronic Chagas' disease, residing in a low endemicity area of Argentina. Rev. Soc. Bras. Med. Trop. 37, 365–375.

Strout, R.G., 1962. A method for concentrating hemoflagellates. J. Parasitol. 48, 100.

Tello, P., Fernandez, P., Sandoval, L., Ampuero, G., Pizarro, T., Schenone, H., 1982. Incidence of *Trypanosoma cruzi* infection in mothers and sons in a section of the northern area of Santiago. Bol. Chil. Parasitol. 37, 23–24.

Torrico, F., Alonso-Vega, C., Suarez, E., Rodriguez, P., Torrico, M.C., Dramaix, M., et al., 2004. Maternal *Trypanosoma cruzi* infection, pregnancy outcome, morbidity, and mortality of congenitally infected and non-infected newborns in Bolivia. Am. J. Trop. Med. Hyg. 70, 201–209.

Torrico, F., Vega, C.A., Suarez, E., Tellez, T., Brutus, L., Rodriguez, P., et al., 2006. Are maternal re-infections with *Trypanosoma cruzi* associated with higher morbidity and mortality of congenital Chagas disease? Trop. Med. Int. Health 11, 628–635.

Tzelepis, F., de Alencar, B.C., Penido, M.L., Gazzinelli, R.T., Persechini, P.M., Rodrigues, M. M., 2006. Distinct kinetics of effector CD8+ cytotoxic T cells after infection with *Trypanosoma cruzi* in naive or vaccinated mice. Infect. Immun. 74, 2477–2481.

Tzelepis, F., de Alencar, B.C., Penido, M.L., Claser, C., Machado, A.V., Bruna-Romero, O., et al., 2008. Infection with *Trypanosoma cruzi* restricts the repertoire of parasite-specific CD8+ T cells leading to immunodominance. J. Immunol. 180, 1737–1748.

Umezawa, E.S., Nascimento, M.S., Kesper, N., Jr., Coura, J.R., Borges-Pereira, J., Junqueira, A.C., et al., 1996. Immunoblot assay using excreted-secreted antigens of *Trypanosoma cruzi* in serodiagnosis of congenital, acute, and chronic Chagas' disease. J. Clin. Microbiol. 34, 2143–2147.

Umezawa, E.S., Nascimento, M.S., Stolf, A.M., 2001. Enzyme-linked immunosorbent assay with *Trypanosoma cruzi* excreted-secreted antigens (TESA-ELISA) for serodiagnosis of acute and chronic Chagas' disease. Diagn. Microbiol. Infect. Dis. 39, 169–176.

Vago, A.R., Macedo, A.M., Oliveira, R.P., Andrade, L.O., Chiari, E., Galvao, L.M., et al., 1996. Kinetoplast DNA signatures of *Trypanosoma cruzi* strains obtained directly from infected tissues. Am. J. Pathol. 149, 2153–2159.

Vekemans, J., Truyens, C., Torrico, F., Solano, M., Torrico, M.C., Rodriguez, P., et al., 2000. Maternal *Trypanosoma cruzi* infection upregulates capacity of uninfected neonate cells To produce pro- and anti-inflammatory cytokines. Infect. Immun. 68, 5430–5434.

Verani, J., Seitz, A., Gilman, R., LaFuente, C., Galdos-Cardenas, G., Kawai, V., et al., 2009. Geographic variation in the sensitivity of recombinant antigen-based rapid tests for chronic *Trypanosoma cruzi* infection. Am. J. Trop. Med. Hyg. 80, 410–415.

Viotti, R., Vigliano, C., Armenti, H., Segura, E., 1994. Treatment of chronic Chagas' disease with benznidazole: clinical and serologic evolution of patients with long-term follow-up. Am. Heart J. 127, 151–162.

Viotti, R., Vigliano, C., Lococo, B., Bertocchi, G., Petti, M., Alvarez, M.G., et al., 2006. Long-term cardiac outcomes of treating chronic Chagas disease with benznidazole versus no treatment: a nonrandomized trial. Ann. Intern. Med. 144, 724–734.

Virreira, M., Torrico, F., Truyens, C., Alonso-Vega, C., Solano, M., Carlier, Y., et al., 2003. Comparison of polymerase chain reaction methods for reliable and easy detection of congenital *Trypanosoma cruzi* infection. Am. J. Trop. Med. Hyg. 68, 574–582.

Virreira, M., Truyens, C., Alonso-Vega, C., Brutus, L., Jijena, J., Torrico, F., et al., 2007. Comparison of *Trypanosoma cruzi* lineages and levels of parasitic DNA in infected mothers and their newborns. Am. J. Trop. Med. Hyg. 77, 102–106.

Wegner, D.H., Rohwedder, R.W., 1972. The effect of nifurtimox in acute Chagas' infection. Arzneimittelforschung 22, 1624–1635.

WHO Expert Committee, 2002. Control of Chagas Disease WHO technical report series number 905. World Health Organization. http://whqlibdoc.who.int/trs/WHO_TRS_905.pdf.

Wincker, P., Bosseno, M.F., Britto, C., Yaksic, N., Cardoso, M.A., Morel, C.M., et al., 1994a. High correlation between Chagas' disease serology and PCR-based detection of *Trypanosoma cruzi* kinetoplast DNA in Bolivian children living in an endemic area. FEMS Microbiol. Lett. 124, 419–423.

Wincker, P., Britto, C., Pereira, J.B., Cardoso, M.A., Oelemann, W., Morel, C.M., 1994b. Use of a simplified polymerase chain reaction procedure to detect *Trypanosoma cruzi* in blood

samples from chronic chagasic patients in a rural endemic area. Am. J. Trop. Med. Hyg. 51, 771–777.
World Health Organization, 2008. The Global Burden of Disease: 2004 Update. World Health Organization, Geneva, Switzerland.
Yadon, Z.E., Schmunis, G.A., 2009. Congenital Chagas disease: estimating the potential risk in the United States. Am. J. Trop. Med. Hyg. 81, 927–933.
Yoshida, N., 2008. *Trypanosoma cruzi* infection by oral route: how the interplay between parasite and host components modulates infectivity. Parasitol. Int. 57, 105–109.
Young, C., Losikoff, P., Chawla, A., Glasser, L., Forman, E., 2007. Transfusion-acquired *Trypanosoma cruzi* infection. Transfusion 47, 540–544.
Zingales, B., Andrade, S.G., Briones, M.R., Campbell, D.A., Chiari, E., Fernandes, O., et al., 2009. A new consensus for *Trypanosoma cruzi* intraspecific nomenclature: second revision meeting recommends TcI to TcVI. Mem. Inst. Oswaldo Cruz 104, 1051–1054.

CHAPTER 3

Cell-Based Therapy in Chagas Disease

Antonio C. Campos de Carvalho,
Adriana B. Carvalho, and **Regina C.S. Goldenberg**

Contents

Abstract

Chagas disease was first described one century ago, yet the mechanisms underlying chagasic cardiomyopathy remain elusive. Disease progression often leads to heart failure and patients with this infectious cardiomyopathy have a poor prognosis. Treatment options for heart failure due to Chagas disease are not different from standard therapy. Over the past decade, cell-based therapies have emerged as a new alternative in the treatment of this disease, not only because of the possibility of replacing lost vessels and cardiomyocytes but also because these cells could potentially influence the microenvironmental changes that perpetuate the disease. In this chapter, we will review current knowledge on cell-based therapies for the treatment of Chagas disease.

Carlos Chagas Filho Institute of Biophysics, Federal University of Rio de Janeiro and National Cardiology Institute, Rio de Janeiro, RJ, Brazil

Advances in Parasitology, Volume 75
ISSN 0065-308X, DOI: 10.1016/B978-0-12-385863-4.00003-4

3.1. INTRODUCTION

Chagas disease in its chronic phase affects primarily the gastrointestinal track resulting in so-called mega-syndromes and the cardiovascular system resulting in cardiomyopathy. Chagasic cardiomyopathy is the most important clinical manifestation of the disease and affects 10–30% of all infected individuals. Endemic in Latin America, this infectious cardiomyopathy is one of the main causes of heart disease in the region, affecting approximately of 1.8–5.4 million people resulting in about 20,000 deaths annually (Salvatella, 2006). Globalization has led to a recent increase in awareness of Chagas disease, since it is an emerging health issue in nonendemic areas with an increase in immigration from endemic areas (Armaganijan and Morillo, 2010; Bern et al., 2007; Rassi et al., 2010).

The cardiomyopathy caused by the parasite *Trypanosoma cruzi* develops years or decades after the primary infection. However, even 100 years after the discovery of the disease by Carlos Chagas (Chagas, 1909), the pathophysiology of this cardiomyopathy is not completely understood. Current knowledge attributes cardiac manifestations to multifactorial causes that include parasite persistence, vascular impairment, destruction of ganglia of the autonomic nervous system, and autoimmunity (Kierszenbaum, 2005). Chronic chagasic cardiomyopathy is characterized by focal or disseminated inflammatory infiltrates, myocytolysis, myonecrosis, and progressive fibrosis (Andrade and Andrade, 1955; Andrade and Lopes, 1963). As a result of damage to the extracellular matrix and the replacement of cardiac myocytes (CMs) and/or vascular cells by fibrous tissue, remodelling of the myocardium and vasculature ensues. This leads to thinning of the left ventricular wall and can result in the formation of apical aneurysms of the left ventricle, a hallmark of chronic chagasic cardiomyopathy. Thromboembolic events are also common as a result of this remodelling process. The intensity of the myocarditis varies considerably from mild cardiac symptoms to intense cardiomyopathy, leading to heart failure and death (Rosenbaum, 1964). Patients with chronic chagasic cardiomyopathy may also have several different types of arrhythmias, causing heart malfunction. The most frequent alterations recorded are ventricular premature beats, complete right bundle branch block, left anterior fascicular block, and atrioventricular block (Moia and Rosenbaum, 1960; Rosenbaum and Alvarez, 1955).

Therapy for chronic chagasic cardiomyopathy is the standard treatment used for congestive heart failure and includes β-blockers, diuretics, angiotensin-converting enzyme inhibitors, and angiotensin receptor blockers. Amiodarone is frequently used to prevent or revert arrhythmias. There is no consensus about the use of anti-trypanosomal agents in chronic chagasic cardiomyopathy; however, while they may decrease progression of disease they do not reverse damage that has already occurred. The BENEFIT study, a large, multicentre, randomized trial designed to address the efficacy of benznidazole in chagasic cardiomyopathy is underway and should provide a definitive answer about the usefulness of anti-trypanosomal agents as a treatment option (ClinicalTrials.gov, BENEFIT: Identifier NCT00123916).

Chronic chagasic cardiomyopathy has been reported to be the main prognostic mortality factor among patients with heart failure of different aetiologies (Freitas et al., 2005). Therefore, as the disease progresses, the prognosis is rather bleak and few therapeutic options are left for the patient other than heart transplantation. Although survival in chagasic heart transplant patients has been reported to be longer than that of patients transplanted for heart disease resulting from other aetiologies (Bocchi and Fiorelli, 2001), the limited number of donors and the complications of immune suppressive therapy, including parasite reactivation, make this therapeutic option a very limited one. New therapeutic interventions are clearly needed (Lanes-Vieira et al., 2010), and cell transplantation has emerged as an addendum to standard therapy in the setting of chronic chagasic cardiomyopathy.

3.2. CELL THERAPY IN CARDIAC DISEASES

3.2.1. Experimental models

The history of cell-based therapies in cardiac diseases dates back to the early 1990s of the past century. The pioneering work of Soonpaa et al. (1995), in which labelled foetal syngeneic CMs were transplanted into adult mouse hearts, proved that exogenous cells could be integrated into the host myocardium. These observations paved the way for many studies utilizing different cell types in various experimental models, which intensified over the past decades. Initially, most of the studies focused on using foetal CM, embryonic stem cell or skeletal myoblast transplantation into hearts that were damaged cryogenically or as a result of myocardial infarction (for a review, see Dimmeler et al., 2005). Skeletal myoblasts and satellite cells do not integrate properly into the host myocardium since they do not form gap junctions with the surrounding CM, thus leading to the development of arrhythmias and precluding further use of these cell types in clinical applications (Menasché, 2009).

Attempts to engraft CMs derived from embryonic stem cells into injured hearts were successful (Hodgson et al., 1994; Klug et al., 1996; Laflamme and Murry, 2005; Laflamme et al., 2005; Ménard et al., 2005). However, the occurrence of teratomas after injection of embryonic stem cells in infarcted animals (Cao et al., 2006) has hampered clinical application of this technique.

An important development in the use of cell therapies to improve cardiac function came as a result of the observations demonstrating that mesenchymal bone marrow cells (BMCs) could be induced to differentiate into CMs *in vitro* (Makino et al., 1999). Tomita et al. (1999) demonstrated that autologous bone marrow mesenchymal cells transplanted into cryoinjured rat hearts improved myocardial function and promoted angiogenesis. Other reports followed, but none demonstrated that the injected stromal BMC were in fact able to differentiate into CMs or blood vessel cells. Orlic et al. (2001) reported that bone marrow c-kit$^+$ haematopoietic stem cells from transgenic mice expressing enhanced green fluorescent protein transplanted into the hearts of syngeneic mice with myocardial infarction differentiated into cardiac muscle and vascular cells. According to the authors, these cells could regenerate the damaged myocardium, promote angiogenesis, and improve cardiac function. Most importantly, they demonstrated complete integration of the transplanted c-kit$^+$ marrow cells, including the formation of gap junctions made of connexin 43 between the newly formed myocardium and the surviving tissue. Other groups demonstrated that haematopoietic and mesenchymal stem cells (MSCs) derived from bone marrow were able to improve cardiac function in models of both cryoinjured and ischaemic heart lesions (Kocher et al., 2001; Olivares et al., 2004; Toma et al., 2002; Wang et al., 2000, 2001). However, heart regeneration by BMC has been questioned. In 2004, three groups failed to reproduce Orlic's data using reporter genes under the control of cardiac specific promoters in c-kit$^+$ positive cells that were transplanted into the hearts of infarcted mice (Balsam et al., 2004; Murry et al., 2004; Nygren et al., 2004). Nevertheless, in the only study where functional measurements were done (Balsam et al., 2004) improvement in heart function was detected after cell transplantation. Since then, the beneficial effects of cell therapies using BMC in heart disease have been increasingly attributed to paracrine effects (Gnecchi et al., 2005; Mangi et al., 2003).

3.2.2. Clinical trials

In the clinical arena, several trials have been performed testing the ability of cell-based therapies to improve cardiac function, mainly in ischaemic heart disease. The first patient was treated in France using skeletal myoblasts (Menasché et al., 2001). However, an efficacy trial failed to demonstrate beneficial effects of this cell type (Menasché et al., 2008), and its use has been discontinued.

Bone marrow-derived cell therapy for ischaemic heart disease has been more intensively studied. By far, the mononuclear fraction of the bone marrow has been the most used cell-based type of therapy, but selected marrow cell populations such as CD34$^+$ and CD133$^+$ have also been tested in small trials (Assmus et al., 2002; Stamm et al., 2003). Results are still somewhat controversial, although metanalyses of randomized trials enrolling almost 700 patients (Lipinsky et al., 2007) and more than 800 patients (Martin-Rendon et al., 2008) have shown a small gain in ejection fraction of patients receiving standard treatment plus cell therapy. More recently, MSCs from bone marrow or adipose tissue origin have been used and, although larger efficacy trials are necessary and underway, initial results do not seem to show improvement beyond that obtained with bone marrow mononuclear fraction (Hare et al., 2009).

3.3. CELL THERAPY IN CHAGAS DISEASE

3.3.1. Experimental models

The mouse has been the most widely used animal model for chronic chagasic cardiomyopathy. Inflammation and fibrosis have been extensively demonstrated in mouse hearts during the chronic phase of Chagas disease (Soares et al., 2004); however, few studies have documented left ventricular dysfunction in these animals, especially using high-resolution imaging modalities, such as dedicated small animal echocardiography equipment and high gradient magnetic resonance imaging (MRI). In fact, for the past 3 years, we have been unable to consistently demonstrate significant left ventricular dysfunction by high-resolution echocardiography using different combinations of mouse and *T. cruzi* strains (unpublished results and Ribeiro dos Santos R., personal communication). In contrast, right ventricular dilatation has been consistently demonstrated by MRI (Goldenberg et al., 2008) and by high-resolution echocardiography (unpublished results). It remains to be explained why the intense inflammation and fibrosis detected in histopathology specimens of the mouse left ventricle fail to induce functional alterations in this ventricular chamber. Based on the above observations, the efficacy of cell-based therapies in the mouse model of chronic chagasic cardiomyopathy can be ascertained by diminished inflammation and fibrosis of the heart or of the right ventricular diameter

Due to the widespread nature of chronic chagasic cardiomyopathy, systemic delivery of cells was chosen for studies in the mouse model of Chagas disease. Thus, as a first step, it was necessary to demonstrate that cells injected intravenously homed into the chagasic hearts. In initial experiments, bone marrow mononuclear cells were labelled with Hoechst 33258 prior to injection into the tail veins of normal and chagasic mice, and cell-treated mice were sacrificed at various time points thereafter. In chagasic mice, Hoechst-labelled cells were observed in the heart 1–7 days after cell injection but were not found in heart sections of normal mice injected with the same cells (Ribeiro dos Santos R., personal communication). As a result of these and other experiments in which BMCs from EGFP transgenic mice were used, it was concluded that bone marrow stem cells home to the chagasic heart, validating systemic injection as a viable approach for cell therapy in this context.

Once homing to the diseased myocardium was established, we demonstrated that bone marrow mononuclear cells from normal syngeneic donors significantly reduced cardiac inflammation and fibrosis in BALB/c and C57BL/6 mice chronically infected with the Colombian strain of *T. cruzi* (Soares et al., 2004). This reduction was long lasting, being observed up to 6 months after cell therapy. Cell dosing experiments demonstrated that a minimum of 10^5 cells were necessary for a significant reduction in the number of inflammatory cells and injection of 10^6 or 10^7 cells induced similar effects (Soares et al., 2004). To translate this therapy into the clinical setting, BMCs from chronically infected mice were used as a source of material for cell therapy, since clinical trials using autologous BMCs would be much easier to conduct. Mononuclear cells derived from bone marrow of chronic chagasic mice were also effective in decreasing inflammation and fibrosis in the hearts of mice with chronic chagasic cardiomiopathy (Soares et al., 2004).

Using a different combination of mouse and *T. cruzi* strains (C129 and Brazil strain), Goldenberg et al. (2008) demonstrated, by cardiac MRI, that 10^7 bone marrow mononuclear cells prevented and reversed right ventricular dilatation induced by *T. cruzi* infection. Another study has reported that repeated injections of granulocyte-colony stimulating factor (G-CSF), which mobilizes stem cells from the bone marrow, decreases inflammation and fibrosis in the hearts of chagasic mice while increasing maximal oxygen consumption during treadmill exercise (Macambira et al., 2009). Furthermore, the combination of mononuclear cells and G-CSF is reported to enhance the effect of the cell therapy in reducing inflammatory infiltrate in chagasic hearts (Ribeiro dos Santos R., personal communication).

In a rat model of chagasic cardiomyopathy, Guarita-Souza et al. (2006) used local left ventricular injection of co-cultured skeletal myoblasts and mesenchymal bone marrow-derived cells. They reported improvement in heart function in chronically infected rats as measured by increased ejection fraction and decreased end-systolic and end-diastolic volumes by echocardiography. These findings suggest that local injection of stem cells may also be effective in chagasic cardiomyopathy, indicating that cells may be able to diffuse from the injection site to reach other regions of the heart.

T. cruzi infection has been shown to induce profound alterations in cardiac transcriptome, both *in vitro* and *in vivo* (Goldenberg et al., 2009; Mukherjee et al., 2003; Soares et al., 2010). Bone marrow-derived mononuclear cell therapy has been extremely effective in reestablishing the normal cardiac transcriptome (84% recovery; Soares et al., 2011), reinforcing the concept that cell-based therapies may indeed contribute as an additional therapeutic option in chronic chagasic cardiomyopathy.

3.4. CLINICAL TRIALS

Based on promising results in animal models and the limitations of currently available therapies for end-stage chagasic cardiomyopahty, a clinical trial was performed to determine the feasibility and safety of autologous BMC transplantation in chagasic patients with congestive heart failure (Vilas-Boas et al., 2006). Due to uncertainties regarding the mechanisms of action of mononuclear cells and the novelty of the procedure, this trial was designed for patients with end-stage congestive heart failure whose only therapeutic option would be heart transplantation. This open label, uncontrolled, single centre clinical trial enrolled 28 patients. Inclusion criteria required patients to be 20–70 years old, of either gender, with congestive heart failure due to Chagas disease, in New York Heart Association (NYHA) class III or IV, with an ejection fraction of less than 40% while on optimized pharmacologic therapy for at least 4 weeks before enrolment (Vilas-Boas et al., 2006). Bone marrow aspiration was performed on the day of cell injection. Bone marrow mononuclear fraction was obtained through Ficoll density gradient centrifugation and, after repeated washes; the mononuclear cell suspension was diluted in 20 ml of saline with 5% autologous serum and injected in the coronary arteries using an angioplasty catheter. Cells were distributed in the coronary circulations as follows: 10 ml in the left descending coronary artery, 5 ml in the circumflex artery, and 5 ml in the right coronary artery. Mean number of cells injected was 270 million. At the 25th day after cell injection, patients received 5 μg/kg of G-CSF for 5 days in order to mobilize progenitor cells from the marrow to the circulation. Patients were followed for 6 months with monthly visits to the outpatient clinic. Since this was a safety trial, special attention was focused on arrhythmias and signs of myocardial injury during the procedure. Fortunately there were no detectable increases in arrhythmias or in troponin I levels during or after the procedure. Evaluation by echocardiography using Simpson's rule indicated that cell therapy induced a small but significant increase in left ventricular ejection fraction, which rose from the mean baseline value of 20–23% after 60 days. Quality of life also improved as determined by the Minnesota Questionnaire and by NYHA class, a result supported by the significant increase in the 6 min walking test. These results were initially observed 1 month after therapy and persisted for the 6-month follow-up period. Authors concluded that bone marrow mononuclear cell therapy by intracoronary delivery was feasible and safe in chronic chagasic cardiomyopathy patients (Vilas-Boas et al., 2006).

Studies using cells labelled with technetium-99m were performed to evaluate cell homing and retention in the chagasic heart. In one patient with chagasic cardiomyopathy, bone marrow mononuclear cells delivered by the intracoronary route were reported to home into diseased, hypoperfused areas of the myocardium at 2 and 6 h after cell injection (Jacob et al., 2007). Another study performed in six chagasic patients using technetium-labelled cells and thallium perfusion images concluded that cells homed preferentially to the perfused areas of the myocardium (Barbosa da Fonseca et al., 2011). Cell retention in this study was estimated by cardiac uptake of the total injected radioactivity at 1, 3, and 24 h after cell injection. Numerical values were 5.4%, 4.3%, and 2.3% respectively, indicating that the majority of the injected cells did not home to the myocardium (Barbosa da Fonseca et al., 2010). In fact, liver and spleen were the preferential retention sites of total radioactivity.

Based on the results of the safety trial, a larger, multicentre, randomized, double-blind, and placebo controlled trial was designed to test for efficacy of the intracoronary delivery of bone marrow-derived mononuclear cells in chronic chagasic cardiomyopathy. The inclusion criteria were diagnosis of heart failure by the Framingham criteria, at least two independent serological diagnoses of Chagas disease, ages between 18 and 75 years, ejection fraction below 35% by echocardiography according to Simpson's rule, to be in classes III or IV of the NYHA and in optimized pharmacologic therapy for at least 6 weeks before the procedure. Main exclusion criteria were valvular diseases (except for functional mitral or tricuspid regurgitation), coronary angiography with significant lesions (more than 50% of obstruction), sustained ventricular tachycardia, abusive use of drugs or alcohol, serum creatinine > 2.5 mg/dl, neoplasia, and other diseases that might impact life expectancy within 2 years. Since all patients had to undergo cardiac catheterization to rule out coronary lesions, randomization was performed during angiography and cell or saline (placebo) were injected while the patient was still in the catheterization laboratory, thus avoiding the need for a second catheterization. However, the double-blind nature of the trial required all patients underwent bone marrow aspiration.

Primary endpoint for the trial was the difference in ejection fraction between the cell and the placebo group as determined by Simpson's rule in echocardiography at baseline and 6-month follow-up. The trial was powered to detect an absolute 5% difference as significant. Secondary endpoints included difference in ejection fraction, life quality assessment by Minnesota Quality of Life Questionnaire, 6 min walking distance, NYHA class and brain natriuretic peptide (BNP) levels at baseline, and 6 and 12 months after therapy. The trial enrolled 234 patients, but two patients abandoned the study and 49 were recruited by centres that were excluded from the study after the first monitoring round, leaving 187 patients who were included and followed in the study (90 randomized to the cell and 93 to the placebo group). Given the baseline values for ejection fraction (26% ± 6%) and the 5% absolute difference between the groups, sample size required for adequate statistical power was 106 patients, considering 16% mortality. Results of 155 patients who completed the initial 6-month follow-up have been communicated to the European Cardiology Society meeting this year by Feitosa et al. (2010, personal communication). Although an increase in left ventricular ejection fraction of 4% was detected in the cell group after 6 months in comparison to baseline, the placebo group also increased ejection fraction by 4% and the difference between the groups did not reach statistical significance. Therefore, the authors concluded that intracoronary injection of bone marrow-derived mononuclear cells does not improve left ventricular ejection fraction in chronic chagasic cardiomyopathy patients with congestive heart failure.

3.5. FUTURE PERSPECTIVES FOR CELL-BASED THERAPIES IN CHAGAS DISEASE

Since the beginning of cell therapy trials in humans, an impressive amount of progress has been achieved in the stem cell field. This opens new perspectives for cell-based therapies in treating cardiac diseases in general, and chagasic cardiomyopathy in particular.

The reported regenerative capacity of the human heart by Frisen's group (Bergmann et al., 2009) has attracted attention to cardiac stem/progenitor cells as an ideal source for cardiac cell therapy. The problem is that there is no consensus as to which cell is the true cardiac stem cell (Barile et al., 2007) and, even for this cell type, engraftment seems very limited after intracardiac injection in experimental models (Wu et al., 2010). Nevertheless, safety clinical trials with different types of cardiac stem cells are currently being performed in heart failure in the United States and in Japan and preliminary results are anxiously awaited (ClinicalTrials.gov, CADUCEUS, Identifier NCT00893360; SCIPIO, Identifier NCT00474461; ALCADIA, Identifier NCT00981006).

The seminal discovery that adult cells can be reverted into a pluripotent state by Takahashi and Yamanaka (2006) has opened new hope for autologous cell therapy using patient specific stem cells. Nonetheless, the induced pluripotent stem cells (iPSCs) are plagued by the same restrictions that embryonic stem cells face for clinical use: the high proliferative and differentiation potential that raises the risk of tumour development. Pre-differentiation of the pluripotent cells into the desired cell type for therapy is an alternative to circumvent this problem and is being used by the Geron Corporation in a phase I trial for spinal cord injury (ClinicalTrials.gov, Identifier NCT01217008). The main problem with this approach is that differentiation protocols for pluripotent cells using defined conditions are still highly ineffective, not reaching yields of more than 50% in the case of cardiomyocytes (Wu et al., 2004).

Another exciting possibility for cell-based therapy in cardiac diseases is direct reprogramming of cells into a cardiac phenotype. This type of approach, recently described by Srivastava's group (Ieda et al., 2010), precludes the need to reprogram the cell to a pluripotent state. Ieda et al. (2010) demonstrated that it is possible to differentiate mouse cardiac and skin derived fibroblasts directly into cardiomyocytes by introducing three transcription factors: Gata4, Mef2c, and Tbx5. This revolutionary concept waits to be demonstrated for human cells, but opens the extraordinary possibility of transforming the fibroblast scar that follows myonecrosis back into cardiac muscle.

All three strategies mentioned above still face important challenges to translate into effective clinical use and, since clinical trials using bone marrow mononuclear cells reported a limited improvement in cardiac function so far, the quest for the ideal stem cell for therapy in chagasic cardiomyopathy remains. A promising candidate is the MSC (Fig. 3.1), a cell type that remains to be tested in chagasic cardiomyopathy experimental models. A growing body of evidence suggests that MSC might have the capacity to modulate immune responses via direct and indirect interactions with a broad range of cell types (Aggarwal and Pittenger, 2005). Based on the knowledge that MSC display immunosuppressive properties, *ex vivo* expanded bone marrow-derived MSC were used to treat patients with steroid refractory graft-versus-host disease (GVHD) in a small scale pilot study (Le Blanc et al., 2004) with promising results. Further, MSC are currently being used in trials of Crohn's disease, type 1 diabetes mellitus and multiple sclerosis (Ankrum and Karp, 2010). While preliminary results look encouraging, there is currently a distinct lack of mechanistic data with regard to how MSC regulate immune cells *in vivo*.

It is believed that in response to tissue injury, MSC home to the site of damage and induce repair through the production of trophic factors, including growth factors, cytokines, and antioxidants (Karp and Leng Teo, 2009), some of which provide the basis for their capacity to modulate immune responses. The paramount goal in cell transplantation in Chagas disease is to decrease myocardial inflammation and fibrosis and to restore cardiac function. Since myocardial inflammation is directly associated to the immune response either to parasite or auto-antigens, the use of the MSC in cell therapy for chagasic cardiomyopathy may induce additional benefits, as modulation of the inflammatory response will lead to decreased fibrosis and, in consequence, to improvement in cardiac function.

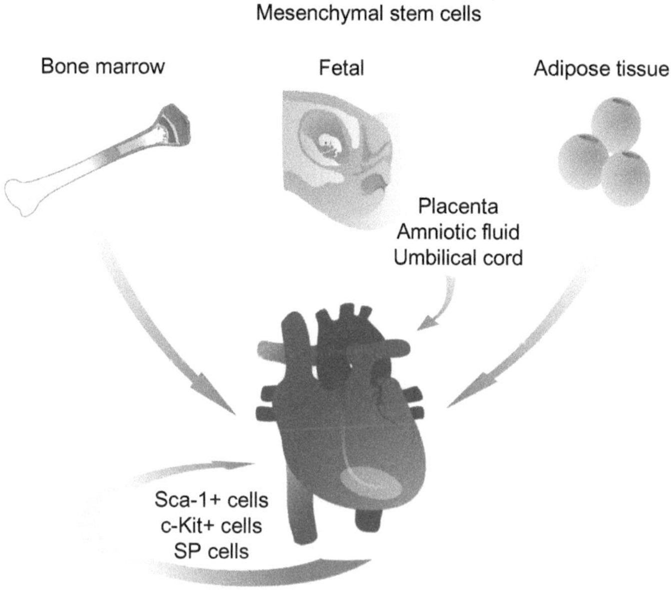

FIGURE 3.1 Chagas disease: cell therapy options for the next decade. Mesenchymal stem cells are a promising alternative for the short-term treatment of chagasic cardiomyopathy. These cells can be obtained from multiple sources, such as bone marrow, extra-embryonic, and adipose tissue. It has been shown that they can modulate the immune system, which is an interesting feature for the treatment of chagasic cardiomyopathy since autoimmunity likely plays an important role in the pathogenesis of the disease. Additionally, it has been shown that MSC exert paracrine effects and can recruit endogenous stem cell populations within the heart.

Autologous cells are clearly the safest option for clinical cell therapy in terms of the relative risk of rejection or graft-versus-host reactions. However, there are circumstances in which healthy autologous, HLA-matched or haploidentical cells will not be available. Moreover, preliminary tests with BMCs from chronic chagasic patients have revealed a diminished colony forming capacity (unpublished results), indicating that these cells are functionally compromised. In this scenario, an allogeneic MSC transplant should be considered for clinical use. In fact, use of allogeneic MSC in ischaemic heart disease patients has been reported and, although it was a safety trial, functional improvement was reported (Hare et al., 2009). Importantly, the injection route used was intravenous, which proved to be safe and is much less invasive. In Brazil, we are currently testing the use of bone marrow-derived MSC in the mouse model of chronic chagasic cardiomyopathy in preparation for a new clinical trial using *ex vivo* expanded autologous and allogeneic MSC in chagasic cardiomyopathy patients.

REFERENCES

Aggarwal, S., Pittenger, M.F., 2005. Human mesenchymal stem cells modulate allogeneic immune cell responses. Blood 105, 1815–1822.

Andrade, Z.A., Andrade, S.G., 1955. Pathogenesis of Chagas chronic myocarditis: importance of ischemic lesions. Arq. Bras. Med. 45, 279–288.

Andrade, Z.A., Lopes, E.A., 1963. A histochemical study of experimental Chagas disease. Rev. Inst. Med. Trop. Sao Paulo 5, 236–242.

Ankrum, J., Karp, J.M., 2010. Mesenchymal stem cell therapy: two steps forward, one step back. Trends Mol. Med. 16, 203–209.

Armaganijan, L., Morillo, C.A., 2010. Chagas disease: 101 years of solitude! Time for action. Stroke 41, 2453–2454.

Assmus, B., Schächinger, V., Teupe, C., Britten, M., Lehmann, R., Döbert, N., et al., 2002. Transplantation of progenitor cells and regeneration enhancement in acute myocardial infarction. Circulation 106, 3009–3017.

Balsam, L.B., Wagers, A.J., Christensen, J.L., Kofidis, T., Weissman, I.L., Robbins, R.C., 2004. Haematopoietic stem cells adopt mature haematopoietic fates in ischaemic myocardium. Nature 428, 668–673.

Barbosa da Fonseca, L.M., Xavier, S.S., Rosado de Castro, P.H., Lima, R.S., Gutfilen, B., Goldenberg, R.C., et al., 2011. Biodistribution of bone marrow mononuclear cells in chronic chagasic cardiomyopathy after intracoronary injection. Int. J. Cardiol. 149 (3), 310–314.

Barile, L., Messina, E., Giacomello, A., Marbán, E., 2007. Endogenous cardiac stem cells. Prog. Cardiovasc. Dis. 50, 31–48.

Bergmann, O., Bhardwaj, R.D., Bernard, S., Zdunek, S., Barnabé-Heider, F., Walsh, S., et al., 2009. Evidence for cardiomyocyte renewal in humans. Science 324, 98–102.

Bern, C., Montgomery, S.P., Herwaldt, B.L., Rassi, A., Jr., Marin-Neto, J.A., Dantas, R.O., et al., 2007. Evaluation and treatment of Chagas disease in the United States: a systematic review. JAMA 298, 2171–2181.

Bocchi, E.A., Fiorelli, A., 2001. The paradox of survival results after heart transplantation for cardiomyopathy caused by *Trypanosoma cruzi*. First Guidelines Group for Heart Transplantation of the Brazilian Society of Cardiology. Ann. Thorac. Surg. 71, 1833–1838.

Cao, F., Lin, S., Xie, X., Ray, P., Patel, M., Zhang, X., et al., 2006. In vivo visualization of embryonic stem cell survival, proliferation, and migration after cardiac delivery. Circulation 113, 1005–1014.

Chagas, C., 1909. Nova tripanosomíase humana: Estudos sobre a morfologia e o ciclo evolutivo do *Schizotrypanum cruzi* n.g., n.sp., agente etiológico de nova entidade mórbida no homem. Mem. Inst. Oswaldo Cruz 1, 159–218.

ClinicalTrials.gov, 2010a. Autologous human cardiac-derived stem cell to treat ischemic cardiomyopathy (ALCADIA), Identifier NCT00981006. http://clinicaltrials.gov.

ClinicalTrials.gov, 2010b. Cardiac stem cell infusion in patients with ischemic cardiomyopathy (SCIPIO), Identifier NCT00474461. http://clinicaltrials.gov.

ClinicalTrials.gov, 2010c. Cardiosphere-derived autologous stem cells to reverse ventricular dysfunction (CADUCEUS), Identifier NCT00893360. http://clinicaltrials.gov.

ClinicalTrials.gov, 2010d. Safety study of GRNOPC1 in spinal cord injury, Identifier NCT01217008. http://clinicaltrials.gov.

ClinicalTrials.gov, 2010e. The BENEFIT Trial: evaluation of the use of an antiparasital drug (Benznidazole) in the treatment of chronic Chagas disease, Identifier NCT00123916. http://clinicaltrials.gov.

Dimmeler, S., Zeiher, A.M., Schneider, M.D., 2005. Unchain my heart: the scientific foundations of cardiac repair. J. Clin. Invest. 115, 572–583.

Freitas, H.F., Chizolla, P.R., Paes, A.T., Lima, A.C., Mansur, A.J., 2005. Risk stratification in a Brazilian hospital-based cohort of 1220 outpatients with heart failure: role of Chagas heart disease. Int. J. Cardiol. 102, 239–247.

Gnecchi, M., He, H., Liang, O.D., Melo, L.G., Morello, F., Mu, H., et al., 2005. Paracrine action accounts for marked protection of ischemic heart by Akt-modified mesenchymal stem cells. Nat. Med. 11, 367–368.

Goldenberg, R.C., Jelicks, L.A., Fortes, F.S., Weiss, L.M., Rocha, L.L., Zhao, D., et al., 2008. Bone marrow cell therapy ameliorates and reverses chagasic cardiomyopathy in a mouse model. J. Infect. Dis. 197, 544–547.

Goldenberg, R.C., Iacobas, D.A., Iacobas, S., Rocha, L.L., Fortes, F.S., Vairo, L., et al., 2009. Transcriptomic alterations in *Trypanosoma cruzi*-infected cardiac myocytes. Microbes Infect. 11, 1140–1149.

Guarita-Souza, L.C., Carvalho, K.A., Woitowicz, V., Rebelatto, C., Senegaglia, A., Hansen, P., et al., 2006. Simultaneous autologous transplantation of cocultured mesenchymal stem cells and skeletal myoblasts improves ventricular function in a murine model of Chagas disease. Circulation 114, I120–I124.

Hare, J.M., Traverse, J.H., Henry, T.H., Dib, N., Strumpf, R.K., Schulman, S.P., et al., 2009. A randomized, double-blind, placebo-controlled, dose-escalation study of intravenous adult human mesenchymal stem cells (Prochymal) after acute myocardial infarction. J. Am. Coll. Cardiol. 54, 2277–2286.

Hodgson, D.M., Behfar, A., Zingman, L.V., Kane, G.C., Perez-Terzic, C., Alekseev, A.E., et al., 1994. Stable benefit of embryonic stem cell therapy in myocardial infarction. Am. J. Heart Circ. Physiol. 287, H471–H479.

Ieda, M., Fu, J.D., Delgado-Olguin, P., Vedantham, V., Hayashi, Y., Bruneau, B.G., et al., 2010. Direct reprogramming of fibroblasts into functional cardiomyocytes by defined factors. Cell 142, 375–386.

Jacob, J.L., Salis, F.V., Ruiz, M.A., Greco, O.T., 2007. Labeled stem cells transplantation to the myocardium of a patient with Chagas disease. Arq. Bras. Cardiol. 89, e10–e11.

Karp, J.M., Leng Teo, G.S., 2009. Mesenchymal stem cell homing: the devil is in the details. Cell Stem Cell 6, 206–216.

Kierszenbaum, F., 2005. Where do we stand on the autoimmunity hypothesis of Chagas disease? Trends Parasitol. 21, 513–516.

Klug, M.G., Soonpaa, M.H., Koh, G.Y., Field, L.J., 1996. Genetically selected cardiomyocytes from differentiating embryonic stem cells forms stable intracardiac grafts. J. Clin. Invest. 98, 216–224.

Kocher, A.A., Schuster, M.D., Szabolcs, M.J., Takuma, S., Burkhoff, D., Wang, J., et al., 2001. Neovascularization of ischemic myocardium by human bone marrow-derived angioblasts prevents cardiomyocyte apoptosis, reduces remodeling and improves cardiac function. Nat. Med. 7, 430–436.

Laflamme, M.A., Murry, C.E., 2005. Regenerating the heart. Nat. Biotechnol. 23, 845–856.

Laflamme, M.A., Gold, J., Xu, C., Hassanipour, M., Rosler, E., Police, S., et al., 2005. Formation of human myocardium in the heart from human embryonic stem cells. Am. J. Pathol. 167, 663–671.

Lanes-Vieira, J., De Araújo-Jorge, T.C., Soeiro, Mde N., Gadelha, P., Corrêa-Oliveira, R., 2010. The centennial of the discovery of Chagas disease: facing the current challenges. PLoS Negl. Trop. Dis. 4, e645.

Le Blanc, K., Rasmusson, I., Sundberg, B., Götherström, C., Hassan, M., Uzunel, M., et al., 2004. Treatment of severe acute graft-versus-host disease with third party haploidentical mesenchymal stem cells. Lancet 363, 1439–1441.

Lipinsky, M.J., Biondi-Zoccai, G.G., Abbate, A., Khianey, R., Sheiban, I., Bartunek, J., et al., 2007. Impact of intracoronary cell therapy on left ventricular function in the setting of acute myocardial infarction: a collaborative systematic review and meta-analysis of controlled clinical trials. J. Am. Coll. Cardiol. 50, 1761–1767.

Macambira, S.G., Vasconcelos, J.F., Costa, C.R., Klein, W., Lima, R.S., Guimarães, P., et al., 2009. Granulocyte colony-stimulating factor treatment in chronic Chagas disease: preservation and improvement of cardiac structure and function. FASEB J. 23, 3843–3850.

Makino, S., Fukuda, K., Miyoshi, S., Konishi, F., Kodama, H., Pan, J., et al., 1999. Cardiomyocytes can be generated from marrow stromal cells in vitro. J. Clin. Invest. 103, 697–705.

Mangi, A.A., Noiseux, N., Kong, D., He, H., Rezvani, M., Ingwall, J.S., et al., 2003. Mesenchymal stem cells modified with Akt prevent remodeling and restore performance of infracted hearts. Nat. Med. 9, 1195–1201.

Martin-Rendon, E., Brunskill, S.J., Hyde, C.J., Stanworth, S.J., Mathur, A., Watt, S.M., 2008. Autologous bone marrow stem cells to treat acute myocardial infarction: a systematic review. Eur. Heart J. 29, 1807–1818.

Ménard, C., Hagège, A., Agbulut, O., Barro, M., Morichetti, M.C., Brasselet, C., 2005. Transplantation of cardiac-committed mouse embryonic stem cells to infarcted sheep myocardium: a preclinical study. Lancet 366, 1005–1012.

Menasché, P., 2009. Stem cell therapy for heart failure: are arrhythmias a real safety concern? Circulation 119, 2735–2740.

Menasché, P., Hagège, A.A., Scorsin, M., Pouzet, B., Desnos, M., Duboc, D., 2001. Myoblast transplantation for heart failure. Lancet 357, 279–280.

Menasché, P., Alfieru, O., Janssens, S., McKenna, W., Reichenspurner, H., Trinquart, L., 2008. The Myoblast Autologous Grafting in Ischemic Cardiomyopathy (MAGIC) trial: first randomized placebo-controlled study of myoblast transplantation. Circulation 117, 1189–1200.

Moia, B., Rosenbaum, M.B., 1960. The electrocardiogram in chronic Chagas myocarditis. Arq. Bras. Cardiol. 13, 236–243.

Mukherjee, S., Belbin, T.J., Spray, D.C., Iacobas, D.A., Weiss, L.M., Kitsis, R.N., 2003. Microarray analysis of changes in gene expression in a murine model of chronic chagasic cardiomyopathy. Parasitol. Res. 91, 187–196.

Murry, C.E., Soonpaa, M.H., Reinecke, H., Nakajima, H., Nakajima, H.O., Rubart, M., et al., 2004. Haematopoietic stem cells do not transdifferentiate into cardiac myocytes in myocardial infarcts. Nature 428, 664–668.

Nygren, J.M., Jovinge, S., Breitbach, M., Sawen, P., Roll, W., Hescheler, J., et al., 2004. Bone marrow-derived hematopoietic cells generate cardiomyocytes at a low frequency through cell fusion, but not transdifferentiation. Nat. Med. 10, 494–501.

Olivares, E.L., Ribeiro, V.P., Werneck-de-Castro, J.P., Ribeiro, K.C., Mattos, E.C., Goldenberg, R.C., et al., 2004. Bone marrow stromal cells improve cardiac performance in healed infracted rat hearts. Am. J. Physiol. Heart Circ. Physiol. 287, H464–H470.

Orlic, D., Kajstura, J., Chimenti, S., Jakoniuk, I., Anderson, S.M., Li, B., et al., 2001. Bone marrow cells regenerate infracted myocardium. Nature 410, 701–705.

Rassi, A., Jr., Rassi, A., Marin-Neto, J.A., 2010. Chagas disease. Lancet 375, 1388–1402.

Rosenbaum, M.B., 1964. Chagasic myocardiopathy. Prog. Cardiovasc. Dis. 7, 199–225.

Rosenbaum, M.B., Alvarez, A.J., 1955. The electrocardiogram in chronic chagasic myocarditis. Am. Heart J. 50, 492–527.

Salvatella, R., 2006. Current Status of Chagas Disease. Pan American Health Organization, Washington, DC.

Soares, M.B., Lima, R.S., Rocha, L.L., Takyia, C.M., Pontes-de-Carvalho, L., de Carvalho, A.C., et al., 2004. Transplanted bone marrow cells repair heart tissue and reduce myocarditis in chronic chagasic mice. Am. J. Pathol. 164, 441–447.

Soares, M.B., de Lima, R.S., Rocha, L.L., Vasconcelos, J.F., Rogatto, S.R., dos Santos, R.R., et al., 2010. Gene expression changes associated with myocarditis and fibrosis in hearts of mice with chronic chagasic cardiomyopathy. J. Infect. Dis. 202, 416–426.

Soares, M.B., Lima, R.S., Souza, B.S.F., Vasconcelos, J.F., Rocha, L.L., dos Santos, R.R., et al., 2011. Reversion of gene expression alterations in hearts of mice with chronic chagasic cardiomyopathy after transplantation of bone marrow cells. Cell Cycle 10 (9), 1448–1455.

Soonpaa, M.H., Daud, A.I., Koh, G.Y., Klug, M.G., Kim, K.K., Wang, H., et al., 1995. Potential approaches for myocardial regeneration. Ann. N. Y. Acad. Sci. 752, 446–454.

Stamm, C., Westphal, B., Kleine, H.D., Petzsch, M., Kittner, H., Schümichen, C., et al., 2003. Autologous bone-marrow stem-cell transplantation for myocardial regeneration. Lancet 361, 45–46.

Takahashi, K., Yamanaka, S., 2006. Induction of pluripotent stem cells from mouse embryonic and adult fibroblast cultures by defined factors. Cell 126, 663–676.

Toma, C., Pittenger, M.F., Cahill, K.S., Byrne, B.J., Kessler, P.D., 2002. Human mesenchymal stem cells differentiate to a cardiomyocyte phenotype in the adult murine heart. Circulation 105, 93–98.

Tomita, S., Li, R.K., Weisel, R.D., Mickle, D.A., Kim, E.J., Sakai, T., et al., 1999. Autologous transplantation of bone marrow cells improves damaged heart function. Circulation 100, II247–II256.

Vilas-Boas, F., Feitosa, G.S., Soares, M.B., Mota, A., Pinho-Filho, J.A., Almeida, A.J., et al., 2006. Early results of bone marrow cell transplantation to the myocardium of patients with heart failure due to Chagas disease. Arq. Bras. Cardiol. 87, 159–166.

Wang, J.S., Shum-Tim, D., Galipeau, J., Chedrawy, E., Eliopoulos, N., Chiu, R.C., 2000. Marrow stromal cells for cellular cardiomyoplasty: feasibility and potential clinical advantages. J. Thorac. Cardiovasc. Surg. 120, 999–1005.

Wang, J.S., Shum-Tim, D., Chedrawy, E., Chiu, R.C., 2001. The coronary delivery of stromal cells for myocardial regeneration: pathophysiologic and therapeutic implications. J. Thorac. Cardiovasc. Surg. 122, 699–705.

Wu, X., Ding, S., Ding, Q., Gray, N.S., Schultz, P.G., 2004. Small molecules that induce cardiomyogenesis in embryonic stem cells. J. Am. Chem. Soc. 126, 1590–1591.

Wu, J.C., Abraham, M.R., Kraitchman, D.L., 2010. Current perspectives on imaging cardiac stem cell therapy. J. Nucl. Med. 51, 128S–136S.

CHAPTER 4

Targeting *Trypanosoma cruzi* Sterol 14α-Demethylase (CYP51)

Galina I. Lepesheva,[*] Fernando Villalta,[†] and **Michael R. Waterman[*]**

Contents

[*] Department of Biochemistry School of Medicine, Vanderbilt University, Nashville, Tennessee, USA
[†] Department of Microbiology and Immunology, Meharry Medical College, Nashville, Tennessee, USA

Advances in Parasitology, Volume 75
ISSN 0065-308X, DOI: 10.1016/B978-0-12-385863-4.00004-6

Abstract

There are at least two obvious features that must be considered upon targeting specific metabolic pathways/enzymes for drug development: the pathway must be essential and the enzyme must allow the design of pharmacologically useful inhibitors. Here, we describe *Trypanosoma cruzi* sterol 14α-demethylase as a promising target for anti-Chagasic chemotherapy. The use of anti-fungal azoles, which block sterol biosynthesis and therefore membrane formation in fungi, against the protozoan parasite has turned out to be highly successful: a broad spectrum anti-fungal drug, the triazole compound posaconazole, is now entering phase II clinical trials for treatment of Chagas disease. This review summarizes comparative information on anti-fungal azoles and novel inhibitory scaffolds selective for *Trypanosomatidae* sterol 14α-demethylase through the lens of recent structure/functional characterization of the target enzyme. We believe our studies open wide opportunities for rational design of novel, pathogen-specific and therefore more potent and efficient anti-trypanosomal drugs.

4.1. INTRODUCTION

Cytochrome P450 (CYP) is the generic name for a superfamily of protoheme containing monooxygenases (Omura and Sato, 1964). There are about 12,000 members of this superfamily which increases in size as more genomes are sequenced (www.http://drnelson.utmem.edu/cytochromeP450.html). P450s can be most generally grouped into two classes, one which inactivates xenobiotics and the other which is necessary for biosynthesis of endogenous compounds. The general reaction catalysed by P450s is seen below, where SH indicates substrate and $2e^-$ indicates reducing equivalents from NADH or NADPH.

$$SH + O_2 + 2e^- \rightarrow SOH + H_2O$$

P450s are found in a large number of organisms through all biological kingdoms. The only specific form found in all biological kingdoms is the sterol 14α-demethylase (CYP51 family), an essential enzyme in sterol biosynthesis and therefore membrane structure. Some investigators have suggested that CYP51 is the oldest of the known P450s (Yoshida et al., 2000).

Inhibition of CYP51 activity has been found to be lethal in organisms requiring sterol biosynthesis for membrane function (Lepesheva and Waterman, 2007). Initial studies of CYP51 inhibitory drugs were carried out topically in fungi and yeast infections on the skin, such as athletes foot. Subsequently, systemic treatment of such infections has been necessary, for example, *Candida albicans* or *Aspergillus* spp. infection in HIV/AIDS or in other immunosuppressed states such those attending cancer chemotherapy or organ transplantation. Effective systemic treatment should be specific for the CYP51 of the infectious pathogen, not the host (human). Our studies have found that members of the genera *Trypanosoma* and *Leishmania* can be killed by CYP51 inhibitors. Three features of inhibition of *Trypanosoma cruzi* are presented in this chapter. First, we will present studies on inhibition of *T. cruzi* CYP51 enzymatic activity. Second, structural studies of CYP51 will be used to explain the way that azole compounds can inhibit *T. cruzi* CYP51 activity. Third, we will summarize results from anti-parasitic effects in *T. cruzi*. Finally, we will show why CYP51 inhibition is such a promising treatment for *T. cruzi* infection and present chemical scaffolds for development of additional drugs.

4.2. STEROL BIOSYNTHESIS

Eukaryotic organisms require sterols (Benveniste, 1986; Schaller, 2003; Schroepfer, 1981). The sterols, such as cholesterol in animals, sitosterol in plants or ergosterol in fungi, are essential structural components of eukaryotic membranes, regulating their fluidity and permeability (Haines, 2001). In addition, sterols serve as precursors for biologically active molecules that regulate growth and development processes. The sterols are either produced solely endogenously (plants, the majority of fungi, *T. cruzi*; Docampo et al., 1981; Beach et al., 1986; Haughan and Goad, 1991; Liendo et al., 1999; *Leishmania*) or must be acquired from the diet (insects, some fungi and protists). Many species, including mammals (humans), yeasts or *Trypanosoma brucei*, can utilize both endogenous and exogenous sources to fulfil the requirement for bulky structural sterols but only endogenously made molecules are further converted into species-specific regulatory sterols (Lepesheva et al., 2010b).

Sterol biosynthesis can be considered as a "eukaryotic extension" of the mavalonate pathway (Rohmer et al., 1979; Volkman, 2005). The mavalonate pathway begins anaerobically, with acetyl-CoA condensation, and proceeds via several intermediates to produce farnesyl pyrophosphate (Fig. 4.1A). Farnesyl pyrophosphate can serve as precursor in various biological processes (Goldstein and Brown, 1990). In the first step of committed sterol biosynthesis, farnesyl pyrophosphate forms squalene (Fig. 4.1B). In the presence of molecular oxygen, the latter is transformed into squalene 2,3-epoxide. Opposite to plants/algae, where squalene 2,3-epoxide is converted into cycloartenol, animals, fungi and *Trypanosomatidae* cyclyse it into lanosterol (Lepesheva and Waterman, 2007). Further, reactions on the lanostane skeleton include demethylations of the sterol core and modifications of the sterol B ring and C20–27 arm.

In *T. cruzi* (Fig. 4.1C), lanosterol is first converted into eburicol (C24-methylene-24, 25-digydrolanosterol), which is the preferred

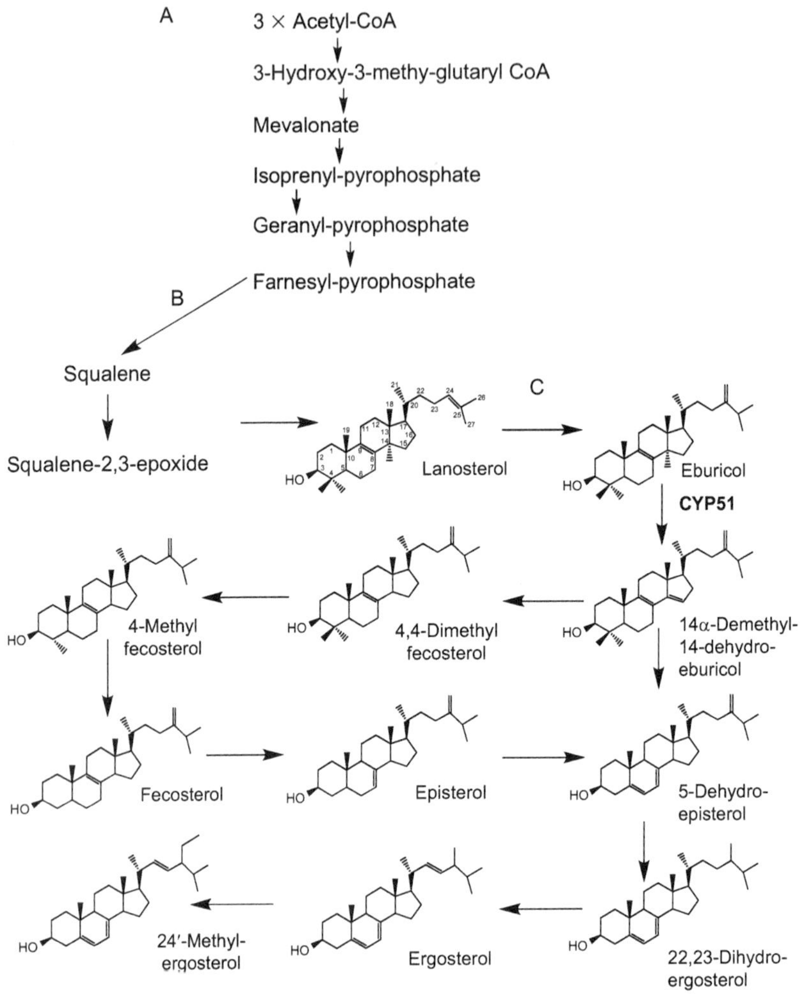

FIGURE 4.1 Sterol biosynthetic pathway in *T. cruzi*. (A) Mevalonate portion. (B) First eukaryote-specific steps. (C) *T. cruzi*-specific steps.

substrate of *T. cruzi* sterol 14α-demethylase (Lepesheva et al., 2006b). The 14α-demethylated product of CYP51 reaction is then reduced to 4,4-dimethyl-fecosterol and C4-demethylated into fecosterol. Rearrangement of the double bond in ring B from ΔC8–9 to ΔC7–8 position produces episterol; introduction of the double bond at C5–6 gives 5-dehydro-episterol. The C24-methylene group of 5-dehydro-episterol is saturated forming 22,23-dihydro-egrosterol; its desaturation at ΔC22–23 results in formation of ergosterol, which together with its C24 methylated analog represent the major final products of the pathway (Urbina et al., 1998, 2003a,b). It has been reported, however, that *T. cruzi* amastigotes lack ΔC5 and ΔC22 desaturase activity and therefore the major sterol products of this intracellular form of the parasite appear to be episterol and two C5–6, C22–23 saturated analogs of ergosterol and 24′-methyl-ergosterol (ergosta-7-en-3*b*-ol and 24′-methyl-ergosta-7-en-3b-ol, respectively; Liendo et al., 1998, 1999).

In higher eukaryotes, sterol biosynthesis occurs in the endoplasmic reticulum, and major sterols are concentrated in the plasma membranes, while in *Trypanosomatidae* the endogenously produced sterols as well as several sterol biosynthetic enzymes are also found in the membranes of glycosomes and mitochondria, suggesting a possibility of multi-organelle location of the sterol biosynthetic pathway in the parasites (Pena-Diaz et al., 2004; Quinones et al., 2004; Rodrigues et al., 2001). The reasons for the possible broader subcellular distribution of the pathway remain to be understood, yet it might support multiple functions of endogenous sterols in these protozoa.

4.3. POTENTIAL DRUG TARGETS IN THE PATHWAY

The fact that *T. cruzi* is entirely dependent on endogenously produced sterols for survival and proliferation and cannot use the supply of host cholesterol makes the sterol biosynthetic pathway in the parasite especially attractive for drug development. There are several enzymes in the pathway that have potential to serve as future targets for anti-trypanosomal chemotherapy. The most apparent examples are HMG-CoA reductase, which in humans is the clinical target for statins (Puccetti et al., 2007), farnesyl diphosphate synthase, the target for bisphosphonates (Kavanagh et al., 2006), squalene synthase, which is inhibited by quinuclidine derivatives (Cammerer et al., 2007), sterol 24-methyltransferase inhibited by azasterols (Gros et al., 2006; Magaraci et al., 2003) and sterol 14α-demethylase (CYP51).

The major advantage of sterol 14α-demethylase is connected with its high druggability. Inhibitors of this enzyme (azoles) are the most efficient anti-fungal agents in clinical medicine and in agriculture (Petrikkos and Skiada, 2007; Zonios and Bennett, 2008). In addition to blocking sterol biosynthesis, the potency of azoles is enhanced by accumulation of toxic methylated sterol precursors that also promote fungal growth arrest and deleterious changes in the membrane permeability (Cournia et al., 2007; Nes, 1974; Yeagle et al., 1977). Anti-parasitic effects of anti-fungal azoles in *T. cruzi* have been observed by multiple investigators, the first reports being published in 1981 (Araujo et al., 2000; Beach et al., 1986; Docampo et al., 1981; Molina et al., 2000; Urbina et al., 1988, 2000). Several of them, including posaconazole, were proven to have curative effect in both acute and chronic forms of Chagas disease in animal models (Apt et al., 1998; Urbina, 2009; Urbina et al., 1996, 2003a,b). Finally, this year, after it cured chronic Chagas disease in an immunosuppressed patient in Barcelona (Pinazo et al., 2010), posaconazole has been reported to enter phase II clinical trial for Chagas disease in Spain (Clayton, 2010). Another azole, ravuconazole, which is currently under phase II clinical trials as an antifungal agent, is considered by the Drug for Neglected Diseases Initiative (DNDi) as an option for clinical development for Chagas disease treatment (Clayton, 2010), even though it only has a suppressive effect on the parasite *in vivo* (Diniz Lde et al., 2010).

Until recently, when it became a global problem due to human migration, blood bank/organ transplant contaminations and HIV coinfections, Chagas disease predominantly threatened lives of the poorest. Therefore, low investment into Chagas drug discovery research, lack of serious interest from pharmaceutical companies, as well as long-term domination of the autoimmune hypothesis of chronic Chagas disease pathogenesis which underscored the notion that causative treatment would not be beneficial (Urbina, 2010) significantly impeded implementation of the therapeutic use of the azoles obtained from antifungal drug development programs let alone development of new *T. cruzi* sterol 14α-demethylase specific therapies. However, the fact that sterol 14α-demethylases from *Trypanosomatidae* have only 22–26% amino acid sequence identity to the fungal CYP51 orthologs (Lepesheva and Waterman, 2011) clearly suggests that more effective inhibitors of the protozoan enzyme remain to be found.

4.4. *TRYPANOSOMA CRUZI* STEROL 14α-DEMETHYLASE (CYP51)

4.4.1. Reaction and catalysis

T. cruzi sterol 14α-demethylase (EC: 1.14.13.70, CYP51 gene family) is a CYP monooxygenase that catalyses removal of the 14α-methyl group from eburicol (Fig. 4.2). As all cytochromes P450, CYP51 contains a haem cofactor (protoporphyrin IX), where the iron in its fifth (axial) coordination position is tethered to the proximal side of the protein via a thiolate ligand derived from a cysteine residue (Cys422 in *T. cruzi* CYP51). This iron-cysteine coordination is responsible for the P450 name that originated from the spectral property of the reduced enzyme to produce a characteristic absorbance maximum at 450 nm upon binding of carbon monoxide (Omura and Sato, 1964). The cysteine is a better electron donor than histidine, the residue that is coordinated to the haem iron in the majority of other haemoproteins, and this allows P450s

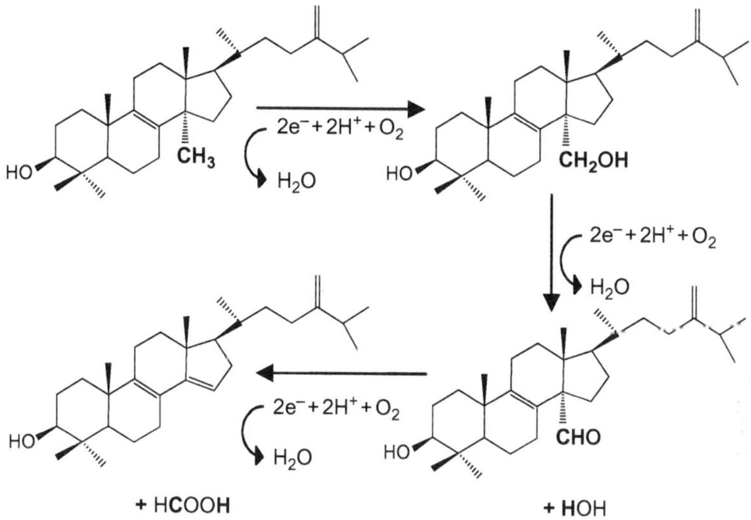

FIGURE 4.2 Three-step catalytic reaction of *T. cruzi* CYP51. Each step requires molecular oxygen, two electrons and two catalytic protons. The 14α-methyl group of eburicol is converted into first the alcohol, second the aldehyde and third removed as formic acid. The substrates of CYP51s from other biological kingdoms are all structurally very similar. Eburicol also serves as the substrate for sterol 14α-demethylases in filamentous fungi. Plant and *T. brucei* orthologs metabolize its C4-monomethylated analog obtusifoliol. Lanosterol and 24,25-dihydrolanosterol, both lacking the methylene group at C24, are the natural substrates for the human (mammalian) enzyme.

to function as monooxygenases catalysing scission of molecular oxygen. As a result of P450 catalysis, one atom of oxygen is incorporated into an organic compound, sterol substrate in the case of CYP51, while another is released as a water molecule.

The CYP51 reaction includes three CYP catalytic cycles. When the sterol substrate, most likely entering through the membrane, binds in the enzyme active site in such a way that the 14α-methyl group is positioned about 5 Å above the haem iron plane, the P450 accepts the first electron from cytochrome P450 reductase (CPR), and its haem iron is reduced from the resting ferric (Fe^{3+}) to the active ferrous (Fe^{2+}) state. Delivery of the first electron enables binding of an oxygen molecule in the sixth coordination position of the reduced iron, perpendicular to the haem plane and in close proximity to the sterol 14α-methyl group. After this, the second electron is transferred by CPR, reducing the haem bound oxygen. Then two catalytic protons arrive from the cytoplasm-exposed protein surface causing the oxygen scission and release of one water molecule while introducing the other atomic oxygen into the methyl group of the sterol (—C—H → —C—O—H). The second cycle of catalysis converts the 14α-alcohol group into the 14α-aldehyde; the third cycle results in release of formic acid and introduction of the Δ14-15-double bond into the sterol ring D.

4.4.2. Spectral responses to ligand binding

4.4.2.1. Ligand-induced shift in the Soret band maximum

Having the haem as an active cofactor, P450s are known to be competitively inhibited by heterocyclic compounds such as pyridine, pyrimidine and especially azole derivatives (Ortiz de Montellano and Correia, 1995). A basic atom from the heterocyclic ring coordinates directly to the haem iron, while the rest of the molecule occupies the active site cavity affecting substrate binding/metabolism. Such interactions can be recorded spectrally, serving as a useful tool to screen for new CYP51 inhibitors (Lepesheva et al., 2007). The principle for the optical screening is as follows: in the substrate-free state the haem in CYP51 is always hexacoordinated, a water molecule being bound to the iron as the sixth ligand (Lepesheva et al., 2010b). When a stronger ligand replaces the water molecule in the iron 6th coordination position, it causes a red shift in the Soret band maximum from 417 to 422–427 nm, also known as type II spectral response.

The same approach can also be used to estimate apparent affinity of the CYP51 interaction with substrate analogs. Although substrates or structurally related compounds do not bind to the haem iron directly, their binding expels the water molecule from the iron coordination sphere. As a result, they induce transition of the iron from the hexacoordinated low spin to the pentacoordinated high-spin state, the interaction being monitored as a blue shift in the Soret band maximum (from 417 to 390 nm), or type I spectral response.

Upon searching for anti-protozoan CYP51 inhibitors, however, we faced two limitations of the spectral titration. First, in some cases, the apparent binding parameters determined by titration do not correlate with the inhibitory effects of the compounds in the reconstituted enzyme reaction (Lepesheva et al., 2007, 2008). Second, especially strong CYP51 inhibitors (tight-binding ligands with the Kds < 0.1 μM) cannot be distinguished at standard conditions.

4.4.2.2. CO binding spectra

As an alternative, to estimate relative affinities of inhibitors to *T. cruzi* CYP51, we suggest to monitor their influence on the formation of the reduced P450-CO complexes (Lepesheva et al., 2010a). This approach appears to be rather sensitive, since it reflects the ability of carbon monoxide to replace the inhibitors from the iron coordination sphere when the enzyme is in the reduced, reactive state. We found that while weaker inhibitors such as fluconazole and ketoconazole decrease the rate of *T. cruzi* CYP51-CO-complex formation, VNI and VNF (see Section 4.5.1, and Fig. 4.3A) completely prevent CO-iron coordination.

4.4.3. Reconstituted activity *in vitro*

Based on our experience, the most reliable method to evaluate potency of a compound as a CYP51 inhibitor is to test its effect on the enzyme activity in the *in vitro* reconstituted CYP51 reaction. Even this approach has its limitations (Lepesheva et al., 2007), the major problem being due to the IC_{50} detection limit. In traditional enzymology, the IC_{50} values were introduced to quantify inhibition of water soluble enzymes, the catalysts that are meant to be used at very low concentrations with very high molar excess of substrate. However, eukaryotic CYP51s are membrane bound highly hydrophobic proteins, which metabolize highly hydrophobic sterol substrates of extremely low solubility in water. An efficient system for reconstitution of CYP51 activity *in vitro* (catalytic turnover of *T. cruzi* CYP51 at these conditions is about 5 nmol/nmol/min) requires (1) the electron donor protein CPR, the Kd for the protein–protein complex being around 1 μM, (2) a phospholipid to incorporate the P450-CPR complex and (3) hydroxypropyl-β-cyclodextrin to dissolve the sterol (Lepesheva et al., 2006b). This, together with the issues of enzyme stability, especially in the reactive, reduced (Fe^{2+}) state restricts the option of decreasing the CYP51 concentration in the reaction. Therefore, we quantify effects of moderate inhibitors as I/E_2 (molar ratio inhibitor/enzyme that causes a twofold decrease in the CYP51 turnover; Lepesheva et al., 2007), while in order to compare the most potent compounds we monitor the time-course of substrate conversion at equimolar ratio inhibitor/enzyme. As described below, the strongest *Trypanosomatidae* CYP51 inhibitors identified in this system prevent any conversion of the substrate over time thus acting not only as tight-binding but essentially as functionally irreversible inhibitors, their anti-parasitic effects in *T. cruzi* cells being in the lower nanomolar range.

4.5. INHIBITORS OF *TRYPANOSOMA CRUZI* CYP51

4.5.1. Anti-fungal drugs and experimental azole derivatives

The inhibitory effects of three anti-fungal drugs, ketoconazole, fluconazole and posaconazole, on the activity of *T. cruzi* CYP51 are included in Fig. 4.3A. Posaconazole (Zonios and Bennett, 2008), the drug soon to be in clinical trial for Chagas disease (Clayton, 2010; Urbina, 2010) is certainly the most potent amongst them. However, posaconazole is a complex

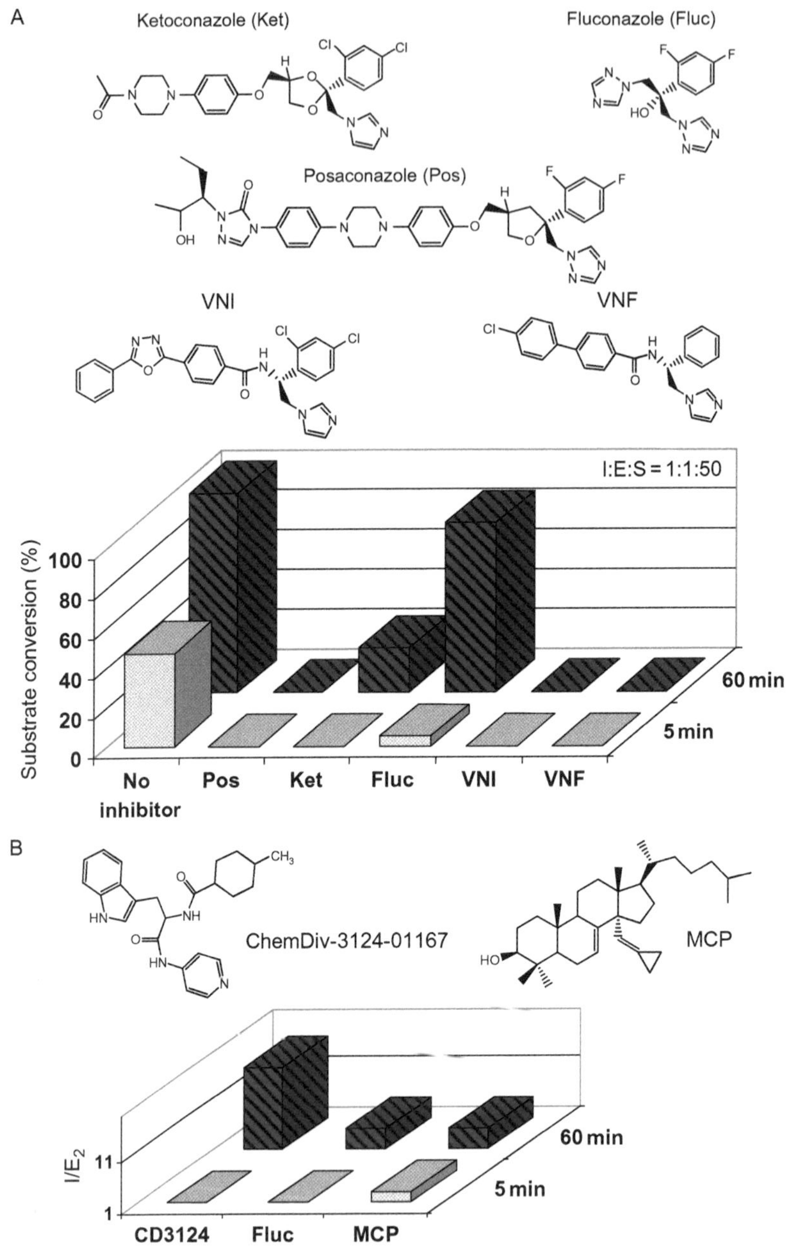

FIGURE 4.3 Selected inhibitors and their effects on *T. cruzi* CYP51 activity. (A) Antifungal and experimental azoles; I : E : S, molar ratio inhibitor/enzyme/substrate. (B) Non-azole compounds; I/E2, inhibitor/enzyme ratio that causes a twofold decrease in activity.

compound, difficult to synthesize and therefore too costly to be expected to cure Chagas disease globally. Besides, it has significant toxicity and limited selectivity (I/E_2 for human CYP51 is about 40; Lepesheva et al., 2010a). Due to its side effects, most common of which include nausea, vomiting, headache, abdominal pain and diarrhoea (Nagappan and Deresinski, 2007; Petrikkos and Skiada, 2007; Schiller and Fung, 2007), posaconazole was approved by the FDA in the United States only in 2006, solely as a salvage therapy for invasive fungal infections in immunocompromised patients. Therefore, the task of finding additional drug candidates, especially those which would be specific to *T. cruzi* CYP51, remains extremely important.

We screened a large number of experimental compounds against purified *T. cruzi* CYP51, the best inhibitory scaffold being identified amongst the set of imidazole derivatives originally synthesized by the Novartis Research Institute (Vienna, Austria) (Lepesheva et al., 2007). These azoles completely inhibit *T. cruzi* CYP51 activity (VNI and VNF in Fig. 4.3A) and also show very high selectivity to CYP51s from other pathogenic organisms. Acting as rather strong inhibitors of the fungal ortholog (*C. albicans*), they do not affect human CYP51, $I/E_2 > 200$ (Lepesheva et al., 2010a,b). Accordingly, we found them to have low general cytotoxicity, $EC_{50} > 50$ μM (human leukaemia cell line HL60), while even at 1 μM they kill more than 99% of *T. cruzi* amastigotes (Lepesheva et al., 2007). Moreover, contrary to posaconazole or fluconazole, they do not enhance the *T. cruzi* CYP51 gene expression and do not require increase in the dosage to maintain constant cellular growth inhibition over time (Lepesheva and Waterman, 2011), which suggest their weaker propensity to induce resistance in the parasite.

Two other inhibitory scaffolds, disubstituted imidazoles and derivatives of the anti-cancer drug tipifarnib (triazole-based), were identified by Buckner et al. (Buckner et al., 2003; Hucke et al., 2005). In this case, the investigators originally observed strong anti-parasitic effects of the compounds with *T. cruzi*; analysis of parasite sterols has shown that they inhibit sterol 14α-demethylase. Testing these azoles in the reconstituted reaction confirmed their high inhibitory potencies and selectivity to the enzyme from *T. cruzi* (Kraus et al., 2009).

4.5.2. Non-azole inhibitors

Although azole derivatives remain the most potent CYP51 inhibitors identified so far, some of other non-azole types of compounds can also be considered as potential leads for the development of alternative therapies targeting *T. cruzi* sterol 14α-demethylase. One such example would be a pyridine derivative ChemDiv-3124-01167, which we identified via high-throughput screening (Lepesheva et al., 2008), the inhibitory effect and the formula can be seen in Fig. 4.3B. The compound shows clear anti-parasitic effects in *T. cruzi*, EC_{50} being ~7 μM (Konkle et al., 2009). Recently, our experiments with this inhibitor were reproduced at UCSF with very similar results (Chen et al., 2009). Furthermore, these authors report some curative effect of ChemDiv-3124-01167 in their murine model of the acute Chagas disease (Doyle et al., 2010).

CYP51 substrate analogs represent another opportunity for drug development. Inhibitory effects of several lanosterol derivatives on mammalian and yeast orthologs were described by several investigators (Aoyama et al., 1987; Cooper et al., 1988; Frye et al., 1993; Trzaskos et al., 1995; Tuck et al., 1991), one such compound was proven to act as a mechanism-based inhibitor of the enzyme (Bossard et al., 1991). So far we have tested only a limited number of substrate analogous compounds with *T. cruzi* CYP51 (Lepesheva et al., 2006b, 2008), Δ7-14α-methylene-cyclopropyl-dihydrolanosterol (MCP), EC_{50} in *T. cruzi* cells ~5 μM being the best we have found (Fig. 4.3B). Recent determination of the structure of the complex of this sterol with CYP51 (PDB code 3P99, unpublished) opens new opportunities to enhance the inhibitory effects of this compound by further modifications. In general, a large number of diverse structures that can act as CYP51 inhibitors further confirm the highly druggable nature of these enzymes (Cheng et al., 2007).

4.6. STRUCTURAL BASIS FOR CYP51 DRUGGABILITY

Although, no doubt, highly potent, even species-specific CYP51 inhibitors can be found empirically, in the absence of a 3D structure of an eukaryotic CYP51 enzyme that functions *in vivo* as a sterol 14α-demethylase, it has been hard to comprehend what makes inhibitors particularly strong, what causes their selectivity or why the CYP51 propensity to be inhibited by azoles is generally much stronger than that of many other, especially drug-metabolizing P450s (Obach et al., 2006; Ortiz de Montellano and Correia, 1995; Wexler et al., 2004). Crystal structures of *Trypanosomatidae* CYP51 are helpful in answering these questions and also outline a general strategy for rational design of novel drugs for anti-trypanosomal chemotherapy.

4.6.1. Overview of the CYP51 structure

Structurally, sterol 14α-demethylase has the characteristic P450 fold (Poulos et al., 1987), which from the distal view of the protein resembles an upside-down triangle (Fig. 4.4A). The set of the secondary structural elements includes 12 main helices, 10 additional, shorter helices between them and 12 β-strands assembled into four anti-parallel β-sheets; the

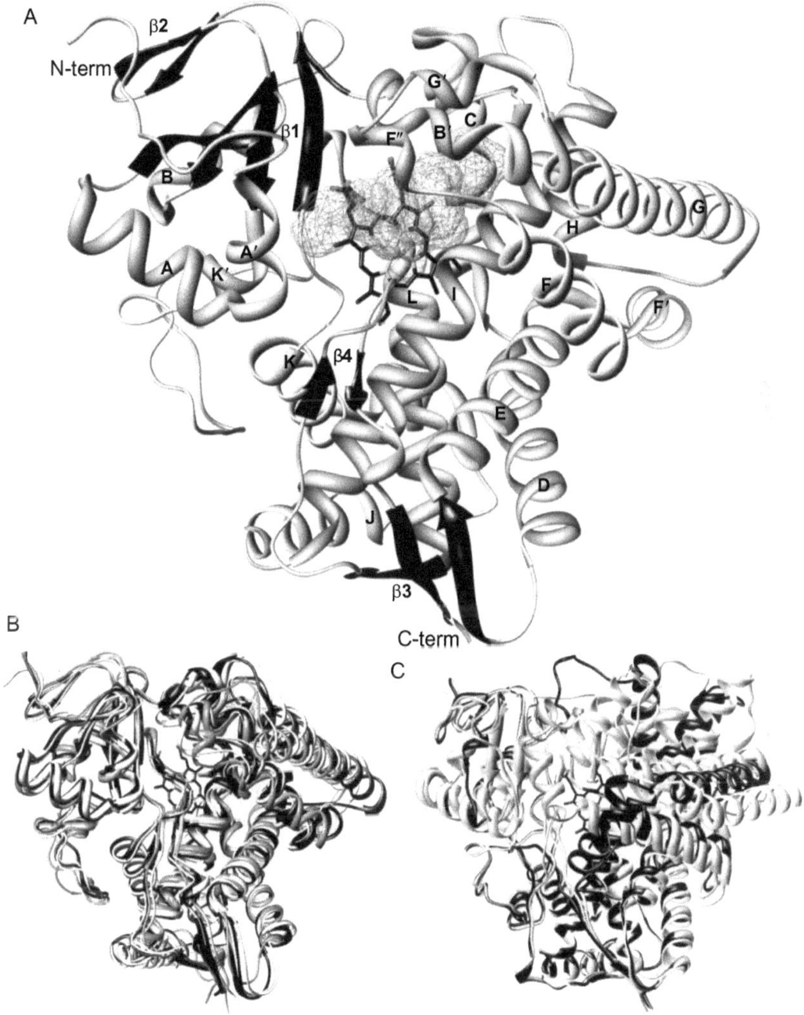

FIGURE 4.4 CYP51 crystal structure. (A) Distal view, helices (grey) and β-sheets bundles (black) are shown in ribbon representation and marked. The haem is shown as a stick model. The active site cavity surface is depicted as the grey mesh. (B) Ligand-free *T. brucei* CYP51 (black) superimposed with VNI-bound *T. brucei* CYP51, posaconazole-bound *T. cruzi* (grey) and ketoconazole-bound human (dark grey) orthologs. Only minor alterations are seen in the CYP51 active site cavity area. (C) An example of a xenobiotic-metabolizing P450, CYP2B4, in ligand-free form (black) and bound to two different ligands, 4-(4-chlorophenyl)imidazole and bifonazole (grey). Large-scale conformational changes significantly alter shape and volume of its active site pocket.

helix/strand/coil ratio being about 50/10/30. Two nearly parallel "CYP core helices", I and L, surround the haem from the distal and proximal sides, respectively. Helices A′, F″ and the top of the β4 hairpin on the upper left side of the distal surface of the protein are forming the entrance into the substrate access channel. *In vivo*, this highly hydrophobic portion of the protein molecule is predicted to be immersed into the endoplasmic reticulum membrane, receiving their sterol substrates through the lipid bilayer (Lepesheva et al., 2010b). About 6 × 9 Å wide at the beginning, the substrate access channel makes an angle of about 50° to the haem plane and runs about 20 Å to the haem iron, gradually broadening into the active site cavity inside the protein globule. The cavity is bordered by the haem (back), B′ helix/B′C loop (top), the N-terminal parts of helices C and I (right), β1-4 strand with the preceding K′/β1-4 loop (left and bottom, respectively) and β4 hairpin (front), the substrate binding surface being composed of 47 residues, including 43 side chains, as described in more detail in Section 4.6.3. The haem propionate side chains form hydrogen bonds with five dissociable amino acid residues, Y103, Y116, R124, R361 and H420, the haem iron is coordinated to C422.

4.6.2. Specific structural features

Perhaps the most characteristic feature of the CYP51 structure is that the active site cavity does not change much, in shape or volume, both upon ligand binding and across species (Fig. 4.4B). The most flexible regions are presented by the GH loop, which is located on the P450 proximal surface, far away from the active site cavity and the FG-loop (including helix F″ that covers the entrance into the channel). In all three cases of azole-bound structures, it can be seen that the middle portion of the I-helix shifts slightly away from the haem, providing space for the heterocyclic ring to coordinate with the iron. On average, the r.m.s. deviation for all Cα atoms in the three *T. cruzi* CYP51 inhibitor complexes ranges only from 0.7 to 1.4 Å, and the r.m.s. deviation between the posaconazole-bound *T. cruzi* and ketoconazole-bound human CYP51s (27% amino acid sequence identity) is only 1.7 Å. Though at first quite surprising, this structural feature of CYP51 family members lead us to the conclusion that CYP51 enzymes appear to maintain their strict functional conservation (including the three-step catalytic reaction) by preserving high similarity at the secondary and tertiary structural levels (Lepesheva and Waterman, 2011).

This elevated rigidity of the substrate binding cavity appears to distinguish the CYP51 family from other CYPs, especially those involved in metabolism of xenobiotics (e.g. drug-metabolizing CYP families), whose structures are known to demonstrate high plasticity, allowing these enzymes to accommodate and metabolize a variety of chemical structures

(CYP2B4 is shown in Fig. 4.4C as an example). On the contrary, CYP51 family members must preserve very strict substrate specificity, regardless of their low amino acid sequence identity across the biological kingdoms. High rigidity of the substrate binding cavity explains why a single amino acid substitution can completely inactivate the enzyme (Lepesheva et al., 2003) or switch its substrate preferences from C4-double- to C4-monomethylated sterols (Lepesheva et al., 2006a). Moreover, to fulfil their catalytic function, the enzymes must maintain their substrate properly oriented during the three steps of catalysis, which could be another reason for the requirement to have a rigid substrate binding site—a real "cavity" instead of flexible "pockets" typical for highly promiscuous CYPs. Most relevant here, the rigidity of the substrate binding cavity might be the basis for the experimentally proven elevated susceptibility of CYP51 to azole inhibitors. Next we will discuss how CYP51 structure can be helpful for drug development, in order to increase their (a) potency and (b) selectivity.

4.6.3. Structural explanation for the potencies of selected inhibitors

CYP51 complexes with the three most potent inhibitors, posaconazole [3K1O], VNI [3GW9] and VNF [3KSW], will be analysed here as examples (Fig. 4.5). As all azole inhibitors, the compounds coordinate to the CYP51 haem iron. It is well known, however, that Fe–N coordination alone is insufficient to make a strong inhibitor: small molecules, like imidazole or phenylimidazole, have very low binding affinity, while elongation of the non-coordinated, usually hydrophobic part of the inhibitor molecule may significantly enhance the interaction, indicating an essential role of the protein moiety in the azole-CYP51 complex formation (Ortiz de Montellano and Correia, 1995).

Interaction with posaconazole in *T. cruzi* CYP51 is strengthened by van der Waals contacts with 25 amino acid residues (Lepesheva et al., 2010a). Thirteen of these residues lie inside the substrate binding cavity, and 12 others are located around the entrance into the substrate access channel, surrounding the remote portion of the posaconazole long arm, which protrudes ~3 Å above the protein surface (Fig. 4.5A). This second binding subsite seems to be unique to the posaconazole-CYP51 interaction, its importance for the drug inhibitory potency being supported by the fact that posaconazole has much stronger anti-parasitic activity than its numerous derivatives of altered arm configuration (the side products of the posaconazole synthesis procedure) (Nomeir et al., 2008). Roughly, 25 van der Waals contacts should contribute up to 7.5 kcal/mol to the energy of the inhibitor–enzyme interaction.

In the complex with *T. brucei* CYP51 (Lepesheva et al., 2010b), VNI is oriented very similarly to posaconazole; however, its arm, being ~8 Å

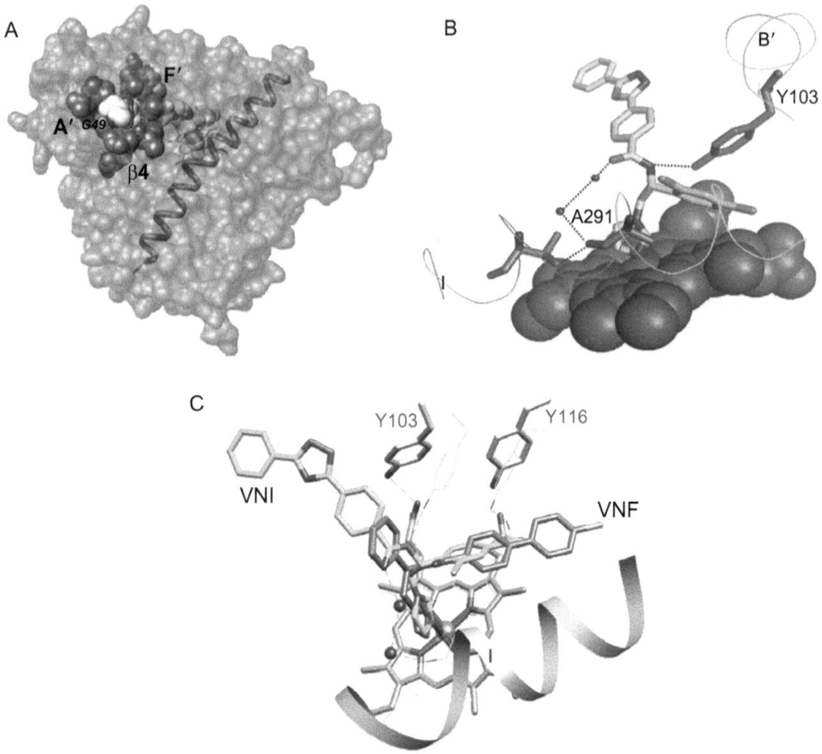

FIGURE 4.5 Specific details of inhibitor-CYP51 complexes. (A) Surface binding subsite in posaconazole-bound *T. cruzi* CYP51 (surface representation, I-helix is shown). (B) The carboxamide fragment of VNI forms a hydrogen-bond network with *T. brucei* CYP51 helices B′ and I. The haem is shown as spheres. (C) VNF binds in the orientation opposite to VNI, its long arm being directed deeper into the active site cavity.

shorter, does not reach the protein surface. Although van der Waals contacts are formed with only 15 protein residues (up to 4.5 kcal/mol), the carboxamide group of VNI provides two hydrogen bonds, which connect the inhibitor molecule with two secondary structural elements of the protein, helices B′ and I (Fig. 4.5B). Such a hydrogen-bond network should add up to 10 kcal/mol to the energy of the inhibitor/enzyme binding. Stronger anti-parasitic effect of VNI compared to posaconazole in *T. cruzi* (unpublished) is in agreement with these calculations.

VNF, which is structurally similar to VNI, binds to *T. cruzi* CYP51 in an opposite orientation (Fig. 4.5C), including 180° rotation of its carboxamide group fragment. Although the electron density for the hydrogen-bond network around VNF cannot be clearly seen at medium resolution, it is quite likely that the comparably strong inhibitory potencies of VNI and VNF can have the same "hydrogen-bond mediated" origin (Lepesheva et al., 2010a). The number of van der Waals contact forming residues in the VNF-CYP51 complex is 14. The longer, two-ring arm of VNF is intercalated between helices B′, C and the N-terminal portion of helix I, which are shifted 1–2 Å away from the haem compared to their position in the posaconazole and VNI-bound structures. The backbone rearrangements can cause some tension pushing the inhibitor back towards the haem plane and also strengthening the interaction.

Structure-directed modifications of the VNI/VNF scaffold are currently in progress, aiming to further enhance the compounds anti-parasitic potency and optimize their pharmacokinetic properties while maintaining their low potential for toxicity.

4.6.4. Towards drug selectivity

Because humans can consume cholesterol from the diet and statins, inhibitors of an early step of sterol biosynthesis (Fig. 4.1), are broadly used as cholesterol-lowering drugs; at first glance, blocking this pathway with anti-microbial azoles does not seem to be essential for humans. However, inhibitors selective for pathogenic sterol 14α-demethylases are still highly desirable, especially in cases of long-term systemic treatment, to prevent formation of harmful methylated sterols in the human body and also to avoid potentially negative effects on biosynthesis of meiosis activating sterols, steroid hormones and bile acids.

As mentioned above, when superimposed, the secondary structural elements which form the active site cavity in *T. cruzi* and human CYP51 have similar location. Very similar positions are occupied by several residues that are identical in all known CYP51 family members, allowing these enzymes to preserve their catalytic role across the kingdoms. However, 22 of the 47 cavity forming residues in *T. cruzi* CYP51 are different from the corresponding residues in the human counterpart (Fig. 4.6). These differences influence active site topology and can direct subtle structure-based modifications of CYP51 inhibitors in order to rationally increase their selectivity against human pathogens as well as to control potential development of CYP51-related resistance.

4.7. ANTI-PARASITIC EFFECTS OF CYP51 INHIBITION IN *TRYPANOSOMA CRUZI*

CYP51 inhibitors clearly affect *T. cruzi* sterol composition (Konkle et al., 2009; Lepesheva et al., 2007; Fig. 4.7A), profoundly damage ultrastructural organization of the parasite membranes (Lepesheva et al., 2008; Fig. 4.7B) and finally kill the pathogen, acting even stronger on its intracellular forms, amastigotes (Lepesheva et al., 2007; Fig. 4.7C). This is in good

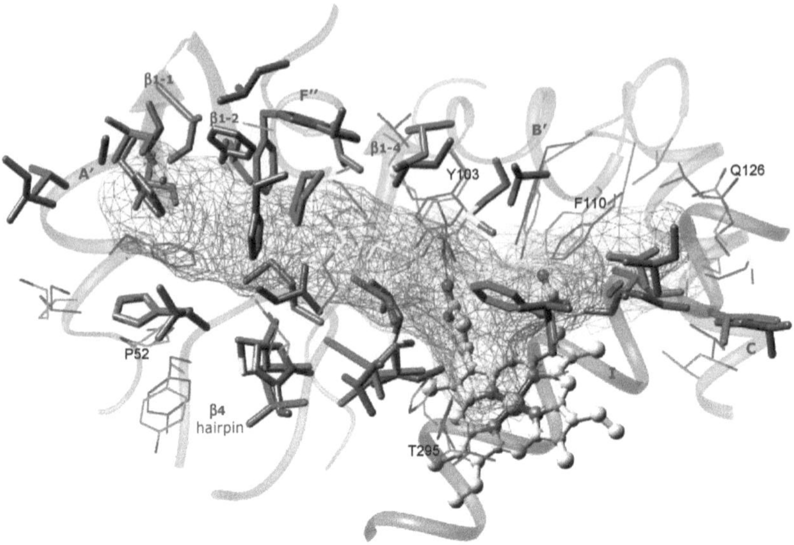

FIGURE 4.6 Active site forming residues in *T. cruzi* (black) and human (grey) CYP51s. The corresponding secondary structural elements in *T. cruzi* are depicted as the transparent ribbon and marked, the haem is seen as ball and stick model. The active site cavity is outlined as grey mesh. The cavity residues which are conserved the human and *T. cruzi* enzymes are shown in line representation. Some of the residues conserved in the whole CYP51 family are marked (*T. cruzi* CYP51 numbering). The active site residues that differ in the two proteins are displayed as stick models.

agreement with the results from the Urbina group (Liendo et al., 1998, 1999; Urbina et al., 1998, 2003a), the first to report that the anti-parasitic effects of anti-fungal azoles are usually much more expressed in the multiplying form of *T. cruzi*. Interestingly, we have found that the CYP51 gene, being expressed in significant amounts at all stages of the *T. cruzi* life-cycle is also upregulated in the multiplying forms of the parasite (Fig. 4.7.D). Altogether, this (1) confirms the importance of sterol biosynthesis to survival of *T. cruzi*, (2) reflects acceleration of the sterol flow in the multiplying stages of the pathogen, and (3) supports the notion (Lepesheva et al., 2010b) of possible requirements for additional sterol production, both structural and regulatory, which appear to be accelerated upon *T. cruzi* multiplication.

Finally, we have found that while posaconazole and fluconazole upregulate CYP51 gene expression in *T. cruzi*, our new carboxamide-containing inhibitory scaffold does not change it (Fig. 4.7E). Besides, contrary to posaconazole, it does not require increase in the concentration in order to maintain the inhibitory effect over time (Fig. 4.7F), which makes this scaffold highly advantageous in terms of its lower potential to cause

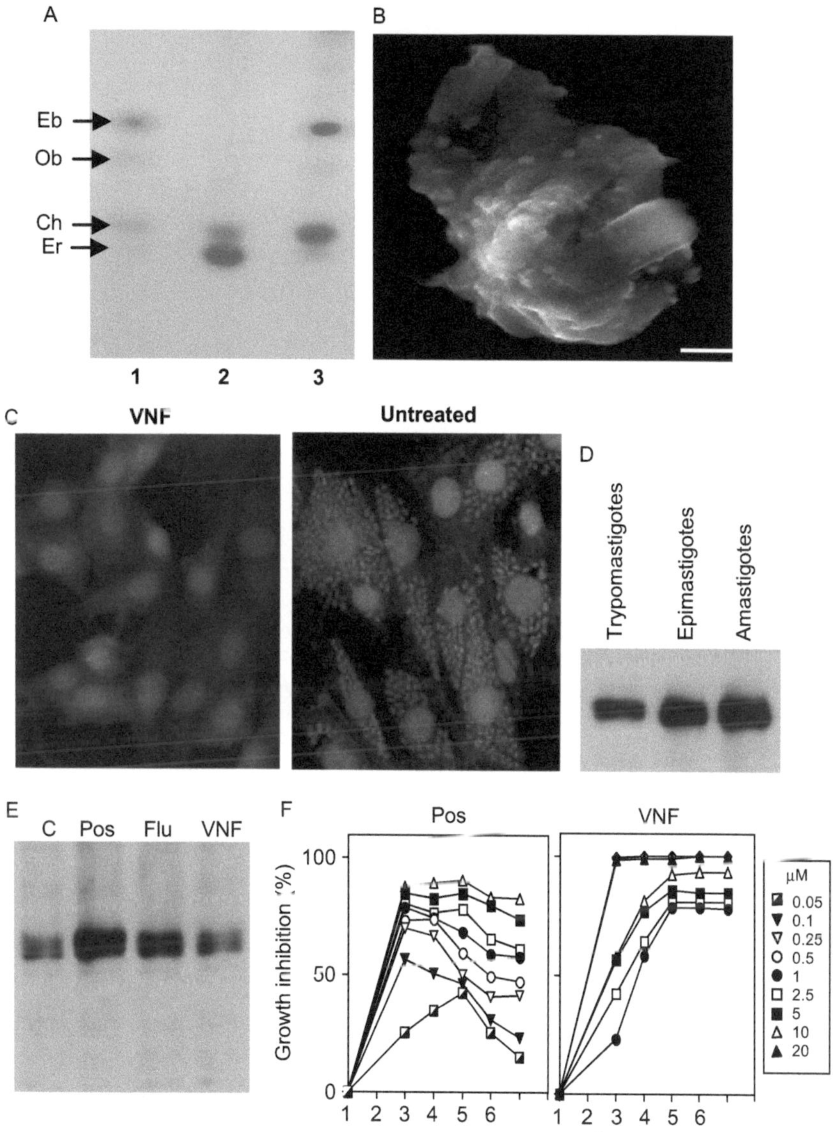

FIGURE 4.7 Cellular effects of VNI/VNF in *T. cruzi*. (A) TLC of sterol standards (1) and unsaponified lipids extracted from *T. cruzi* amastigotes, untreated (2) and treated with 1 μM VNI (3). Eb, eburicol; Ob, obtusifoliol; Ch, cholesterol (exogenous); Er, ergosterol. (B) Scanning electron microscopy of *T. cruzi* amastigotes treated with 1 μM VNI; bar = 1 μm. Membrane disruption is seen as blebs on the surface. (C) Anti-parasitic effect of VNF (1 μM) on *T. cruzi* amastigotes within cardiomyocytes (GFP-expressing transgenic *T. cruzi*) is seen as small light dots, cardiomyocytes nuclei are seen as circles. (D) CYP51 gene expression in *T. cruzi*, immunoblotting. (E) CYP51 gene expression upon treatment of *T. cruzi* with 1 μM CYP51 inhibitors. C, control. (F) Inhibition of *T. cruzi* growth with different concentrations of posaconazole and VNF.

resistance. Our most recent work has shown that at low drug concentration the anti-parasitic effect of VNI in *T. cruzi* is stronger than that of posaconazole ($EC_{50} = 1.2$ nM vs. $\sim$5 nM, respectively (unpublished)). Testing of these compounds in animal models of Chagas disease as well as investigation of their pharmacokinetic properties is currently underway with the hope to bring new effective drugs for the chronic phase of the infection.

ACKNOWLEDGEMENTS

The authors are grateful for support by the National Institute of Health grants GM067871 (M. R. W. and G. I. L.) and AI 080580 (F. V) and Vanderbilt Institute of Chemical Biology Pilot Project grant 2011 (G. I. L.).

REFERENCES

Aoyama, Y., Yoshida, Y., Sonoda, Y., Sato, Y., 1987. 7-Oxo-24,25-dihydrolanosterol: a novel lanosterol 14 alpha-demethylase (P-45014DM) inhibitor which blocks electron transfer to the oxyferro intermediate. Biochim. Biophys. Acta 922, 270–277.

Apt, W., Aguilera, X., Arribada, A., Perez, C., Miranda, C., Sanchez, G., et al., 1998. Treatment of chronic Chagas' disease with itraconazole and allopurinol. Am. J. Trop. Med. Hyg. 59, 133–138.

Araujo, M.S., Martins-Filho, O.A., Pereira, M.E., Brener, Z., 2000. A combination of benznidazole and ketoconazole enhances efficacy of chemotherapy of experimental Chagas' disease. J. Antimicrob. Chemother. 45, 819–824.

Beach, D.H., Goad, L.J., Holz, G.G., Jr., 1986. Effects of ketoconazole on sterol biosynthesis by *Trypanosoma cruzi* epimastigotes. Biochem. Biophys. Res. Commun. 136, 851–856.

Benveniste, P., 1986. Sterol biosynthesis. Annu. Rev. Plant Physiol. Plant Mol. Biol. 37, 275–308.

Bossard, M.J., Tomaszek, T.A., Gallagher, T.F., Metcalf, B.W., Adams, J.L., 1991. Steroidal acetylenes—mechanism-based inactivators of lanosterol 14-alpha-demethylase. Bioorg. Chem. 19, 418–432.

Buckner, F., Yokoyama, K., Lockman, J., Aikenhead, K., Ohkanda, J., Sadilek, M., et al., 2003. A class of sterol 14-demethylase inhibitors as anti-*Trypanosoma cruzi* agents. Proc. Natl. Acad. Sci. USA 100, 15149–15153.

Cammerer, S.B., Jimenez, C., Jones, S., Gros, L., Lorente, S.O., Rodrigues, C., et al., 2007. Quinuclidine derivatives as potential antiparasitics. Antimicrob. Agents Chemother. 51, 4049–4061.

Chen, C.K., Doyle, P.S., Yermalitskaya, L.V., Mackey, Z.B., Ang, K.K., McKerrow, J.H., et al., 2009. Trypanosoma cruzi CYP51 inhibitor derived from a Mycobacterium tuberculosis screen hit. PLoS Negl. Trop. Dis. 3, e372.

Cheng, A.C., Coleman, R.G., Smyth, K.T., Cao, Q., Soulard, P., Caffrey, D.R., et al., 2007. Structure-based maximal affinity model predicts small-molecule druggability. Nat. Biotechnol. 25, 71–75.

Clayton, J., 2010. Chagas disease: pushing through the pipeline. Nature 465, S12–S15.

Cooper, A.B., Wright, J.J., Ganguly, A.K., Desai, J., Loebenberg, D., Parmegiani, R., et al., 1988. Synthesis and anti-fungal properties of 14-aminomethyl-substituted lanosterol derivatives. Ann. N. Y. Acad. Sci. 544, 109–112.

Cournia, Z., Ullmann, G.M., Smith, J.C., 2007. Differential effects of cholesterol, ergosterol and lanosterol on a dipalmitoyl phosphatidylcholine membrane: a molecular dynamics simulation study. J. Phys. Chem. B 111, 1786–1801.

Diniz Lde, F., Caldas, I.S., Guedes, P.M., Crepalde, G., de Lana, M., Carneiro, C.M., et al., 2010. Effects of ravuconazole treatment on parasite load and immune response in dogs experimentally infected with Trypanosoma cruzi. Antimicrob. Agents Chemother. 54, 2979–2986.

Docampo, R., Moreno, S.N., Turrens, J.F., Katzin, A.M., Gonzalez-Cappa, S.M., Stoppani, A.O., 1981. Biochemical and ultrastructural alterations produced by miconazole and econazole in *Trypanosoma cruzi*. Mol. Biochem. Parasitol. 3, 169–180.

Doyle, P.S., Chen, C.K., Johnston, J.B., Hopkins, S.D., Leung, S.S., Jacobson, M.P., et al., 2010. A nonazole CYP51 inhibitor cures Chagas' disease in a mouse model of acute infection. Antimicrob. Agents Chemother. 54, 2480–2488.

Frye, L.L., Cusack, K.P., Leonard, D.A., 1993. 32-Methyl-32-oxylanosterols: dual-action inhibitors of cholesterol biosynthesis. J. Med. Chem. 36, 410–416.

Goldstein, J.L., Brown, M.S., 1990. Regulation of the mevalonate pathway. Nature 343, 425–430.

Gros, L., Castillo-Acosta, V.M., Jimenez Jimenez, C., Sealey-Cardona, M., Vargas, S., Manuel Estevez, A., et al., 2006. New azasterols against *Trypanosoma brucei*: role of 24-sterol methyltransferase in inhibitor action. Antimicrob. Agents Chemother. 50, 2595–2601.

Haines, T.H., 2001. Do sterols reduce proton and sodium leaks through lipid bilayers? Prog. Lipid Res. 40, 299–324.

Haughan, P.A., Goad, L.J., 1991. Lipid biochemistry of trypanosomatids. In: Coombs, G., North, M. (Eds.), Biochemical Protozoology. Taylor & Francis, London, pp. 312–328.

Hucke, O., Gelb, M.H., Verlinde, C.L., Buckner, F.S., 2005. The protein farnesyltransferase inhibitor Tipifarnib as a new lead for the development of drugs against Chagas disease. J. Med. Chem. 48, 5415–5418.

Kavanagh, K.L., Guo, K., Dunford, J.E., Wu, X., Knapp, S., Ebetino, F.H., et al., 2006. The molecular mechanism of nitrogen-containing bisphosphonates as anti-osteoporosis drugs. Proc. Natl. Acad. Sci. USA 103, 7829–7834.

Konkle, M.E., Hargrove, T.Y., Kleshchenko, Y.Y., von Kries, J.P., Ridenour, W., Uddin, M.J., et al., 2009. Indomethacin amides as a novel molecular scaffold for targeting *Trypanosoma cruzi* sterol 14 alpha-demethylase. J. Med. Chem. 52, 2846–2853.

Kraus, J.M., Verlinde, C.L., Karimi, M., Lepesheva, G.I., Gelb, M.H., Buckner, F.S., 2009. Rational modification of a candidate cancer drug for use against Chagas disease. J. Med. Chem. 52, 1639–1647.

Lepesheva, G.I., Waterman, M.R., 2007. Sterol 14alpha-demethylase cytochrome P450 (CYP51), a P450 in all biological kingdoms. Biochim. Biophys. Acta 1770, 467–477.

Lepesheva, G.I., Waterman, M.R., 2011. Structural basis for conservation in the CYP51 family. Biochim. Biophys. Acta 1814, 88–93.

Lepesheva, G.I., Virus, C., Waterman, M.R., 2003. Conservation in the CYP51 family. Role of the B′ helix/BC loop and helices F and G in enzymatic function. Biochemistry 42, 9091–9101.

Lepesheva, G.I., Hargrove, T.Y., Ott, R.D., Nes, W.D., Waterman, M.R., 2006a. Biodiversity of CYP51 in trypanosomes. Biochem. Soc. Trans. 34, 1161–1164.

Lepesheva, G.I., Zaitseva, N.G., Nes, W.D., Zhou, W., Arase, M., Liu, J., et al., 2006b. CYP51 from Trypanosoma cruzi: a phyla-specific residue in the B′ helix defines substrate preferences of sterol 14alpha-demethylase. J. Biol. Chem. 281, 3577–3585.

Lepesheva, G.I., Ott, R.D., Hargrove, T.Y., Kleshchenko, Y.Y., Schuster, I., Nes, W.D., et al., 2007. Sterol 14 alpha-demethylase as a potential target for anti-trypanosomal therapy: enzyme inhibition and parasite cell growth. Chem. Biol. 14, 1283–1293.

Lepesheva, G., Hargrove, T., Kleshchenko, Y., Nes, W., Villalta, F., Waterman, M., 2008. CYP51: a major drug target in the cytochrome P450 superfamily. Lipids 43, 1117–1125.

Lepesheva, G.I., Hargrove, T.Y., Anderson, S., Kleshchenko, Y., Furtak, V., Wawrzak, Z., et al., 2010a. Structural insights into inhibition of sterol 14 alpha-demethylase in the human pathogen *Trypanosoma cruzi*. J. Biol. Chem. 285, 25582–25590.

Lepesheva, G.I., Park, H.W., Hargrove, T.Y., Vanhollebeke, B., Wawrzak, Z., Harp, J.M., et al., 2010b. Crystal structures of *Trypanosoma brucei* sterol 14 alpha-demethylase and implications for selective treatment of human infections. J. Biol. Chem. 285, 1773–1780.

Liendo, A., Lazardi, K., Urbina, J.A., 1998. In-vitro anti-proliferative effects and mechanism of action of the bis-triazole D0870 and its S(−) enantiomer against *Trypanosoma cruzi*. J. Antimicrob. Chemother. 41, 197–205.

Liendo, A., Visbal, G., Piras, M.M., Piras, R., Urbina, J.A., 1999. Sterol composition and biosynthesis in *Trypanosoma cruzi* amastigotes. Mol. Biochem. Parasitol. 104, 81–91.

Magaraci, F., Jimenez, C.J., Rodrigues, C., Rodrigues, J.C., Braga, M.V., Yardley, V., et al., 2003. Azasterols as inhibitors of sterol 24-methyltransferase in Leishmania species and *Trypanosoma cruzi*. J. Med. Chem. 46, 4714–4727.

Molina, J., Martins-Filho, O., Brener, Z., Romanha, A.J., Loebenberg, D., Urbina, J.A., 2000. Activities of the triazole derivative SCH 56592 (posaconazole) against drug-resistant strains of the protozoan parasite Trypanosoma (Schizotrypanum) cruzi in immunocompetent and immunosuppressed murine hosts. Antimicrob. Agents Chemother. 44, 150–155.

Nagappan, V., Deresinski, S., 2007. Reviews of anti-infective agents: posaconazole: a broad-spectrum triazole anti-fungal agent. Clin. Infect. Dis. 45, 1610–1617.

Nes, W.R., 1974. Role of sterols in membranes. Lipids 9, 596–612.

Nomeir, A.A., Pramanik, B.N., Heimark, L., Bennett, F., Veals, J., Bartner, P., et al., 2008. Posaconazole (Noxafil, SCH 56592), a new azole anti-fungal drug, was a discovery based on the isolation and mass spectral characterization of a circulating metabolite of an earlier lead (SCH 51048). J. Mass Spectrom. 43, 509–517.

Obach, R.S., Walsky, R.L., Venkatakrishnan, K., Gaman, E.A., Houston, J.B., Tremaine, L.M., 2006. The utility of in vitro cytochrome P450 inhibition data in the prediction of drug-drug interactions. J. Pharmacol. Exp. Therapeut. 316, 336–348.

Omura, T., Sato, R., 1964. The carbon monoxide-binding pigment of liver microsomes. I. Evidence for its hemoprotein nature. J. Biol. Chem. 239, 2370–2378.

Ortiz de Montellano, P.R., Correia, M.A., 1995. Inhibition of cytochrome P450 enzymes. In: Ortiz de Montellano, P.R. (Ed.), Cytochrome P450: Structure, Mechanism, and Biochemistry. Plenum Publishing Corporation, New York, pp. 305–364.

Pena-Diaz, J., Montalvetti, A., Flores, C.L., Constan, A., Hurtado-Guerrero, R., De Souza, W., et al., 2004. Mitochondrial localization of the mevalonate pathway enzyme 3-Hydroxy-3-methyl-glutaryl-CoA reductase in the Trypanosomatidae. Mol. Biol. Cell 15, 1356–1363.

Petrikkos, G., Skiada, A., 2007. Recent advances in anti-fungal chemotherapy. Int. J. Antimicrob. Agents 30, 108–117.

Pinazo, M.J., Espinosa, G., Gallego, M., Lopez-Chejade, P.L., Urbina, J.A., Gascon, J., 2010. Successful treatment with posaconazole of a patient with chronic Chagas disease and systemic lupus erythematosus. Am. J. Trop. Med. Hyg. 82, 583–587.

Poulos, T.L., Finzel, B.C., Howard, A.J., 1987. High-resolution crystal-structure of cytochrome-P450cam. J. Mol. Biol. 195, 687–700.

Puccetti, L., Acampa, M., Auteri, A., 2007. Pharmacogenetics of statins therapy. Recent Pat. Cardiovasc. Drug Discov. 2, 228–236.

Quinones, W., Urbina, J.A., Dubourdieu, M., Luis Concepcion, J., 2004. The glycosome membrane of *Trypanosoma cruzi* epimastigotes: protein and lipid composition. Exp. Parasitol. 106, 135–149.

Rodrigues, C.O., Catisti, R., Uyemura, S.A., Vercesi, A.E., Lira, R., Rodriguez, C., et al., 2001. The sterol composition of *Trypanosoma cruzi* changes after growth in different culture media and results in different sensitivity to digitonin-permeabilization. J. Eukaryot. Microbiol. 48, 588–594.

Rohmer, M., Bouvier, P., Ourisson, G., 1979. Molecular evolution of biomembranes: structural equivalents and phylogenetic precursors of sterols. Proc. Natl. Acad. Sci. USA 76, 847–851.

Schaller, H., 2003. The role of sterols in plant growth and development. Prog. Lipid Res. 42, 163–175.

Schiller, D.S., Fung, H.B., 2007. Posaconazole: an extended-spectrum triazole anti-fungal agent. Clin. Ther. 29, 1862–1886.

Schroepfer, G.J., Jr., 1981. Sterol biosynthesis. Annu. Rev. Biochem. 50, 585–621.

Trzaskos, J.M., Ko, S.S., Magolda, R.L., Favata, M.F., Fischer, R.T., Stam, S.H., et al., 1995. Substrate-based inhibitors of lanosterol 14 alpha-methyl demethylase: I. Assessment of inhibitor structure-activity relationship and cholesterol biosynthesis inhibition properties. Biochemistry 34, 9670–9676.

Tuck, S.F., Patel, H., Safi, E., Robinson, C.H., 1991. Lanosterol 14 alpha-demethylase (P45014DM): effects of P45014DM inhibitors on sterol biosynthesis downstream of lanosterol. J. Lipid Res. 32, 893–902.

Urbina, J.A., 2009. Ergosterol biosynthesis and drug development for Chagas disease. Mem. Inst. Oswaldo Cruz 104 (Suppl. 1), 311–318.

Urbina, J.A., 2010. New insights in Chagas' disease treatment. Drugs Future 35, 409–419.

Urbina, J.A., Lazardi, K., Aguirre, T., Piras, M.M., Piras, R., 1988. Anti-proliferative synergism of the allylamine SF 86–327 and ketoconazole on epimastigotes and amastigotes of Trypanosoma (Schizotrypanum) cruzi. Antimicrob. Agents Chemother. 32, 1237–1242.

Urbina, J.A., Payares, G., Molina, J., Sanoja, C., Liendo, A., Lazardi, K., et al., 1996. Cure of short- and long-term experimental Chagas' disease using D0870. Science 273, 969–971.

Urbina, J.A., Payares, G., Contreras, L.M., Liendo, A., Sanoja, C., Molina, J., et al., 1998. Anti-proliferative effects and mechanism of action of SCH 56592 against Trypanosoma (Schizotrypanum) cruzi: in vitro and in vivo studies. Antimicrob. Agents Chemother. 42, 1771–1777.

Urbina, J.A., Lira, R., Visbal, G., Bartroli, J., 2000. In vitro anti-proliferative effects and mechanism of action of the new triazole derivative UR-9825 against the protozoan parasite Trypanosoma (Schizotrypanum) cruzi. Antimicrob. Agents Chemother. 44, 2498–2502.

Urbina, J.A., Payares, G., Sanoja, C., Lira, R., Romanha, A.J., 2003a. In vitro and in vivo activities of ravuconazole on *Trypanosoma cruzi*, the causative agent of Chagas disease. Int. J. Antimicrob. Agents 21, 27–38.

Urbina, J.A., Payares, G., Sanoja, C., Molina, J., Lira, R., Brener, Z., et al., 2003b. Parasitological cure of acute and chronic experimental Chagas disease using the long-acting experimental triazole TAK-187. Activity against drug-resistant *Trypanosoma cruzi* strains. Int. J. Antimicrob. Agents 21, 39–48.

Volkman, J.K., 2005. Sterols and other triterpenoids: source specificity and evolution of biosynthetic pathways. Org. Geochem. 36, 139–159.

Wexler, D., Courtney, R., Richards, W., Banfield, C., Lim, J., Laughlin, M., 2004. Effect of posaconazole on cytochrome P450 enzymes: a randomized, open-label, two-way cross over study. Euro. J. Pharmaceut. Sci. 21, 645–653.

Yeagle, P.L., Martin, R.B., Lala, A.K., Lin, H.K., Bloch, K., 1977. Differential effects of cholesterol and lanosterol on artificial membranes. Proc. Natl. Acad. Sci. USA 74, 4924–4926.

Yoshida, Y., Aoyama, Y., Noshiro, M., Gotoh, O., 2000. Sterol 14-demethylase P450 (CYP51) provides a breakthrough for the discussion on the evolution of cytochrome P450 gene superfamily. Biochem. Biophys. Res. Commun. 273, 799–804.

Zonios, D.I., Bennett, J.E., 2008. Update on azole anti-fungals. Semin. Respir. Crit. Care Med. 29, 198–210.

CHAPTER 5

Experimental Chemotherapy and Approaches to Drug Discovery for *Trypanosoma cruzi* Infection

Frederick S. Buckner

Contents

Abstract

In the 100 years since the discovery of Chagas disease, only two drugs have been developed and introduced into clinical practice, and these drugs were introduced over 40 years ago. The tools of drug discovery have improved dramatically in the interim; however, this has not translated into new drugs for Chagas disease. This has been largely because the main practitioners of drug discovery are pharmaceutical companies who are not financially motivated to

Department of Medicine, University of Washington, Seattle, Washington, USA

Advances in Parasitology, Volume 75
ISSN 0065-308X, DOI: 10.1016/B978-0-12-385863-4.00005-8

invest in Chagas disease and other "orphan" diseases. As a result, it has largely been up to academic groups to bring drug candidates through the discovery pipeline and to clinical trials. The difficulty with drug discovery in academia has been the challenge of bringing together the diverse expertise in biology, chemistry, and pharmacology in concerted efforts towards a common goal of developing therapeutics. Funding is often inadequate, but lack of coordination amongst academic investigators with different expertise has also contributed to the slow progress. The purpose of this chapter is to provide an overview of approaches that can be accomplished in academic settings for preclinical drug discovery for Chagas disease. The chapter addresses methods of drug screening against *Trypanosoma cruzi* cultures and in animal models and includes general topics on compound selection, testing for drug-like properties (including oral bioavailability), investigating the pharmacokinetics and toxicity of compounds, and finally providing parameters to help with triaging compounds.

5.1. INTRODUCTION

The primary purpose of laboratory testing of chemical compounds against *Trypanosoma cruzi* is to identify compounds with potential to be advanced into clinical trials as drug candidates for Chagas disease. The laboratory models need to take under consideration the ultimate goals of chemotherapy for human *T. cruzi* infection. Establishing these goals is not trivial due to the complex pathophysiology of Chagas disease. In individuals with asymptomatic infection (indeterminate stage), the ultimate goal is to completely prevent the occurrence of the disease manifestations of Chagas disease. Whether or not this requires complete parasitological cure is unknown. However, it would be necessary for the drug to give parasitological cures if it were to eliminate the risk of disease transmission from these individuals, be it by maternal–foetal routes, vectorial spread, or through blood products. In the case of immune compromised individuals (e.g. persons with AIDS or solid organ transplants), it would be preferable to achieve cures because of the high risk of parasite recrudescence when non-curative chemotherapy is used. With respect to persons manifesting symptoms of Chagas disease, the goal of antiparasitic chemotherapy should be to prevent disease progression, and perhaps help reverse symptoms when the disease is not exceedingly advanced. There is some evidence that chronic patients treated with benznidazole, while not necessarily parasitologically cured, benefit in terms of reduction in the occurrence of electrocardiographic changes and lower frequency of clinical deterioration (Viotti et al., 1994). Thus, reduction in parasite burden without cure may improve clinical outcomes. However, because of the potential public health benefits of curing patients, most would agree that a curative drug should be the goal. Moreover, a drug that has a trypanocidal (as opposed to trypanostatic) mechanism of action is more likely to cure individuals who lack normal immune systems. A curative drug acting by a trypanocidal mechanism is the preferred goal and will guide the discussion of laboratory testing described in this chapter. While striving for this goal, if a drug is discovered that is safe, easy to use, and ameliorates disease, this would be an advance over current drugs, even if it was not curative in many cases.

A research program to introduce new drugs for clinical testing against Chagas disease requires having a target product profile (TPP) in mind. Specifically, it is necessary to have a clear vision of the properties of the final drug to direct the activities of the drug discovery campaign. A TPP for Chagas disease has only occasionally been articulated in the literature (Urbina, 1999, 2009). A recent article by the scientists at Drugs for Neglected Diseases Initiative has defined a TPP that is worth reproducing here (Table 5.1; Ribeiro et al., 2009). Naturally, the TPP is a matter of opinion, thus, various points will be addressed here. The TPP is divided between the "ideal" and the "acceptable" profiles. In both cases, the "label" (or indication) includes early chronic/indeterminate phase Chagas disease. By implication, the drug would be expected to be effective for acute stage disease since existing drugs demonstrate that cures are more easily achieved during acute infection than during chronic infection (Bern et al., 2007). Treatment for patients with late chronic infections has been left out of the TPP. This seems reasonable due to the apparent irreversibility of much of the organ damage during late chronic infection. Under the "ideal" TPP, immunocompromised patients with reactivations are included. Since this represents a small population compared to immune competent patients with indeterminate or early chronic disease, it makes sense to aim for this challenging goal only under ideal circumstances.

The quoted TPP includes activity of the drug on the two sub-species of *T. cruzi* (TcI and TcII) (Ribeiro et al., 2009). Recently, a new intraspecific nomenclature for *T. cruzi* has been introduced that divides the species into six discrete typing units (TcI to TcVI) (Zingales et al., 2009); thus, the TPP should be updated to account for this change. The important point is that new drugs should have activity against the spectrum of clinically significant *T. cruzi* strains. This matters because drug susceptibility has been shown to be variable between different *T. cruzi* isolates (Filardi and Brener, 1987).

A new drug should certainly be effective for adults as indicated in the "Acceptable" column in the TPP, but many would argue that treatment should also be available for school age children. It would be desirable to target this population in public health campaigns since this would facilitate treatment of young individuals with indeterminate infection at a time

TABLE 5.1 Target product profile for a Chagas drug—chronic indeterminate phase (Ribeiro et al., 2009)

Product feature	Acceptable	Ideal
Target label	Early chronic/ indeterminate Chagas disease	Early chronic/ indeterminate Chagas disease plus reactivations (immunocompromised)
T. cruzi sub-species	TcI + TcII	TcI + TcII
Distribution	All areas	All areas
Target population	Immunocompetent	Immunocompetent and immunocompromised
Adult/children	Adult	All
Clinical efficacy	Superiority over benznidazole in all endemic regions (parasitological)	70% (parasitological and serological)
Resistance	Active against nitrofuran- and nitroimidazole-resistant *T. cruzi* strains	Active against nitrofuran- and nitroimidazole-resistant *T. cruzi* strains
Safety	Superiority to benznidazole 3 clinical evaluations + 2 standard laboratory evaluations during treatment	Superiority to benznidazole No monitoring needed during treatment
Contraindications	Pregnancy, lactation	None
Precautions	No genotoxicity, no prolongation of QTc interval	No genotoxicity, no teratogenicity, no negative inotropic effects, no prolongation of QTc interval
Interactions	No clinically significant interactions with antihypertensive, anti-arrhythmic, or anticoagulant drugs	None
Presentation	Oral	Oral
Stability	3 years, climatic zone IV	5 years, climatic zone IV
Dosing regimen	Comparable to systemic antifungal treatments	Two times a day for 60 days

when they can be easily screened and supervised. Since it would be important to treat relatively young people before they have disease manifestations, this would include females of reproductive age. A drug targeting this group is particularly desirable because of the importance of preventing vertical transmission of Chagas disease. Consequently, a new drug that was unsafe in pregnancy or lactation would complicate utilization of the drug in resource-limited settings and would be a serious drawback.

Due to the frequent abnormalities in the cardiac conduction system in Chagas disease patients, it makes sense to avoid drugs that could exacerbate arrhythmias by prolonging the QT_C interval. Furthermore, finding a drug with low risk for drug–drug interactions is highly desirable because of the potential for patients to be on other medications that are used to manage heart rhythm, blood pressure, or risk of thromboembolic disease. The simplest approach to reducing the risks of drug-drug interactions translates to finding compounds with minimal effects on hepatic CYP450 enzymes.

Based on clinical experience with nitroaromatic compounds and experimental research with numerous classes of compounds, it is probable that any new drug will require a lengthy course (>30 days) of therapy to give rise to parasitological cures. (*Note*: recommended treatment courses for adults are benznidazole twice a day for 60 days or nifurtimox three times a day for 90 days; Bern et al., 2007.) As a consequence, it is essential that the drug be administered orally (not parenterally) so that it will be practical in resource-limited settings. It is unrealistic to try to administer a parenteral drug over a time scale of weeks due to costs, inconvenience, and safety. In order to ensure reasonable compliance, the drug should be orally administered no more than twice a day and be well tolerated by the vast majority of individuals. Treatment monitoring (particularly blood testing) should be unnecessary to keep costs down. Since treatment will commonly be targeted to asymptomatic individuals (indeterminate phase), a drug is needed with minimal side effects to maximize patient compliance.

How does one organize a drug discovery program for Chagas disease that enables the research team to identify compounds that fit the TPP described above? The rest of this chapter focuses on this question, with a subsection at the end briefly summarizing recent advancements in compound classes in development for treating Chagas disease.

5.2. COMPOUND SELECTION

Two basic approaches are employed in early drug discovery for antimicrobial chemotherapy. The first is whole-cell screening in which compounds or semi-purified natural products are tested for phenotypic effects on the pathogen grown in culture. Typically, the quantified endpoint is growth inhibition which is usually reported as an IC_{50} or MIC. The second approach is target-based screening in which a biochemical target from the pathogen is screened for compounds or natural products that bind to it (and usually inhibit its function). Both approaches have their advocates and detractors. Historically, most antibiotic drug discovery has been accomplished by whole-cell (or even animal model) screening followed by traditional medicinal chemistry approaches for hit to lead optimization. In these cases, the biochemical target of the drug candidates was usually not understood during the drug development process. With the advent of molecular biology and modern instrumentation, the pendulum swung towards target-based drug discovery. This approach has the potential to exploit the power of structure-based drug design when protein–ligand structures are available. Clearly target-based drug discovery has its success stories in infectious diseases such as with the development of HIV protease inhibitors (Wlodawer, 2002) and with influenza neuraminidase inhibitors (Liu et al., 2007). However, the failures of target-based drug design for infectious diseases have been well documented (Payne et al., 2007). As a result, the pendulum seems to have swung back towards whole-cell screening as evidenced by recent high-throughput screening campaigns against bacterial pathogens (Ananthan et al., 2009; Cheng et al., 2010) and several pathogenic protozoa (Bettiol et al., 2009; Guiguemde et al., 2010; Mackey et al., 2006; Sharlow et al., 2009). A high-throughput screen against *T. cruzi* amastigotes of more than 300,000 compounds was recently performed at the Broad Institute with results available online at PubChem (http://www.ncbi.nlm.nih.gov/pcassay?term=1885).

In the case of target-based drug discovery, it is likely that focused small-molecule libraries or even selected individual compounds are more likely to give screening hits than diverse chemical libraries. For example, compound libraries can be purchased that are enriched for protein kinase inhibitors (EMD4Biosciences, http://www.emdchemicals.com/life-science-research/products/EMD_BIO-539744/p_uuid), and such libraries have been effectively used to discover hits for antiparasitic drug discovery (Corey et al., 1996; Ojo et al., 2008). The approach of "piggy-back" drug development takes advantage of individual compounds that are well advanced in drug development for another indication. For example, protein farnesyltransferase (PFT) inhibitors that were under development for cancer chemotherapy were observed to have potent inhibitory activity on PFT enzymes from Plasmodium and Trypanosomes (Gelb et al., 2000). Since some of the compounds (e.g. tipifarnib) were already in clinical trials, the research had an advantage of starting with well-characterized compounds already endowed with drug-like properties (Gelb et al., 2003).

Whether compounds are selected individually, as focused libraries, or in diverse libraries, it is important that they can be developed within the parameters of the TPP. Since an orally delivered drug is required, the compounds should generally conform to Lipinski's "rule of five" (Table 5.2). These are chemical properties that are associated with orally administered drugs (Lipinski et al., 2001). Molecules that are substrates for biological transporters, as seen with many natural product drugs, are exceptions to the rule. Additional guidelines have been described that are associated with oral bioavailability, in particular, Veber rules (Veber et al., 2002; Table 5.2). Aqueous solubility which is directly related to the Log P (included in Lipinski rules) is an important consideration as highly insoluble molecules are difficult to use for *in vitro* biological assays and are often poorly (or erratically) absorbed by the GI tract.

Additional structural features help predict the likelihood of toxicity and chemical reactivity (Table 5.2). Some chemical features specifically associated with toxicity include alkylating agents (Lawley, 1980), anilines (Bomhard and Herbold, 2005), epoxides (Wade et al., 1978),

TABLE 5.2 Guidelines for profiling compounds from structures

	Structural features to use caution with or avoid	
Predictors of oral bioavailability	>5 H-bond donors (expressed as the sum of all OHs and NHs) MW > 500 Log P > 5 >10 H-bond acceptors (expressed as the sum of all Ns and Os)	Lipinksi Rules of 5
	>10 rotatable bonds >140 Å polar surface area or >12 total hydrogen bonds (acceptors plus donors)	Veber Rules
Structural alerts for toxicity or metabolic activitation	Alkylating agents, anilines, epoxides, alkyl halides, nitroaromatics, DNA intercalators, and more	
Chemical tractability	Structures for which analogs cannot be easily made	
Factors affecting cost of goods	Expensive starting materials Costly catalysts >1 chiral centre	

nitroaromatics (Boelsterli et al., 2006), DNA intercalators (Ferguson and Denny, 2007), and others (Baell and Holloway, 2010; Brun et al., 1996; Williams and Naisbitt, 2002). Although there are examples of drugs in clinical use that contain these features, for example, nifurtimox and benznidazole are nitroaromatics (Santos et al., 1994), it is advisable to avoid these types of molecules as they increase the risk of failure during the drug development process. Sometimes the biological activity of a hit may not be dependent on the toxic side group; thus, if the molecule is otherwise desirable, it may be worth synthesizing the analogue without the toxic side group to see if the scaffold retains activity.

Chemical tractability needs to be in the forefront when considering hit compounds for further investigation. Chemical scaffolds that allow for the easy synthesis of analogues enable the chemistry team to quickly study structure–activity relationships and more readily optimize compounds. In addition, drugs for the developing world need to be inexpensive, so early attention to cost of goods is imperative. This requires that chemistry schemes use inexpensive starting materials requiring relatively few steps and inexpensive catalysts. Furthermore, chiral compounds present the risk of significantly increasing the cost of goods as chiral synthesis or chiral separation can dramatically complicate the production of the molecules.

5.3. *IN VITRO* EFFICACY TESTING

The following discussion will focus on whole-cell screening against *T. cruzi*. For information on target-based screening methods, such as high-throughput enzyme assays, the reader is referred to other sources (Seethala and Fernandes, 2001) including the NIH website at http://www.ncgc.nih.gov/guidance/section4.html. For general safety guidelines to work with live *T. cruzi* cultures, the reader is directed to the following resources (Hudson, 1983; US Department of Health and Human Services, 2009).

5.3.1. *Trypanosoma cruzi* growth inhibition assays

The natural life cycle of *T. cruzi* involves the parasite inhabiting the gut of triatomine insects and surviving within the blood and tissues of diverse mammalian hosts. Epimastigotes (the form that replicates in the invertebrate host) can be easily grown *in vitro* as freely dividing (axenic) cultures usually using liver infusion tryptone (LIT) medium that includes hemin and serum (Miles, 1993). Depending on the *T. cruzi* strain, epimastigotes have replication doubling times of 22.5–58.4 h when growing in mid-log phase (Engel et al., 1985). The strain used for the *T. cruzi* genome project,

CL Brener, has a doubling time of 58 ± 13 h as epimastigotes (Zingales et al., 1997). Cultures can achieve densities up to ~3–4 × 10^7 mL^{-1} (Lauria-Pires et al., 1997), which is useful for biochemical studies requiring large quantities of cellular material. Growth inhibition assays using epimastigotes are widely reported in the *T. cruzi* literature; however, substantial biochemical differences between the insect-stages and mammalian stages raise concerns that the results from epimastigote assays may not accurately predict activity against mammalian stages. Significant differences in IC_{50} values for certain compounds between epimastigotes and mammalian stages of *T. cruzi* are documented (Neal and Van Bueren, 1988), raising further concerns about depending on epimastigotes for drug screening.

T. cruzi has the capacity to infect and replicate in a wide range of host cells including cardiac muscle cells, smooth muscle cells, skeletal muscle cells, fibroblasts, neurons, adipocytes, macrophages, dendritic cells, epithelial cells, endothelial cells, and others (Alves and Mortara, 2009; Buckner et al., 1999; Combs et al., 2005; Mukherjee et al., 2004). Based on *in vitro* studies, infectious trypomastigotes attach to and invade mammalian host cells through an active process that takes ~5–10 min (Rodriguez et al., 1996). After entering the host cell, parasites are found in an acidic membrane-bound compartment referred to as the parasitophorous vacuole (Burleigh and Andrews, 1998). Within 1–2 h (for tissue culture derived trypomastigotes; Alves and Mortara, 2009), the parasites escape the parasitophorous vacuole to reside in the host cell cytoplasm where they differentiate to replicative amastigotes. The lag period from host cell penetration to reproduction as amastigotes is ~18–34 h depending on the strain (Dvorak and Poore, 1974; Engel et al., 1985). Doubling times of amastigotes in host cells range from 9 to 22 h (Engel et al., 1985). After 6–9 rounds of replication (Engel et al., 1985), amastigotes transform to trypomastigotes and rupture the host cell. The total duration of the intracellular cycle usually ranges from 96 to 215 h (i.e. 4–9 days; Engel et al., 1985). The complexity and timing of the mammalian stage life cycle is clearly important when considering the duration of exposure to chemical inhibitors while conducting drug screening experiments.

The most widely used *in vitro* methods for testing compounds for anti-*T. cruzi* activity depend on quantifying parasite growth in co-culture with mammalian host cells. Less frequently, direct observation of free (non-replicative) trypomastigotes is used to evaluate anti-*T. cruzi* effects of compounds (Yardley and Croft, 1999). In intracellular growth assays, there are several variables to take into account, the first being the duration of the assay. Most reported assay methods quantify the growth of *T. cruzi* after they have been co-cultured with mammalian cells for 4–8 days (Bettiol et al., 2009; Buckner et al., 1996; Neal and Van Bueren, 1988; Urbina et al., 1993). This amount of time allows most strains to complete one intracellular life cycle (trypomastigotes → amastigotes amplification → trypomastigotes) with the number of *T. cruzi* increasing by a factor >100 (assuming 7–9 rounds of replication). This degree of parasite amplification provides excellent signal-to-noise discrimination when compounds are tested for growth inhibition. Typically, *T. cruzi* are allowed to pre-incubate with host cells before test compounds are added to the medium to ensure that compounds are acting on intracellular parasites. However, this method misses compounds that specifically interfere with the invasion process, particularly if the assay is run for a short enough period of time that the parasites do not enter a second round of invasion and replication. Experiments to specifically assay inhibition of invasion obviously have to be designed differently.

The next variable to consider for *in vitro T. cruzi* drug assays is the type of host cells to be used. Many different mammalian cell types for co-culture with *T. cruzi* have been described (Table 5.3). It is generally preferable to use adherent cells with large cytoplasmic volumes (to accommodate intracytoplasmic replication of amastigotes) and for the host cells to divide relatively slowly so that they do not deplete the nutrients in the medium in the time frame of a typical 4–8-day experiment. Amongst the cell types that foster robust intracellular growth of *T. cruzi*, it is possible that some cell lines have different permeability

TABLE 5.3 Host cells used for culturing mammalian stages of *T. cruzi*

Cell name	Host/tissue	References
Vero	African green monkey kidney epithelial cells	Bertelli and Brener (1980)
HeLa	Human epithelial cervical cancer cells	Andrews and Colli (1982)
L929	Mouse fibroblast cells	McCabe et al. (1984b)
L6	Rat skeletal muscle cells	von Kreuter et al. (1988)
3T3	Mouse fibroblast cells	Andrews and Colli (1982), Buckner et al. (1996)
LLC-MK2	Rhesus monkey kidney epithelial cells	Andrews and Colli (1982)
Bovine embryonic skeletal muscle cells	Cow skeletal muscle cells	Bertelli and Brener (1980)
Murine peritoneal macrophages	Mouse peritoneal macrophages	McCabe et al. (1984b), Yardley and Croft (1999)

characteristics for chemical compounds, particularly if they express different levels of Pgp efflux pumps or other membrane transporters. Different susceptibility of the same *T. cruzi* strain grown in different host cells has been observed (Grosso et al., 2010), making this more than a theoretical consideration. Another factor relating to the host cell is whether or not it may interfere with the assay readout. For example, mammalian macrophages express relatively high amounts of β-galactosidase which can interfere with assays utilizing *β-galactosidase* transfected parasites (Buckner and Wilson, 2005).

T. cruzi strain selection is another important variable for compound screening. Numerous strains have been collected from invertebrate and vertebrate hosts that demonstrate substantial phenotypic and genetic diversity (Devera et al., 2003). Tissue tropism among strains varies as exemplified by some showing myotropism, some showing macrophage tropism, and some showing tropism for other tissues (nervous, reproductive systems, and others) (Devera et al., 2003). Drug susceptibility is another phenotypic feature with significant variability amongst different *T. cruzi* strains (Brener and Chiari, 1967; Brener et al., 1976; Neal and Van Bueren, 1988). This variability has repeatedly been observed with the nitroaromatic drugs (benznidazole and nifurtimox); strains such as the Colombian are resistant (Camandaroba et al., 2003). Selection of specific strains is complicated by observations that strain phenotypes can change dramatically during laboratory propagation. Virulence attenuation has been described with long-term maintenance of *T. cruzi* in tissue culture (Chiari, 1974; Contreras et al., 1994) and in laboratory animals (Brener et al., 1974; Veloso et al., 1996). Moreover, long-term *in vitro* culturing has been associated with changes in isoenzyme patterns and RFLP of the kDNA profiles (Devera et al., 2003). Remarkably, separate clones from the same parental stock have been observed to exhibit dramatically different growth phenotypes *in vitro* (Lauria-Pires et al., 1997). As a result, it is profoundly challenging to establish a panel of laboratory strains that accurately represent circulating strains responsible for disease. Nonetheless, it seems logical to focus on strains isolated from human cases (or vectors associated with human disease transmission), strains from different geographic regions, and strains representing different tissue tropisms and drug sensitivities. In principle, it makes sense to include strains from all six discrete typing units (*T. cruzi* I–VI) (Zingales et al., 2009), although the emphasis should obviously be on strains responsible for the largest burden of human cases. Due to the labour and costs of testing compounds, some laboratories use a single strain for screening then follow up the results by testing a more diverse set of strains to ensure that the hits are reproducible across various strains (Buckner et al., 2001). Because of the efficiency of using a strain with a reporter gene (discussed below), the *β-galactosidase*-expressing Tulahuen strain has been recommended as a strain for initial screening (Romanha et al., 2010). It seems wise to include strains such as Y and Colombian in the testing algorithm (Neal and Van Bueren, 1988; Romanha et al., 2010) as these strains have partial or complete resistance to drugs in clinical use (Filardi and Brener, 1987). Panels of well-characterized laboratory strains representing diverse genotypes and phenotypes have been reported (Engel et al., 1985; Filardi and Brener, 1987; Moreno et al., 2010; Neal and Van Bueren, 1988).

The final variable for testing compounds on *T. cruzi* is the readout. Typically, the readout is a measurement of growth inhibition or killing activity of the test compounds. The traditional low-throughput methods involve parasite quantification using microscopy. This typically involves culturing the parasites and host cells on glass slides, staining the samples, and scoring the numbers of parasites using light (Harth et al., 1993; Yardley and Croft, 1999). The methods are labour intensive, tedious, and potentially subject to bias when the microscopists are un-blinded.

Image-based high-throughput screening (sometimes known as high-content screening) has recently been described for intracellular *T. cruzi* (Engel et al., 2010; Nohara et al., 2010). Infected mammalian cells are stained with DAPI and software connected to fluorescent microscopy is able to quantify the number of amastigotes per cell (Engel et al., 2010). The method eliminates the human observer, thus improving efficiency and presumably accuracy. A benefit of the method is that no genetic manipulation of the parasites is required for expression of reporter genes; hence, potentially more strains can be included in the assays. One could imagine the method being used for performing drug susceptibility assessments on clinical isolates. The disadvantage of this method is that the technology is expensive and not available to most laboratories.

Methods involving reporter genes in genetically transfected *T. cruzi* were developed in response to the difficulties with low-throughput microscopy methods. The first reporter-gene system developed for drug screening utilized the *E. coli β-galactosidase* gene (Buckner et al., 1996). The *LacZ* gene was targeted to a portion of the calmodulin–ubiquitin locus in the genome that had no apparent effect on *T. cruzi* growth or behaviour. By having the reporter gene chromosomally integrated, the expression level is stable and not dependent on ongoing drug pressure for the selection marker that would be required to maintain an episomal vector. The reporter-gene expression is maintained by *T. cruzi* during infection in mice, even for as long as 10 months post-infection (Buckner et al., 1999). Expression of the β-galactosidase is evident in amastigotes, trypomastigotes, and epimastigotes (Buckner et al., 1996). Several strains of *T. cruzi* have been transfected including Tulahuen, CL, Peru, Sonja, and VL2067, and are available at the American Type Culture Collection (ATCC) (Buckner et al., 1996, 2001). This reporter-gene method has been particularly useful for growth inhibition assays of mammalian stages of *T. cruzi* cultured with host cells, since the quantification of parasite growth by metabolic labelling is complicated by the activity of the host cells. Growth of the parasites at the end of the assay is measured by adding a β-galactosidase substrate and quantifying the signal using an absorbance or fluorescence/luminescence plate reader. Chlorophenolred-β-D-galactopyranoside (CPRG) gives a colorimetric change from yellow to red that can be quantified at OD_{570} with a signal that is proportional to the number of parasites present in the well. The parasites need to be grown in medium without the phenol red colour indicator so as to avoid interference with the CPRG readout. The assay is amenable to 96-well plate conditions and has been shown to give excellent reproducibility with Z'-factor of 0.834 ($\pm$0.018) for independent experiments performed in sextuplicate on three different days (Bettiol et al., 2009). It has also been adapted to a 384-well plate format with the use of a chemiluminescence substrate (Galscreen™, Applied Biosystems). The latter method was recently used by the Broad Institute to screen a library of 303,221 compounds in the first truly high-throughput screen on *T. cruzi* that has been reported (http://pubchem.ncbi.nlm.nih.gov/assay/assay.cgi?aid=1885&loc=ea_ras).

Other reporter genes have been introduced into *T. cruzi*, including luciferase (Weston et al., 1999) and fluorescent proteins (Guevara et al., 2005), although their application for drug screening has not been widely used. However, a recent study describes the use of luciferase for the purpose of *T. cruzi* amastigote drug screening (Bot et al., 2010). Similarly, the use of fluorescent td Tomato protein for quantification of epimastigote or intracellular amastigote growth *in vitro* was recently reported (Canavaci et al., 2010). In the latter case, the readout did not involve lysis of the cells; hence, real-time monitoring of growth could be performed over the 4-day period of the assay. This has the potential to provide additional information relating to the speed at which compounds exert their antiproliferative effects on *T. cruzi* and could be useful for identifying compounds with more rapid trypanocidal or trypanostatic effects.

5.3.2. Testing for trypanocidal versus trypanostatic activity

Definitions for "trypanocidal" and "trypanostatic" have not been established in the *T. cruzi* literature, although the terms are frequently used (Bot et al., 2010; Chen et al., 2010; Ferreira et al., 2010; Molina et al., 2000). In general, compounds are considered "trypanocidal" when they lead to irreversible cell growth arrest *in vitro*. This is usually determined by "washout" experiments in which parasite cultures are exposed for a period of time to a test compound and then observed for another interval after the compound has been removed. For example, one group cultures *T. cruzi* in macrophages then observes them for 40 days to elucidate if the inhibitors clear infection from the host cells or just delay the outgrowth of parasites (Chen et al., 2010). A number of variables will affect whether or not an inhibitor is judged to be trypanocidal including the concentration of the compound used, the duration of the exposure to the compound, the number of parasites used in the starting culture, and the time of observation after the inhibitor is removed. Note that even a compound with rapid killing activity will appear to be trypanostatic if the concentration used or exposure time is insufficient. Since the field has not established definitions for the terms "trypanocidal" or "trypanostatic" (which will ultimately be arbitrary), it behooves investigators to provide the appropriate details of the experimental conditions as well as comparison drugs, such that the relative "cidal" or "static" nature of the study compounds can be compared. Since compounds have different EC_{50} values, it seems logical to characterize the "trypanocidal" concentration of the drug in reference to its EC_{50} as determined at a set time point (e.g. 4–6 days). For example, "*T. cruzi* exposed to drug X at eight times its EC_{50} for 5 days did not recover over a 14-day observation period". Additional research and consensus building need to take place in order to establish definitions for these terms so that they can be used consistently and meaningfully.

5.3.3. Testing compounds in combinations

Combination chemotherapy has become conventional and necessary for many infectious diseases including viral infections (e.g. HIV), bacterial infections (e.g. tuberculosis), and parasitic diseases (e.g. malaria). It seems likely that combination chemotherapy may play a role in future treatment regimens for Chagas disease (Buckner and Navabi, 2010; Coura, 2009; Ribeiro et al., 2009). Combination therapy offers several potential benefits over monotherapy. First, it may provide greater efficacy through the additive or synergistic activity of drug combinations on the microbial pathogen. Second, by providing greater antimicrobial activity, the duration of treatment may be reduced. This is particularly important because of the experience with existing drugs for Chagas disease that very lengthy treatment courses are necessary for efficacy. Third, the doses of drugs used in combination may be reduced from the doses used in monotherapy, potentially reducing side effects. Fourth, combination chemotherapy mitigates the induction or breakthrough of resistant organisms. As a result, *in vitro* methods to test compounds in combinations against *T. cruzi* are discussed below.

Compound interaction studies are typically performed as checkerboard assays (Canfield et al., 1995) or by using the "fixed ratio" method (Ohrt et al., 2002). Either method gives fractional inhibitory concentrations (FICs) that are calculated for each drug based on the equation shown below in which $IC_{50}A_{(B)}$ is the 50% inhibitory concentration of drug A in the presence of drug B:

$$\text{FIC Drug A} = \frac{IC_{50}A_{(B)}}{IC_{50}A}$$

The data are used to plot isobolograms based on calculations of the sum of FICs (Berenbaum, 1978). In the malaria field, definitions for antagonism and synergism have been defined as $\sum$ FICs > 2.0 and <5.0, respectively (Fidock et al., 2004; Gupta et al., 2002). Compound interaction studies, primarily involving the checkerboard method, have been reported for *T. cruzi* epimastigotes (Benaim et al., 2006; Santa-Rita et al., 2005; Urbina et al., 1993) and amastigotes (Benaim et al., 2006; Buckner et al., 2001). For example, it was shown that amiodarone and posaconazole interact synergistically in culture (Benaim et al., 2006). Alone, amiodarone is not extremely potent, but it appears to potentiate the effects of posaconazole, presumably through its common mechanism of inhibiting sterol biosynthesis. Since successful chemotherapy may ultimately depend on using combinations of drugs, it is imperative that synergy testing becomes widely used in drug discovery programs for Chagas disease.

5.4. TOXICITY TESTING

The preclinical evaluation of compounds for Chagas disease requires particular attention to toxicity testing due to the importance of safety and tolerability as discussed earlier in Section 5.1. Cytotoxicity testing involves assessing the effects of compounds on mammalian cells and is often done in parallel with assays measuring the activity on *T. cruzi* cultures. Cytoxicity testing is required when *T. cruzi* inhibition assays are done with amastigotes grown in mammalian cells, as it is necessary to establish that the inhibitory effects of test compounds are due to specific antiparasitic activity and not merely due to toxicity to the host cell on which the parasites depend (Buckner et al., 1996). Usually cytotoxicity testing is done against the same mammalian cells used in the intracellular *T. cruzi* assay such as those listed in Table 5.3. In addition, it is common to assess cytotoxicity against a panel of cell lines representing a broad variety of tissue types. An example of a panel of six cell lines of different tissue origins is shown in Table 5.4. By including a variety of cell types, compounds that may have tissue specific cytotoxicity are more likely to be flagged.

Cytotoxicity is assessed by growth inhibition of the mammalian cells which can be quantified in a variety of ways. Methods that are amenable to microtiter plates and that do not require radiolabelled or expensive

TABLE 5.4 Example of panel of mammalian cells for cytotoxicity testing

Cell line	Tissue type	Origin	Growth type	References
CRL-8155	Lymphoblast	Spleen	Suspension	Levy et al. (1968)
HL-60	Promyeloblast	Acute promyelocytic leukaemia	Suspension	Collins (1987)
HT-1080	Connective tissue	Fibrosarcoma	Adherent	Rasheed et al. (1974)
HCC-2998	Adenocarcinoma	Colon carcinoma	Adherent	Shoemaker (2006)
SF-539	Neural cell	Gliosarcoma	Adherent	Maletinska et al. (2000)
Hep G2	Liver	Hepatocellular carcinoma	Suspension	Miret et al. (2006)

substrates are desirable. The resazurin (e.g. Alamar Blue™ or Upti-Blue™) method is frequently used since it is simple, safe, and relatively inexpensive (Anoopkumar-Dukie et al., 2005). Resazurin is a REDOX indicator that both fluoresces and changes colour in response to chemical reduction of growth medium resulting from cell growth. Another popular method for measuring cytotoxicity is testing for adenosine triphosphate (ATP) which will be depleted if the cells become nonviable (Miret et al., 2006). The ATP method is amenable to luminescence readouts when using the firefly luciferase enzyme and luciferin as substrates. The ratio of the IC_{50} of the test compound against mammalian cells versus the IC_{50} against *T. cruzi* is calculated to give a selectivity index. There is no hard and fast rule, but a selectivity index >10 is a commonly used cut-off to triage compounds.

A detailed discussion of toxicity testing in animal models is beyond the scope of this chapter. Any compounds intended for clinical studies require formal toxicity testing under Good Laboratory Practice conditions using rodent and large animal models to receive regulatory approval. However, the *in vivo* efficacy testing discussed in Section 5.5 provides the opportunity to assess for toxicity while administering the test compounds. It has been recommended that the investigators first establish the maximum tolerated dose (MTD) of compounds in mice to guide the dosing regimen for the efficacy experiments (Romanha et al., 2010). However, this may not always be realistic as MTD studies imply determining the dose that does not cause overt toxicity in a 90-day experiment in laboratory mice or rats (Rodricks et al., 1991). An alternative for getting a snapshot of toxicity is to include an extra arm in efficacy studies in which an uninfected group of mice receives the highest dose of the test compound. These mice can be weighed daily, observed for physical signs of toxicity, and undergo blood testing (haematology and chemistries). By including this extra group, toxicity of the compounds on the mice can be assessed independently of the effects of the *T. cruzi* infection.

5.5. *IN VIVO* EFFICACY TESTING

Mice are readily infected with *T. cruzi* and provide an excellent model for testing the effects of drug candidates in a mammalian host. Unfortunately, there is little uniformity amongst the numerous literature reports on the specific methods used. The variables include:

- Mouse strain, age, sex
- *T. cruzi* strain, life cycle stage
- Inoculum size, route of delivery
- Incubation period before drug treatment
- Treatment: vehicle, dose, route of administration, duration
- Outcome measures: parasitaemia, tests of cure, organ pathology

The use of different combinations of these variables has led to numerous mouse models that produce different outcomes. In models of "acute infection" (Romanha et al., 2010), mouse and parasite strains are matched to give high levels of parasitaemia typically associated with death of the animals within 2–4 weeks of the infection. A well-characterized example is the use of the CL Brener strain in Balb/c mice which leads to 100% mortality by day 16 post-infection (Zingales et al., 1997). Models of acute infection have been widely used for decades to test for activity of drug candidates, including the early studies on benznidazole (Grunberg et al., 1967). Since *T. cruzi* infection in humans is infrequently fatal in the acute stage, the models that result in rapidly fatal outcomes do not accurately reflect the natural course of infection observed in most humans. Chronic infection in mice can be established using small numbers of parasites to infect mice (Molina et al., 2000) or by treating mice with sub-curative doses of drugs during the acute phase (Bustamante et al., 2008). Mice with chronic infection can survive 1–2 years and manifest a variety of tissue pathologies depending on the mouse and parasite strains that are used (Araujo et al., 2000; Buckner et al., 1999; Marinho et al., 2009; Molina et al., 2000). For drug testing, the chronic models require at least 4 months to get the mice ready for the experiment, then often involve treatment courses lasting weeks, making the models expensive and time consuming. Determining the endpoints in the chronic models, such as parasitological cures, can be challenging as will be discussed more below. Some additional models have been developed that give rise to organ damage that more closely approximates Chagas disease in humans. For example, a low virulence model of Chagas disease uses the Sylvio X10/4 *T. cruzi* strain in C3H/He mice (Marinho et al., 2009). This model has been primarily used for studies on immunopathogenesis because it induces chronic cardiac lesions incorporating several pathological features of human disease and does not cause patent acute disease.

Although it makes sense to find a model that most closely resembles the disease as it occurs in humans, there is not enough data to tell us which model best predicts outcomes of drug treatment in humans. The chronic model has a serious drawback in that it takes over 6 months to complete a single experiment, thus providing feedback on new experimental compounds too slowly. The acute model has the advantage of providing results relatively quickly. In the typical acute models, treatment of mice with test compounds is initiated within 1 day of the infection (Maldonado et al., 1993; McCabe et al., 1984a). This approach probably leads to results that exaggerate the activity of the test compounds since the parasites have not had an opportunity to establish themselves in the host, a situation that infrequently occurs in the clinic except in cases where post-exposure prophylaxis is needed. If the infection and the inhibitor treatment occur by the same route (e.g. intraperitoneal), then the parasites may be exposed to very high levels of the compound in a way that does not reflect a realistic situation. The compromise model is the "established" model of *T. cruzi* infection in which the mice are infected for a period of 5–7 days before the test compound is administered (Araujo et al., 2000; Suryadevara et al., 2009). Since this allows sufficient time for dissemination of the parasite to multiple organ sites, the test compound needs to be active throughout the body to affect the levels of parasitism.

The measured outcome of treatment is a particularly important parameter to consider. Microscopic quantification of parasitaemia (usually with a haemacytometer) gives a measure of parasite suppression, but is insufficient to demonstrate parasitological cure as parasites can circulate at low levels in the blood or remain present in tissues (Canavaci et al., 2010). Methods such as xenodiagnosis, blood culture, or polymerase chain reaction (PCR) on blood or tissue are more sensitive, but negativity is not firmly associated with parasitological cures (Canavaci et al., 2010). Seroconversion is another treatment outcome that has been frequently used, but conversion to negative may not occur even when parasitological measurements appear negative (Andrade et al., 1985). The most sensitive measure of cure is probably obtained by subjecting mice to immunosuppressive therapy after the mice have completed the drug treatment. With immunosuppressive therapy, such as cyclophosphamide, mice develop rebound parasitaemia that can be readily detected microscopically (Pereira et al., 1996), by PCR (Bustamante et al., 2008; Dos Santos et al., 2008), or blood culture (Dos Santos et al., 2008). The idea is that with the removal of immune control, any residual parasites have the opportunity to proliferate and become detectable by commonly used methods. With the paradigm that parasitological cures are the goal (Urbina, 1999), it is recommended that outcome measurements be employed that have the ability to convincingly demonstrate that the experimental animals have been cured.

For initial screening of candidate compounds for the purpose of prioritization, a streamlined *in vivo* protocol has been recommended (Romanha et al., 2010). Briefly, Swiss mice are infected with Y strain *T. cruzi*, the infection is established for 5 days, then treatment is given at three different doses for 5 consecutive days. Microscopic parasitaemia is monitored at 5, 8, and 10 days post-infection and survival is monitored out to 30 days. Results from each compound are compared to control groups receiving vehicle or benznidazole. Compounds that pass the initial screening experiments can then be subjected to more rigorous *in vivo* investigations that assess for parasitological cures. This second level test again involves Swiss mice with "established" infection with the *T. cruzi* Y strain. The mice are treated with the test compounds for 20 consecutive days. After another 10 days, the animals without visible parasitaemia are subjected to immunosuppression with three cycles of cyclophosphamide and monitored for parasitaemia until 5 days after completion of the cyclophosphamide treatment (Dos Santos et al., 2008; Romanha et al., 2010). A third level of *in vivo* testing was further recommended to test for activity of the drug candidate against the benznidazole resistant Columbian strain (Romanha et al., 2010).

Recently, new methods have been reported using the IVIS luminescence system for monitoring *T. cruzi* infection in mice (Canavaci et al., 2010). Mice were infected in the footpads with luciferase expressing *T. cruzi* then visualized under anaesthesia at time intervals for a fluorescent signal after injection with luciferin. Mice receiving effective antiparasitic treatments lose the fluorescent signal and those with ineffective treatment retain the signal. It appears necessary to monitor the infection in the footpad, so it is not currently possible to determine if the disseminated infection has been cleared. In addition, the method may not be sensitive enough to discriminate between parasite suppression and complete clearance in the footpads. Nonetheless, this is a powerful new tool for rapid throughput *in vivo* compound screening.

5.6. TESTING FOR DRUG-LIKE PROPERTIES AND SAFETY

Beyond demonstrating antiparasitic activity of test compounds *in vitro*, it is necessary to establish that the compounds avoid liabilities that would make them unsuitable as candidates for drug development. A brief discussion of methods to experimentally characterize compounds follows, however, the reader is directed elsewhere for more comprehensive reviews on this subject (Kerns and Di 2008).

The physical–chemical properties, particularly the solubility and lipophilicity, should be assessed early. Compounds that lack aqueous solubility are problematic for *in vitro* studies and generally have low oral bioavailability. It is common to test solubility in aqueous solutions at various pHs that reflect the blood (pH 7.4), stomach (pH 1.5), and small intestines (pH 6.5). Kinetic solubility methods involve first dissolving the compound in organic solvent (e.g. DMSO) and then diluting it serially in aqueous buffers and assessing for precipitation using light scattering (nephelometric method) (Bevan and Lloyd, 2000). The following solubility classification ranges have been suggested for medicinal chemists (Kerns and Di 2008):

- <10 μg/mL low solubility
- 10–60 μg/mL moderate solubility
- >60 μg/mL high solubility

Lipophilicity is a property that is critical to the pharmacological activity of compounds due to effects on absorption, distribution, metabolism, excretion, and toxicity (ADMET). Liphophilicity is the tendency of a compound to partition into nonpolar lipid matrix (i.e. octanol) as opposed to aqueous matrix. When the aqueous buffer is set at a pH where all the compound molecules are in neutral form, the partitioning value is termed Log P. Computer algorithms are widely available to calculate this value (cLog P). Alternatively, partitioning can be experimentally measured at a specified pH at which a portion of the compound molecules may be in the ionic form, and this is termed Log D. Higher Log P and Log D values indicate greater lipophilicity (i.e. poor aqueous solubility). Compounds with exceedingly high Log P values are insoluble and frequently have poor oral absorption. As indicated by Lipinski Rules (Table 5.2), a Log P > 5 is associated with low oral bioavailability. Compounds with very low Log P values are unable to pass through lipid bilayers, and thus also have low oral bioavailability. Optimal Log P values for oral drugs are between 0 and 3 (Kerns and Di, 2008).

The ability of compounds to permeate through biological membranes is central to their ADMET properties. Methods for measuring permeability typically involve a set up in which compound is added to one side of a membrane or cell monolayer, then samples are collected from the other side and quantified for concentration of the compound. The PAMPA (parallel artificial membrane permeability assay) utilizes an artificial membrane and is widely used in industry (Kansy et al., 1998). Caco-2 or MDCK cell are widely used in trans-well assays to measure permeability through cell monolayers (Kerns and Di, 2008). A special line of cells, MDR1-MDCK, have been transfected a Pgp1 transporter, that allows for additional evaluation of the potential of compounds to be substrates for efflux pumps that can interfere with absorption (Tang et al., 2002). In general, it is necessary to perform liquid-chromatrography/mass-spectrometry to quantify compounds in the assay samples.

Another assessment that is frequently made early in drug discovery is metabolic stability of compounds. *In silico* methods to predict metabolic stability are not particularly accurate, however, *in vitro* methods are heavily relied upon in the pharmaceutical industry (Kerns and Di 2008). The simplest *in vitro* method utilizes liver microsomes that contain the CYP enzymes and flavin monooxygenases (Baranczewski et al., 2006; Masimirembwa et al., 2003). Compounds are incubated with liver microsomes and sampled at time intervals to quantify the rate of loss of the parent compound due to metabolic transformation. Microsomes from various species (mouse, rat, monkey, human) can be purchased commercially. Stability in plasma is another assessment that is frequently done in parallel (Di et al., 2005). Using these methods, groups of compounds can be rapidly tested and prioritized based on their potential for metabolic stability in mammalian hosts. Additional, but more costly, studies employ hepatocytes or S9 fractions that encompass a broader range of metabolizing enzymes found in the whole animal (Kerns and Di, 2008). Experiments on metabolic stability also make it possible to identify the predominate metabolites and hence understand the vulnerable regions of the molecules that can be modified in iterative rounds of optimization.

Protein binding is important property that can impact ADMET. High protein binding reduces the free fraction in solution that is available for penetration into the tissues/cells, thus reducing the concentration at the therapeutic target. On the other hand, highly protein bound compounds are less available to the liver and kidney for metabolism and elimination, thus increasing serum half-life. Protein binding can be measured by a variety of methods including the equilibrium dialysis method, ultrafiltration method, ultracentrifugation method, microdialysis method, and others (Kerns and Di, 2008).

Two other *in vitro* assessments that are particularly relevant for Chagas drug development are CYP inhibition assays and hERG studies. The former is important because cytochrome P450 inhibition is a major cause of drug–drug interactions. CYP enzymes of multiple isoforms along with appropriate substrates can be purchased commercially in kits that include control drugs (Rodrigues and Lin, 2001). Significant inhibitory activity on CYP enzymes is a potential liability if the compound enters clinical use. Similarly, it is important to consider the potential of a candidate drug to block cardiac K^+ (hERG) channels. This is a safety issue because compounds that block hERG channels can induce cardiac arrythmias, a problem to which *T. cruzi* infected patients are already predisposed. The "gold standard" for measuring hERG channel inhibition is the patch-clamp method (Kerns and Di, 2008; Wood et al., 2004). Additional methods that provide further detail utilize rabbit Purkinje fibres or rabbit left ventricular wedge preparations (Lu et al., 2006). Compounds with significant inhibitory activity on hERG channels should probably be avoided in Chagas drug discovery; thus an assessment for this potential liability should be performed relatively early on candidate compounds.

In vivo pharmacokinetic (PK) studies have the potential to be expensive particularly when involving cannulated rats or large animals. However, relatively simple PK studies can be performed that provide a tremendous amount of valuable data during the early evaluation of new compounds. For example, "snapshot" PK studies can be done in which groups of three mice are given a test compound (usually ~50 mg/kg) by oral route, and plasma samples are collected at time intervals (e.g. 0.5, 1, 2, 4, and 8 h) for LC–MS analysis (Kraus et al., 2009). If reasonable compound blood levels are detected at early time points, it can be assumed that the compound is absorbed and not subject to extensive first-pass metabolism. If the compound sustains reasonable levels over the ~8 hour course of the experiment, then it is likely that it is not overly vulnerable to hepatic metabolism or other forms of elimination. In addition, these studies provide an opportunity to look for acute toxicity that can draw early attention to potential liabilities. More formal PK studies usually require the use of rats (and later large animals) to make it possible to draw off adequate volumes and numbers of blood samples for the numerous time points. PK studies allow for quantification of plasma clearance (CL), area under the curve (AUC), maximum concentration (C_{max}), time to maximum concentration (T_{max}), plasma half-life ($T_{½}$), oral bioavailability (FA), volume of distribution (V_d), and other parameters. Although rat PK studies do not necessarily predict the PK behaviour in humans, they are necessary in the preclinical evaluation of compounds. The goal of the PK evaluation is to identify compounds that have good potential to fit the defined TPP of the drug (Table 5.1). For Chagas disease, this means an oral drug with once or twice a day administration schedule. Thus, the preclinical PK studies will be used to discover compounds with good oral bioavailability (i.e. FA >20%) (Nwaka et al., 2009) and a reasonably long terminal half-life (at least >6 h in the rat). In addition, the preclinical compounds should have a reasonably large volume of distribution to help ensure that they achieve the high tissue penetration that is necessary to treat the tissue parasites (Urbina, 2010). Further discussion of PKs (and pharmacodynamics) can be found in standard textbooks (Brunton et al., 2011; Gabrielsson and Weiner, 2007). Additional criteria used in lead optimization and candidate selection for neglected diseases can be found in Nwaka et al. (2009).

5.7. ADVANCES IN EXPERIMENTAL CHEMOTHERAPY FOR *TRYPANOSOMA CRUZI* INFECTION

Numerous compounds with anti-*T. cruzi* activity have been reported in the literature in the past decade. The most advanced compound is the cysteine protease inhibitor, K-777, which is expected to go into early clinical studies in the next year (McKerrow et al., 2009). The repurposing of the antifungal drug, posaconazole, may lead to a late-phase clinical trial for Chagas disease in the near future (Clayton, 2010). Similarly, another antifungal drug, E1224, is being positioned for a clinical trial coordinated by Drugs for Neglected Diseases Initiative (Clayton, 2010). A number of other drug classes are in preclinical development including new nitroaromatic compounds (Cabrera et al., 2009), diamidines (Soeiro et al., 2008), non-peptidic cruzain inhibitors (Brak et al., 2010), sterol 14α-demethylase inhibitors (Buckner, 2008; Doyle et al., 2010; Urbina, 2009), bisphosphonates (Garzoni et al., 2004), PFT inhibitors (Buckner et al., 2002), a variety of natural products (Buckner and Navabi, 2010), and others. Several recent review articles summarize the small-molecules and natural products in preclinical drug development for Chagas disease (Buckner and Navabi, 2010; Clayton, 2010; Coura, 2009; Dujardin et al., 2010;

McKerrow et al., 2009; Moreira et al., 2009; Ribeiro et al., 2009; Rivera et al., 2009; Soeiro et al., 2009; Urbina, 2009, 2010). Some promising compounds are in the pipeline, but many have liabilities of potential toxicity, low oral bioavailability, poor PKs, or high cost of goods. A recent high-throughput screen (Bettiol et al., 2009) of a large compound library against *T. cruzi* revealed numerous hits that provide a starting point for new projects to develop novel chemical scaffolds for Chagas disease (see NCBI website: http://www.ncbi.nlm.nih.gov/sites/entrez?db=pcassay&term=1885). Another area that is ripe for further research relates to testing combinations of compounds, possibly with existing drugs, for efficacy in *T. cruzi* models (Coura, 2009; Ribeiro et al., 2009).

5.8. CONCLUSIONS

Research into drug discovery for Chagas disease largely takes place in academic institutions. A track record of no new drugs in clinical trials for 40 years speaks to the deficiencies of this model. The appearance of private–public partnerships (e.g. Drugs for Neglected Diseases Initiative) helps address the problem, although their role may largely relate to late preclinical studies and clinical trials for the most promising drug candidates. As such, it remains in the purview of academia to discovery new chemical entities that will be candidates for future clinical research. Academic scientists need to form multidisciplinary groups comprised of biologists, chemists, computational scientists, and pharmacologists that more closely resemble the organization of drug companies. The scientists need to be cognizant of the chemical properties that make molecules "drug-like" and rapidly phase out compound series that present insurmountable liabilities. With close attention to the TPP for Chagas disease, multidisciplinary teams of academic scientists are the best hope for bringing desperately needed new drugs to scores of patients infected with *T. cruzi*.

ACKNOWLEDGEMENTS

The author acknowledges the helpful feedback of Ranae Pefley, Matthew Hulverson, and Christophe Verlinde in the preparation of the chapter.

REFERENCES

Alves, M.J., Mortara, R.A., 2009. A century of research: what have we learned about the interaction of *Trypanosoma cruzi* with host cells? Mem. Inst. Oswaldo Cruz 104 (Suppl. 1), 76–88.

Ananthan, S., Faaleolea, E.R., Goldman, R.C., Hobrath, J.V., Kwong, C.D., Laughon, B.E., et al., 2009. High-throughput screening for inhibitors of Mycobacterium tuberculosis H37Rv. Tuberculosis (Edinb.) 89 (5), 334–353.

Andrade, S.G., Magalhaes, J.B., Pontes, A.L., 1985. Evaluation of chemotherapy with benznidazole and nifurtimox in mice infected with *Trypanosoma cruzi* strains of different types. Bull. World Health Organ. 63 (4), 721–726.

Andrews, N.W., Colli, W., 1982. Adhesion and interiorization of *Trypanosoma cruzi* in mammalian cells. J. Protozool. 29 (2), 264–269.

Anoopkumar-Dukie, S., Carey, J.B., Conere, T., O'sullivan, E., van Pelt, F.N., Allshire, A., 2005. Resazurin assay of radiation response in cultured cells. Br. J. Radiol. 78 (934), 945–947.

Araujo, M.S., Martins-Filho, O.A., Pereira, M.E., Brener, Z., 2000. A combination of benznidazole and ketoconazole enhances efficacy of chemotherapy of experimental Chagas' disease. J. Antimicrob. Chemother. 45 (6), 819–824.

Baell, J.B., Holloway, G.A., 2010. New substructure filters for removal of pan assay interference compounds (PAINS) from screening libraries and for their exclusion in bioassays. J. Med. Chem. 53 (7), 2719–2740.

Baranczewski, P., Stanczak, A., Sundberg, K., Svensson, R., Wallin, A., Jansson, J., et al., 2006. Introduction to in vitro estimation of metabolic stability and drug interactions of new chemical entities in drug discovery and development. Pharmacol. Rep. 58 (4), 453–472.

Benaim, G., Sanders, J.M., Garcia-Marchan, Y., Colina, C., Lira, R., Caldera, A.R., et al., 2006. Amiodarone has intrinsic anti-*Trypanosoma cruzi* activity and acts synergistically with posaconazole. J. Med. Chem. 49 (3), 892–899.

Berenbaum, M.C., 1978. A method for testing for synergy with any number of agents. J. Infect. Dis. 137 (2), 122–130.

Bern, C., Montgomery, S.P., Herwaldt, B.L., Rassi, A., Jr., Marin-Neto, J.A., Dantas, R.O., et al., 2007. Evaluation and treatment of chagas disease in the United States: a systematic review. JAMA 298 (18), 2171–2181.

Bertelli, M.S., Brener, Z., 1980. Infection of tissue culture cells with bloodstream trypomastigotes of *Trypanosoma cruzi*. J. Parasitol. 66 (6), 992–997.

Bettiol, E., Samanovic, M., Murkin, A.S., Raper, J., Buckner, F., Rodriguez, A., 2009. Identification of Three Classes of Heteroaromatic Compounds with Activity against Intracellular *Trypanosoma cruzi* by Chemical Library Screening. PLoS Negl. Trop. Dis. 3 (2), e384.

Bevan, C.D., Lloyd, R.S., 2000. A high throughput screening method for the determination of aqueous drug solubility using laser nephelometry in microtiter plates. Anal. Chem. 72 (8), 1781–1787.

Boelsterli, U.A., Ho, H.K., Zhou, S., Leow, K.Y., 2006. Bioactivation and hepatotoxicity of nitroaromatic drugs. Curr. Drug Metab. 7 (7), 715–727.

Bomhard, E.M., Herbold, B.A., 2005. Genotoxic activities of aniline and its metabolites and their relationship to the carcinogenicity of aniline in the spleen of rats. Crit. Rev. Toxicol. 35 (10), 783–835.

Bot, C., Hall, B.S., Bashir, N., Taylor, M.C., Helsby, N.A., Wilkinson, S.R., 2010. Trypanocidal activity of aziridinyl nitrobenzamide prodrugs. Antimicrob. Agents Chemother. 54 (10), 4246–4252.

Brak, K., Kerr, I.D., Barrett, K.T., Fuchi, N., Debnath, M., Ang, K., et al., 2010. Nonpeptidic tetrafluorophenoxymethyl ketone cruzain inhibitors as promising new leads for Chagas disease chemotherapy. J. Med. Chem. 53 (4), 1763–1773.

Brener, Z., Chiari, E., 1967. Susceptibility of different strains of *Trypanosoma cruzi* to various chemotherapeutic agents. Rev. Inst. Med. Trop. Sao Paulo 9 (4), 197–207.

Brener, Z., Chiari, E., Alvarenga, N.J., 1974. Observations on *Trypanosoma cruzi* strains maintained over an 8-year period in experimentally inoculated mice. Rev. Inst. Med. Trop. Sao Paulo 16 (1), 39–46.

Brener, Z., Costa, C.A., Chiari, C., 1976. Differences in the susceptibility of *Trypanosoma cruzi* strains to active chemotherapeutic agents. Rev. Inst. Med. Trop. Sao Paulo 18 (6), 450–455.

Brun, R., Buhler, Y., Sandmeier, U., Kaminsky, R., Bacchi, C.J., Rattendi, D., et al., 1996. In vitro trypanocidal activities of new S-adenosylmethionine decarboxylase inhibitors. Antimicrob. Agents Chemother. 40 (6), 1442–1447.

Brunton, L.L., Chabner, B.A., Knollmann, B.C., 2011. Goodman and Gilman's The Pharmacological Basis of Therapeutics, 12th ed. McGraw Hill Medical, New York.

Buckner, F.S., 2008. Sterol 14-demethylase inhibitors for *Trypanosoma cruzi* infections. Adv. Exp. Med. Biol. 625, 61–80.

Buckner, F.S., Navabi, N., 2010. Advances in Chagas disease drug development: 2009-2010. Curr. Opin. Infect. Dis. 23 (6), 609–616.

Buckner, F.S., Wilson, A.J., 2005. Colorimetric assay for screening compounds against Leishmania amastigotes grown in macrophages. Am. J. Trop. Med. Hyg. 72 (5), 600–605.

Buckner, F.S., Verlinde, C.L.M.J., La Flamme, A.C., Van Voorhis, W.C., 1996. Efficient technique for screening drugs for activity against *Trypanosoma cruzi* using parasites expressing β-galactosidase. Antimicrob. Agents Chemother. 40 (11), 2592–2597.

Buckner, F.S., Wilson, A.J., Van Voorhis, W.C., 1999. Detection of live *Trypanosoma cruzi* in tissues of mice using histochemical stain for β-galactosidase. Infect. Immun. 67, 403–409.

Buckner, F.S., Griffin, J.H., Wilson, A.J., Van Voorhis, W.C., 2001. Potent anti-*Trypanosoma cruzi* activities of oxidosqualene cyclase inhibitors. Antimicrob. Agents Chemother. 45 (4), 1210–1215.

Buckner, F.S., Yokoyama, K., Lockman, J.W., Ohkanda, J., Eastman, R., Van Voorhis, W.C., et al., 2002. Protein Farnesyltransferase Inhibitors for Therapy of Trypanosomatid Infections. Keystone Symposia 2002 Abstract Book.

Burleigh, B.A., Andrews, N.W., 1998. Signaling and host cell invasion by *Trypanosoma cruzi*. Curr. Opin. Microbiol. 1 (4), 461–465.

Bustamante, J.M., Bixby, L.M., Tarleton, R.L., 2008. Drug-induced cure drives conversion to a stable and protective CD8+ T central memory response in chronic Chagas disease. Nat. Med. 14 (5), 542–550.

Cabrera, E., Murguiondo, M.G., Arias, M.G., Arredondo, C., Pintos, C., Aguirre, G., et al., 2009. 5-Nitro-2-furyl derivative actives against *Trypanosoma cruzi*: preliminary in vivo studies. Eur. J. Med. Chem. 44 (10), 3909–3914.

Camandaroba, E.L., Reis, E.A., Goncalves, M.S., Reis, M.G., Andrade, S.G., 2003. *Trypanosoma cruzi*: susceptibility to chemotherapy with benznidazole of clones isolated from the highly resistant Colombian strain. Rev. Soc. Bras. Med. Trop. 36 (2), 201–209.

Canavaci, A.M., Bustamante, J.M., Padilla, A.M., Perez Brandan, C.M., Simpson, L.J., Xu, D., et al., 2010. In vitro and in vivo high-throughput assays for the testing of anti *Trypanosoma cruzi* compounds. PLoS Negl. Trop. Dis. 4 (7), e740.

Canfield, C.J., Pudney, M., Gutteridge, W.E., 1995. Interactions of atovaquone with other antimalarial drugs against Plasmodium falciparum in vitro. Exp. Parasitol. 80 (3), 373–381.

Chen, Y.T., Brinen, L.S., Kerr, I.D., Hansell, E., Doyle, P.S., McKerrow, J.H., et al., 2010. In vitro and in vivo studies of the trypanocidal properties of WRR-483 against *Trypanosoma cruzi*. PLoS. Negl. Trop. Dis. 4 (9), e825.

Cheng, T.J., Wu, Y.T., Yang, S.T., Lo, K.H., Chen, S.K., Chen, Y.H., et al., 2010. High-throughput identification of antibacterials against methicillin-resistant Staphylococcus aureus (MRSA) and the transglycosylase. Bioorg. Med. Chem. 18 (24), 8512–8529.

Chiari, E., 1974. Infectivity of *Trypanosoma cruzi* metacyclic trypomastigotes from cultures kept in laboratory for different periods of time. Rev. Inst. Med. Trop. Sao Paulo 16 (2), 61–67.

Clayton, J., 2010. Chagas disease: pushing through the pipeline. Nature 465, S12–S15.

Collins, S.J., 1987. The HL-60 promyelocytic leukemia cell line: proliferation, differentiation, and cellular oncogene expression. Blood 70 (5), 1233–1244.

Combs, T.P., Nagajyothi, Mukherjee, S., de Almeida, C.J., Jelicks, L.A., Schubert, W., et al., 2005. The adipocyte as an important target cell for *Trypanosoma cruzi* infection. J. Biol. Chem. 280 (25), 24085–24094.

Contreras, V.T., Araque, W., Delgado, V.S., 1994. *Trypanosoma cruzi*: metacyclogenesis in vitro—I. Changes in the properties of metacyclic trypomastigotes maintained in the laboratory by different methods. Mem. Inst. Oswaldo Cruz 89 (2), 253–259.

Corey, E.J., Matsuda, S.P., Baker, C.H., Ting, A.Y., Cheng, H., 1996. Molecular cloning of a *Schizosaccharomyces pombe* cDNA encoding lanosterol synthase and investigation of conserved tryptophan residues. Biochem. Biophys. Res. Commun. 219 (2), 327–331.

Coura, J.R., 2009. Present situation and new strategies for Chagas disease chemotherapy: a proposal. Mem. Inst. Oswaldo Cruz 104 (4), 549–554.

Devera, R., Fernandes, O., Coura, J.R., 2003. Should *Trypanosoma cruzi* be called "cruzi" complex? a review of the parasite diversity and the potential of selecting population after in vitro culturing and mice infection. Mem. Inst. Oswaldo Cruz 98 (1), 1–12.

Di, L., Kerns, E.H., Hong, Y., Chen, H., 2005. Development and application of high throughput plasma stability assay for drug discovery. Int. J. Pharm. 297 (1–2), 110–119.

Dos Santos, F.M., Caldas, S., Assis Cau, S.B., Crepalde, G.P., de Lana, M., Machado-Coelho, G.L., et al., 2008. *Trypanosoma cruzi*: induction of benznidazole resistance in vivo and its modulation by in vitro culturing and mice infection. Exp. Parasitol. 120 (4), 385–390.

Doyle, P.S., Chen, C.K., Johnston, J.B., Hopkins, S.D., Leung, S.S., Jacobson, M.P., et al., 2010. A nonazole CYP51 inhibitor cures Chagas' disease in a mouse model of acute infection. Antimicrob. Agents Chemother. 54 (6), 2480–2488.

Dujardin, J.C., Gonzalez-Pacanowska, D., Croft, S.L., Olesen, O.F., Spath, G.F., 2010. Collaborative actions in anti-trypanosomatid chemotherapy with partners from disease endemic areas. Trends Parasitol. 26 (8), 395–403.

Dvorak, J.A., Poore, C.M., 1974. *Trypanosoma cruzi*: interaction with vertebrate cells in vitro. IV. Environmental temperature effects. Exp. Parasitol. 36 (1), 150–157.

Engel, J.C., Doyle, P.S., Dvorak, J.A., 1985. *Trypanosoma cruzi*: biological characterization of clones derived from chronic chagasic patients. II. Quantitative analysis of the intracellular cycle. J. Protozool. 32 (1), 80–83.

Engel, J.C., Ang, K.K., Chen, S., Arkin, M.R., McKerrow, J.H., Doyle, P.S., 2010. Image-based high-throughput drug screening targeting the intracellular stage of *Trypanosoma cruzi*, the agent of Chagas' disease. Antimicrob. Agents Chemother. 54 (8), 3326–3334.

Ferguson, L.R., Denny, W.A., 2007. Genotoxicity of non-covalent interactions: DNA intercalators. Mutat. Res. 623 (1–2), 14–23.

Ferreira, D.S., Esperandim, V.R., Toldo, M.P., Saraiva, J., Cunha, W.R., de Albuquerque, S., 2010. Trypanocidal activity and acute toxicity assessment of triterpene acids. Parasitol. Res. 106 (4), 985–989.

Fidock, D.A., Rosenthal, P.J., Croft, S.L., Brun, R., Nwaka, S., 2004. Antimalarial drug discovery: efficacy models for compound screening. Nat. Rev. Drug Discov. 3 (6), 509–520.

Filardi, L.S., Brener, Z., 1987. Susceptibility and natural resistance of *Trypanosoma cruzi* strains to drugs used clinically in Chagas' disease. Trans. R. Soc. Trop. Med. Hyg. 81, 755–759.

Gabrielsson, J., Weiner, D., 2007. Pharmacokinetic and Pharmacodynamic Data Analysis Concepts and Applications, fourth ed. Swedish Pharmaceutical Press, Stockholm.

Garzoni, L.R., Waghabi, M.C., Baptista, M.M., de Castro, S.L., Meirelles, M.N., Britto, C.C., et al., 2004. Antiparasitic activity of risedronate in a murine model of acute Chagas' disease. Int. J. Antimicrob. Agents 23 (3), 286–290.

Gelb, M.H., Buckner, F.S., Yokoyama, K., Ohkanda, J., Hamilton, A., Hguyen, L., et al., 2000. Protein prenylation in Trypanosomatids: a new piggy-back medicinal chemistry target for the development of agents against tropical diseases. In: Sebti, S.M. (Ed.),

Farnesyltransferase and Geranylgeranyltransferase-I: Targets for Cancer and Cardiovascular Therapy. Humana Press, Totowa, New Jersey.
Gelb, M.H., Van Voorhis, W.C., Buckner, F.S., Yokoyama, K., Eastman, R., Carpenter, E.P., et al., 2003. Protein farnesyl and N-myristoyl transferases: piggy-back medicinal chemistry targets for the development of antitrypanosomatid and antimalarial therapeutics. Mol. Biochem. Parasitol. 126 (2), 155–163.
Grosso, N.L., Bua, J., Perrone, A.E., Gonzalez, M.N., Bustos, P.L., Postan, M., et al., 2010. *Trypanosoma cruzi*: biological characterization of a isolate from an endemic area and its susceptibility to conventional drugs. Exp. Parasitol. 126 (2), 239–244.
Grunberg, E., Beskid, G., Cleeland, R., DeLorenzo, W.F., Titsworth, E., Scholer, H.J., et al., 1967. Antiprotozoan and antibacterial activity of 2-nitroimidazole derivatives. Antimicrob. Agents Chemother (Bethesda) 7, 513–519.
Guevara, P., Dias, M., Rojas, A., Crisante, G., Abreu-Blanco, M.T., Umezawa, E., et al., 2005. Expression of fluorescent genes in *Trypanosoma cruzi* and Trypanosoma rangeli (Kinetoplastida: Trypanosomatidae): its application to parasite-vector biology. J. Med. Entomol. 42 (1), 48–56.
Guiguemde, W.A., Shelat, A.A., Bouck, D., Duffy, S., Crowther, G.J., Davis, P.H., et al., 2010. Chemical genetics of Plasmodium falciparum. Nature 465 (7296), 311–315.
Gupta, S., Thapar, M.M., Mariga, S.T., Wernsdorfer, W.H., Bjorkman, A., 2002. Plasmodium falciparum: in vitro interactions of artemisinin with amodiaquine, pyronaridine, and chloroquine. Exp. Parasitol. 100 (1), 28–35.
Harth, G., Andrews, N., Mills, A.A., Engel, J.C., Smith, R., McKerrow, J.H., 1993. Peptide-fluoromethyl ketones arrest intracellular replication and intercellular transmission of *Trypanosoma cruzi*. Mol. Biochem. Parasitol. 58 (1), 17–24.
Hudson, L., 1983. Suggested guidelines for work with live *Trypanosoma cruzi*. Trans. R. Soc. Trop. Med. Hyg. 77 (3), 416–419.
Kansy, M., Senner, F., Gubernator, K., 1998. Physicochemical high throughput screening: parallel artificial membrane permeation assay in the description of passive absorption processes. J. Med. Chem. 41 (7), 1007–1010.
Kerns, E.H., Di, L., 2008. Drug-Like Properties: Concepts. Structure Design and Methods Academic Press, Burlington, MA.
Kraus, J.M., Verlinde, C.L., Karimi, M., Lepesheva, G.I., Gelb, M.H., Buckner, F.S., 2009. Rational modification of a candidate cancer drug for use against Chagas disease. J. Med. Chem. 52 (6), 1639–1647.
Lauria-Pires, L., Santana, J.M., Tavares, F.S., Teixeira, A.R., 1997. Diversity of *Trypanosoma cruzi* stocks and clones derived from Chagas disease patients: I—behavioral characterization in vitro. Rev. Soc. Bras. Med. Trop. 30 (3), 187–192.
Lawley, P.D., 1980. DNA as a target of alkylating carcinogens. Br. Med. Bull. 36 (1), 19–24.
Levy, J.A., Virolainen, M., Defendi, V., 1968. Human lymphoblastoid lines from lymph node and spleen. Cancer 22 (3), 517–524.
Lipinski, C.A., Lombardo, F., Dominy, B.W., Feeney, P.J., 2001. Experimental and computational approaches to estimate solubility and permeability in drug discovery and development settings. Adv. Drug Deliv. Rev. 46 (1–3), 3–26.
Liu, Y., Zhang, J., Xu, W., 2007. Recent progress in rational drug design of neuraminidase inhibitors. Curr. Med. Chem. 14 (27), 2872–2891.
Lu, H.R., Vlaminckx, E., Van de, W.A., Rohrbacher, J., Hermans, A., Gallacher, D.J., 2006. In-vitro experimental models for the risk assessment of antibiotic-induced QT prolongation. Eur. J. Pharmacol. 553 (1–3), 229–239.
Mackey, Z.B., Baca, A.M., Mallari, J.P., Apsel, B., Shelat, A., Hansell, E.J., et al., 2006. Discovery of trypanocidal compounds by whole cell HTS of *Trypanosoma brucei*. Chem. Biol. Drug Des. 67 (5), 355–363.

Maldonado, R.A., Molina, J., Payares, G., Urbina, J.A., 1993. Experimental chemotherapy with combinations of ergosterol biosynthesis inhibitors in murine models of Chagas' disease. Antimicrob. Agents Chemother. 37 (6), 1353–1359.

Maletinska, L., Blakely, E.A., Bjornstad, K.A., Deen, D.F., Knoff, L.J., Forte, T.M., 2000. Human glioblastoma cell lines: levels of low-density lipoprotein receptor and low-density lipoprotein receptor-related protein. Cancer Res. 60 (8), 2300–2303.

Marinho, C.R., Nunez-Apaza, L.N., Bortoluci, K.R., Bombeiro, A.L., Bucci, D.Z., Grisotto, M.G., et al., 2009. Infection by the Sylvio X10/4 clone of *Trypanosoma cruzi*: relevance of a low-virulence model of Chagas' disease. Microbes Infect. 11 (13), 1037–1045.

Masimirembwa, C.M., Bredberg, U., Andersson, T.B., 2003. Metabolic stability for drug discovery and development: pharmacokinetic and biochemical challenges. Clin. Pharmacokinet. 42 (6), 515–528.

McCabe, R.E., Remington, J.S., Araujo, F.G., 1984a. Ketoconazole inhibition of intracellular multiplication of *Trypanosoma cruzi* and protection of mice against lethal infection with the organism. J. Infect. Dis. 150 (4), 594–601.

McCabe, R.E., Remington, J.S., Araujo, F.G., 1984b. Mechanisms of invasion and replication of the intracellular stage in *Trypanosoma cruzi*. Infect. Immun. 46 (2), 372–376.

McKerrow, J.H., Doyle, P.S., Engel, J.C., Podust, L.M., Robertson, S.A., Ferreira, R., et al., 2009. Two approaches to discovering and developing new drugs for Chagas disease. Mem. Inst. Oswaldo Cruz 104 (Suppl. 1), 263–269.

Miles, M.A., 1993. Culturing and biological cloning of *Trypanosoma cruzi*. Methods Mol. Biol. 21, 15–28.

Miret, S., De Groene, E.M., Klaffke, W., 2006. Comparison of in vitro assays of cellular toxicity in the human hepatic cell line HepG2. J. Biomol. Screen. 11 (2), 184–193.

Molina, J., Martins-Filho, O., Brener, Z., Romanha, A.J., Loebenberg, D., Urbina, J.A., 2000. Activities of the triazole derivative SCH 56592 (posaconazole) against drug-resistant strains of the protozoan parasite Trypanosoma (Schizotrypanum) cruzi in immunocompetent and immunosuppressed murine hosts. Antimicrob. Agents Chemother. 44 (1), 150–155.

Moreira, D.R., Leite, A.C., dos Santos, R.R., Soares, M.B., 2009. Approaches for the development of new anti-*Trypanosoma cruzi* agents. Curr. Drug Targets 10 (3), 212–231.

Moreno, M., D'avila, D.A., Silva, M.N., Galvao, L.M., Macedo, A.M., Chiari, E., et al., 2010. Trypanosoma cruzi benznidazole susceptibility in vitro does not predict the therapeutic outcome of human Chagas disease. Mem. Inst. Oswaldo Cruz 105 (7), 918–924.

Mukherjee, S., Huang, H., Petkova, S.B., Albanese, C., Pestell, R.G., Braunstein, V.L., et al., 2004. Trypanosoma cruzi infection activates extracellular signal-regulated kinase in cultured endothelial and smooth muscle cells. Infect. Immun. 72 (9), 5274–5282.

Neal, R.A., Van Bueren, J., 1988. Comparative studies of drug susceptibility of five strains of *Trypanosoma cruzi* in vivo and in vitro. Trans. R. Soc. Trop. Med. Hyg. 82 (5), 709–714.

Nohara, L.L., Lema, C., Bader, J.O., Aguilera, R.J., Almeida, I.C., 2010. High-content imaging for automated determination of host-cell infection rate by the intracellular parasite *Trypanosoma cruzi*. Parasitol. Int. 59 (4), 565–570.

Nwaka, S., Ramirez, B., Brun, R., Maes, L., Douglas, F., Ridley, R., 2009. Advancing drug innovation for neglected diseases-criteria for lead progression. PLoS Negl. Trop. Dis. 3 (8), e440.

Ohrt, C., Willingmyre, G.D., Lee, P., Knirsch, C., Milhous, W., 2002. Assessment of azithromycin in combination with other antimalarial drugs against Plasmodium falciparum in vitro. Antimicrob. Agents Chemother. 46 (8), 2518–2524.

Ojo, K.K., Gillespie, J.R., Riechers, A.J., Napuli, A.J., Verlinde, C.L., Buckner, F.S., et al., 2008. Glycogen synthase kinase 3 is a potential drug target for African trypanosomiasis therapy. Antimicrob. Agents Chemother. 52 (10), 3710–3717.

Payne, D.J., Gwynn, M.N., Holmes, D.J., Pompliano, D.L., 2007. Drugs for bad bugs: confronting the challenges of antibacterial discovery. Nat. Rev. Drug Discov. 6 (1), 29–40.

Pereira, M.E., Santos, L.M., Araujo, M.S., Brener, Z., 1996. Recrudescence induced by cyclophosphamide of chronic *Trypanosoma cruzi* infection in mice is influenced by the parasite strain. Mem. Inst. Oswaldo Cruz 91 (1), 71–74.

Rasheed, S., Nelson-Rees, W.A., Toth, E.M., Arnstein, P., Gardner, M.B., 1974. Characterization of a newly derived human sarcoma cell line (HT-1080). Cancer 33 (4), 1027–1033.

Ribeiro, I., Sevcsik, A.M., Alves, F., Diap, G., Don, R., Harhay, M.O., et al., 2009. New, improved treatments for Chagas disease: from the R&D pipeline to the patients. PLoS Negl. Trop. Dis. 3 (7), e484.

Rivera, G., Bocanegra-Garcia, V., Ordaz-Pichardo, C., Nogueda-Torres, B., Monge, A., 2009. New therapeutic targets for drug design against *Trypanosoma cruzi*, advances and perspectives. Curr. Med. Chem. 16 (25), 3286–3293.

Rodricks, J.V., Starr, T.B., Taylor, M.R., 1991. Evaluating the safety of carcinogens in food—current practices and emerging developments. Food Drug Cosmet. Law J. 46 (5), 513–552.

Rodrigues, A.D., Lin, J.H., 2001. Screening of drug candidates for their drug–drug interaction potential. Curr. Opin. Chem. Biol. 5 (4), 396–401.

Rodriguez, A., Samoff, E., Rioult, M.G., Chung, A., Andrews, N.W., 1996. Host cell invasion by trypanosomes requires lysosomes and microtubule/kinesin-mediated transport. J. Cell Biol. 134 (2), 349–362.

Romanha, A.J., Castro, S.L., Soeiro, M.N., Lannes-Vieira, J., Ribeiro, I., Talvani, A., et al., 2010. In vitro and in vivo experimental models for drug screening and development for Chagas disease. Mem. Inst. Oswaldo Cruz 105 (2), 233–238.

Santa-Rita, R.M., Lira, R., Barbosa, H.S., Urbina, J.A., de Castro, S.L., 2005. Anti-proliferative synergy of lysophospholipid analogues and ketoconazole against *Trypanosoma cruzi* (Kinetoplastida: Trypanosomatidae): cellular and ultrastructural analysis. J. Antimicrob. Chemother. 55 (5), 780–784.

Santos, S.J., Takahashi, C.S., Natarajan, A.T., 1994. Cytogenetic effects of the antichagasic benznidazole on human cells in vitro. Mutat. Res. 320 (4), 305–314.

Seethala, R., Fernandes, P., 2001. Handbook of Drug Screening. Marcel Dekker, Inc., New York, NY.

Sharlow, E.R., Close, D., Shun, T., Leimgruber, S., Reed, R., Mustata, G., et al., 2009. Identification of potent chemotypes targeting Leishmania major using a high-throughput, low-stringency, computationally enhanced, small molecule screen. PLoS Negl. Trop. Dis. 3 (11), e540.

Shoemaker, R.H., 2006. The NCI60 human tumour cell line anticancer drug screen. Nat. Rev. Cancer 6 (10), 813–823.

Soeiro, M.N., de Castro, S.L., de Souza, E.M., Batista, D.G., Silva, C.F., Boykin, D.W., 2008. Diamidine activity against trypanosomes: the state of the art. Curr. Mol. Pharmacol. 1 (2), 151–161.

Soeiro, M.N., Dantas, A.P., Daliry, A., da Silva, C.F., Batista, D.G., de Souza, E.M., et al., 2009. Experimental chemotherapy for Chagas disease: 15 years of research contributions from in vivo and in vitro studies. Mem. Inst. Oswaldo Cruz 104 (Suppl. 1), 301–310.

Suryadevara, P.K., Olepu, S., Lockman, J.W., Ohkanda, J., Karimi, M., Verlinde, C.L., et al., 2009. Structurally simple inhibitors of lanosterol 14alpha-demethylase are efficacious in a rodent model of acute Chagas disease. J. Med. Chem. 52 (12), 3703–3715.

Tang, F., Horie, K., Borchardt, R.T., 2002. Are MDCK cells transfected with the human MDR1 gene a good model of the human intestinal mucosa? Pharm. Res. 19 (6), 765–772.

Urbina, J.A., 1999. Parasitological cure of Chagas disease: is it possible? Is it relevant? Mem. Inst. Oswaldo Cruz 94 (Suppl 1), 349–355.

Urbina, J.A., 2009. Ergosterol biosynthesis and drug development for Chagas disease. Mem. Inst. Oswaldo Cruz 104 (Suppl. 1), 311–318.

Urbina, J.A., 2010. Specific chemotherapy of Chagas disease: relevance, current limitations and new approaches. Acta Trop. 115 (1–2), 55–68.

Urbina, J.A., Lazardi, K., Marchan, E., Visbal, G., Aguirre, T., Piras, M.M., et al., 1993. Mevinolin (lovastatin) potentiates the antiproliferative effects of ketoconazole and terbinafine against Trypanosoma (Schizotrypanum) cruzi: in vitro and in vivo studies. Antimicrob. Agents Chemother. 37 (3), 580–591.

US Department of Health and Human Services, 2009. Biosafety in Microbiological and Biomedical Laboratories, fifth ed. Government Printing Office, Washington, DC.

Veber, D.F., Johnson, S.R., Cheng, H.Y., Smith, B.R., Ward, K.W., Kopple, K.D., 2002. Molecular properties that influence the oral bioavailability of drug candidates. J. Med. Chem. 45 (12), 2615–2623.

Veloso, V.M., Tafuri, W.L., Lana, M., Chiari, E., Torres, J.A., Araujo, F.M.G., et al., 1996. Changes on the behaviour of *Trypanosoma cruzi* populations after infection for long periods of time in dogs. Mem. Inst. Oswaldo Cruz 91 (Suppl.), 220–228.

Viotti, R., Vigliano, C., Armenti, H., Segura, E., 1994. Treatment of chronic Chagas' disease with benznidazole: clinical and serological evolution of patients with long-term follow-up. Am. Heart J. 127 (1), 151–162.

von Kreuter, B.F., Sadigursky, M., Santos-Buch, C.A., 1988. Complementary surface epitopes, myotropic adhesion and active grip in *Trypanosoma cruzi*-host cell recognition. Mol. Biochem. Parasitol. 30 (3), 197–208.

Wade, D.R., Airy, S.C., Sinsheimer, J.E., 1978. Mutagenicity of aliphatic epoxides. Mutat. Res. 58 (2–3), 217–223.

Weston, D., La Flamme, A.C., Van Voorhis, W.C., 1999. Expression of *Trypanosoma cruzi* surface antigen FL-160 is controlled by elements in the 3′ untranslated, the 3′ intergenic, and the coding regions. Mol. Biochem. Parasitol. 102 (1), 53–66.

Williams, D.P., Naisbitt, D.J., 2002. Toxicophores: groups and metabolic routes associated with increased safety risk. Curr. Opin. Drug Discov. Devel. 5 (1), 104–115.

Wlodawer, A., 2002. Rational approach to AIDS drug design through structural biology. Annu. Rev. Med. 53, 595–614.

Wood, C., Williams, C., Waldron, G.J., 2004. Patch clamping by numbers. Drug Discov. Today 9 (10), 434–441.

Yardley, V., Croft, S.L., 1999. *In vitro* and *in vivo* activity of amphotericin B-lipid formulations against experimental *Trypanosoma cruzi* infections. Am. J. Trop. Med. Hyg. 61 (2), 193–197.

Zingales, B., Pereira, M.E., Almeida, K.A., Umezawa, E.S., Nehme, N.S., Oliveira, R.P., et al., 1997. Biological parameters and molecular markers of clone CL Brener—the reference organism of the *Trypanosoma cruzi* genome project. Mem. Inst. Oswaldo Cruz 92 (6), 811–814.

Zingales, B., Andrade, S.G., Briones, M.R., Campbell, D.A., Chiari, E., Fernandes, O., et al., 2009. A new consensus for *Trypanosoma cruzi* intraspecific nomenclature: second revision meeting recommends TcI to TcVI. Mem. Inst. Oswaldo Cruz 104 (7), 1051–1054.

CHAPTER 6

Vaccine Development Against *Trypanosoma cruzi* and Chagas Disease

Juan C. Vázquez-Chagoyán,[*] Shivali Gupta,[†] and **Nisha Jain Garg[†,‡,§]**

Contents

Abstract

The pathology of Chagas disease presents a complicated and diverse picture in humans. The major complications and destructive evolutionary outcomes of chronic infection by *Trypanosoma cruzi*

[*] Centro de Investigación y Estudios Avanzados en Salud Animal, Facultad de Medicina Veterinaria y Zootecnia, Universidad Autónoma de Estado de México, Toluca, Mexico
[†] Department of Microbiology and Immunology, University of Texas Medical Branch, Galveston, Texas, USA
[‡] Department of Pathology, University of Texas Medical Branch, Galveston, Texas, USA
[§] Member of the Institute for Human Infections and Immunity, University of Texas Medical Branch, Galveston, Texas, USA

Advances in Parasitology, Volume 75
ISSN 0065-308X, DOI: 10.1016/B978-0-12-385863-4.00006-X

in humans include ventricular fibrillation, thromboembolism and congestive heart failure. Studies in animal models and human patients have revealed the pathogenic mechanisms during disease progression, pathology of disease and features of protective immunity. Accordingly, several antigens, antigen-delivery vehicles and adjuvants have been tested to elicit immune protection to *T. cruzi* in experimental animals. This review summarizes the research efforts in vaccine development against Chagas disease during the past decade.

6.1. VECTOR, PARASITE AND DISEASE BURDEN

The vectors of *Trypanosoma cruzi* are insects of the order *Hemiptera*, family *Reduviidae* and subfamily *Triatominae* (Vallejo et al., 2009). *T. cruzi* is a hemoflagellate protozoan of the *Kinetoplastida* order, *Trypanosomatidae* family. Though vectorial transmission is the major mode of acute exposure to *T. cruzi* in endemic countries, trypomastigotes may also be transferred by transplacental transmission, blood transfusion, oral uptake of infected triatomines or food or by laboratory accident (Schofield et al., 2006; WHO, 2010). *T. cruzi* isolates are grouped into six major phylogenetic groups, that is, I–VI, on the basis of zymodemes and several genetic markers (Zingales et al., 2009). No direct correlation between Chagas disease severity and parasite lineage has yet been established.

In mammalian hosts, *T. cruzi* cycles between a trypomastigote stage that circulates in the blood and infects all cell types, and an amastigote stage that replicates in the cytoplasm of infected host cells. Infection by *T. cruzi* is rarely lethal in immunocompetent hosts. Only very few (<5%) acute patients exhibit sudden death due to congestive heart failure and/or may suffer gastrointestinal and neurological damage. In the majority of cases, patients become parasitemic and exhibit flu-like symptoms, but this stage of infection subsides within a few weeks with activation of a potent immune response capable of controlling acute parasite burden, and patients seek no treatment. In 10–30 years after initial exposure, 30–40% of the infected individuals enter the chronic stage when they develop systemic changes, commonly in the heart, oesophagus and rectosigmoid colon, and less often in the central nervous system (Rassi et al., 2010; Tanowitz et al., 2009). Typical manifestations of chronic disease are thromboembolism in the brain, limbs or lungs, congestive heart failure and sudden death—mainly due to ventricular fibrillation. Echocardiography, serial chest radiographs and electrocardiography are the commonly employed methods for detecting myocardial involvement in chagasic patients (Dubner et al., 2008; Rocha et al., 2003).

Chagas disease is prevalent in almost all Latin American countries, including Mexico and Central America. Currently, the World Health Organization (WHO) estimates that 11–18 million individuals are infected worldwide and ~13,000 children and adults die annually because of the clinical complications of *T. cruzi*-induced heart disease and lack of effective treatments (WHO, 2006, 2010). Upto 100 million, that is, 25% of the Latin America population, are believed to be at risk of infection in endemic countries. Additionally, 2–5% of foetuses carried by infected mothers in endemic areas are either spontaneously aborted or born with congenital Chagas disease (Oliveira et al., 2010). The vectorial, autochthonous and congenital transmission of *T. cruzi* exists in the United States (Bern and Montgomery, 2009), where >300,000 infected individuals can potentially transfer infection through blood or organ donation (CDC, 2006, 2007). The continuous immigration from Latin America, as well as increased business and tourism interests in endemic areas, has further increased the exposure risk of the U.S. population to *T. cruzi* (Garraud et al., 2007; Leiby et al., 2002). When considered from a global perspective, Chagas disease represents the third greatest tropical disease burden after malaria and schistosomiasis.

6.2. TREATMENT

The currently available drugs for the treatment of *T. cruzi* infection, benznidazole and nifurtimox, are effective in curing acute or recent cases of infection (Coura, 1996; de Andrade et al., 1996). However, both of these drugs have serious and frequent side effects and are not available to most patients because either they are not registered in those countries or prices are high. Anti-parasitic drugs are not effective once the patients enter the chronic phase of infection and disease progression (Rodriques-Coura and de Castro, 2002). Several other drugs, for example, posaconazole, amiodarone, Tak-187, K777 and albaconazole have shown promise in experimental models and preclinincal studies (Ribeiro et al., 2009) but have not been employed in large-scale clinical trials for evaluation of their efficacy against Chagas disease (Duschak and Couto, 2007). Rather, treatment of chronic patients focuses on cardiac management that requires specialized clinical infrastructure, is very expensive and is often beyond the reach of the patient.

6.3. A CASE FOR VACCINE DEVELOPMENT AGAINST *TRYPANOSOMA CRUZI*

Vaccines or immunotherapies for prevention and treatment of *T. cruzi* infection are practically non-existent. This is, at least, partially due to the fact that considerable debate exists regarding the pathophysiologic mechanisms that are involved in Chagas disease development. No universally accepted model exists to explain the long latency period between infection and disease development, why a subset of individuals progress to chronic disease or what instigates or perpetuates the damage in the heart that ultimately results in chagasic disease symptoms. Results of preclinical and clinical studies have led to the suggestion that consistent inflammatory immune responses play a role in the development and/or propagation of pathological lesions in chagasic hearts. Two mechanisms, autoimmunity and parasite persistence, are proposed to sustain the pathological inflammatory responses in chagasic hearts. The autoimmune theory asserts that humoral and cellular immune reactions, elicited in response to *T. cruzi* infection, recognize self-antigens, are potentially harmful to the host and contribute to the development and/or propagation of pathological lesions in chagasic myocarditis (Bonney and Engman, 2008; Leon and Engman, 2003). The lack of evidence that *T. cruzi*-induced self-reactive antibodies or T-cells can induce disease upon transfer into a naïve host precludes us from defining chronic chagasic cardiomyopathy as an autoimmune disease. Instead, a systematic review of the literature shows that most researchers now agree that the pathogenesis of the chronic chagasic heart disease is dependent on a low-grade, systemic infection with documented immune-adverse reactions (Marin-Neto et al., 2007). This shift in views is primarily because of the recently enhanced ability to demonstrate parasite persistence during chronic stage. Researchers using modern techniques, for example, PCR, immunohistochemistry and confocal microscopy, have detected parasite DNA or antigens in blood and heart tissue biopsies of experimental animals and chronic human patients (Gutierrez et al., 2009). Others have reported transmission of *T. cruzi* via blood transfusion and transplantation of infected organs obtained from asymptomatic individuals (CDC, 2007; Leiby et al., 2000; Schmunis and Cruz, 2005). The reactivation of acute parasitaemia in chronic individuals, following immunosuppression after heart transplantation (Campos et al., 2008), AIDS (Cordova et al., 2008) or drug therapy (D'Almeida et al., 1996), further illustrated that parasites persist in previously undiagnosed individuals for years after initial infection. It is, thus, accepted that parasite persistence provides sufficient, consistent antigens that work as a trigger for a hypersensitive response against myocardial fibres, leading to pathologic tissue injury and, subsequently, to cardiac insufficiency.

Our work has led to a suggestion that chagasic myocardium sustain oxidative stress associated with mitochondrial dysfunction. Cardiac tissue is extraordinarily dependent upon oxidative phosphorylation for energy to perform its functions. A functional decline in the respiratory chain and increased generation of reactive oxygen species (ROS), coupled with an inability to efficiently scavenge mitochondrial free radicals, predisposed chagasic hearts to oxidative insult during infection and disease development (Garg, 2005; Gupta et al., 2009b; Zacks et al., 2005). The sustained occurrence of DNA, protein and lipid oxidative adducts was shown in the myocardium of experimental models of Chagas disease (Wen et al., 2004, 2008) and in the peripheral blood of rodents and human chagasic subjects (de Oliveira et al., 2007; Dhiman et al., 2008; Wen et al., 2006b). Oxidative damage during Chagas disease may not only be due to increased ROS formation but was also exacerbated by inefficient antioxidant capacity, as was noted in infected mice (Wen et al., 2004, 2006a) and human subjects (Perez-Fuentes et al., 2003; Wen et al., 2006b). Treatment of experimental animals with phenylbutylnitrone antioxidant (Wen et al., 2006a, 2010) and human chagasic patients with Vitamin C and Vitamin E antioxidants (Macao et al., 2007; Ribeiro et al., 2010) was shown to be effective in reducing the oxidative insult-associated pathology in Chagas disease. Recent studies demonstrating ROS signalling of cytokine and chemokine production in infected cardiomyocytes and murine hearts (Ba et al., 2010; Gupta et al., 2009a; Wen et al., 2010) and ROS-dependent activation and proliferation of lymphocytes in infected mice (unpublished observations) have provided a potential mechanistic link between ROS generation and acute and/or chronic inflammation in chagasic cardiomyopathy. We surmise that the contributions of parasite persistence, mitochondrial dysfunction, oxidative stress, parasite strain or clonal variation and host genetics are not mutually exclusive and could contribute in part and/or act at distinct time points during *T. cruzi* infection to initiate and sustain the observed, multifaceted cardiac pathology. The sum of these factors may also determine the degree of pathophysiology the infection may evoke and the severity of chronic disease.

An important implication of these studies is that preventing infection or controlling the acute parasite load below a threshold level would be effective in decreasing the tissue damage imposed by multiple pathogenic mechanisms and lead to decreased disease severity. These observations provide an impetus for vaccine development against *T. cruzi*, also favoured by the fact that the effector mechanisms capable of controlling parasite burden have been delineated. Thus, we propose vaccines would be the most practical tool for prevention and control of any form of *T. cruzi* infection and transmission. A cheap, safe, effective and reliable vaccine will also help alleviate the costs for vector control and drugs used to dispel this infection in endemic countries.

6.4. IMMUNITY TO *TRYPANOSOMA CRUZI*

The comparison in responses exhibited by susceptible and resistant experimental models has contributed to an understanding of protective immune responses to *T. cruzi*. Natural killer (NK) cells appear to be the first source of IFN-γ that augments IL-12, TNF-α and other cytokines synthesized by inflammatory macrophages (Aliberti et al., 2001; Almeida and Gazzinelli, 2001; Almeida et al., 2000). These cytokines signal reactive oxidants (oxidative burst) and nitric oxide production by activated macrophages (Cardoni et al., 1997; Martins et al., 1998; Melo et al., 2003; Munoz-Fernandez et al., 1992a,b) and myeloperoxidase-dependent chloramine production by neutrophils (Dhiman et al., 2009), the essential components of the innate immune system for killing of intra- and extracellular *T. cruzi*. It is suggested that IFN-γ of NK origin and IL-12 of macrophage origin skew the differentiation of parasite-specific T-helper cells towards a protective Th1 phenotype (Abrahamsohn and Coffman, 1996; Duthie and Kahn, 2005, 2006). Parasite-specific $CD4^+$ T cells are desirable, as they assist in the control of *T. cruzi* through secretion of Th1 cytokines (IFN-γ, IL-2), amplification of the phagocytic activity of macrophages, stimulation of B cell proliferation and antibody production and differentiation and activation of $CD8^+$ T cells (Brener and Gazzinelli, 1997). *T. cruzi* antigen-specific $CD8^+$ T cells are frequently present in infected mice and humans (Padilla et al., 2009) and contribute to *T. cruzi* control, either by cytolysis of the infected cells or by secretion of Th1 cytokines (IFN-γ) that induce trypanocidal activity (DosReis, 1997; Miyahira, 2008; Padilla et al., 2009). A strong lytic antibody response enhanced the opsonization, phagocytosis and complement-dependent killing of the parasites (Krautz et al., 2000). The evidence is provided from the experimental models and natural human infections, demonstrating that absence or reduction in any of these immune responses through targeted depletion, immunosuppressive treatments or infection-induced immunosuppression can result in an exacerbation of parasitaemia (D'Almeida et al., 1996; Sartori et al., 1995; Tarleton et al., 1996). To sum up, these studies conclude that parasite persistence is associated with delayed kinetics of $CD8^+$ T cells and mixed type 1/type 2 cytokine responses. An efficient protective response to *T. cruzi* would require elicitation of Th1 cytokines, lytic antibodies, and the concerted activities of phagocytes, T-helper cells and cytotoxic T lymphocytes.

6.5. VACCINE DEVELOPMENT AGAINST *TRYPANOSOMA CRUZI*

There are two stages of the parasite against which developing a vaccine is envisioned. Vaccines against trypomastigotes as they enter host cells following the bite of an infected triatomine or the burst of an infected cell will prevent the initiation or persistence of infection and limit the parasitaemia. Vaccines against intracellular replicative amastigotes would arrest the propagation of parasites in a host and prevent the parasite from entering the blood. Both types of vaccines would arrest or attenuate disease development in humans and the reservoir mammalian host. In addition, vaccines against either stage of the parasite would prevent triatomine infection and, thus, interrupt or reduce parasite transmission in both human and reservoir populations, as well as in insects.

Accordingly, early efforts in developing vaccines against *T. cruzi* tested heat-killed parasites or subcellular fractions of *T. cruzi* in various animal models, including mice, guinea pigs, dogs and monkeys (Bhatia and Garg, 2005; Bhatia et al., 2009). These approaches utilized epimastigotes, the insect stage of the parasite, that was later identified as expressing different antigens from those found in the infective and intracellular stages of *T. cruzi.* A suboptimal content of immunogenic proteins in epimastigotes, or a loss of protective epitopes during inactivation and fractionation, was believed to be the cause for the limited success met in these attempts in vaccine development.

The next series of efforts tested live vaccines having constituents of *T. cruzi* strains attenuated by treatment with pharmacological agents, serial passage *in vitro* cultures or genetic knockouts with a loss of potentially virulent genes (Bhatia and Garg, 2005; Bhatia et al., 2009). These vaccines were tested for their potency in murine and dog models and found to be largely effective in controlling subsequent infections by virulent strains. However, such vaccines were rendered impractical because of the danger of reversion of the attenuated strains to a virulent form and the likelihood of increased virulence of attenuated strains in immunocompromised individuals. These studies, however, showed that a prophylactic vaccine capable of eliciting protective immunity with a minimal risk of biological reversion to virulent phenotype would be useful in controlling *T. cruzi* infection and disease, and provided a foundation for the identification of target antigens of the immune responses and the development of subunit vaccines.

The complexity of the *T. cruzi* genome, estimated to contain >12,000 genes (El-Sayed et al., 2005), necessitated the development of logical strategies to determine which parasite proteins are the likely choice for immune activation. We dealt with this challenge by expressing a classical antigen (ovalbumin) in different cellular compartments of *T. cruzi* and finding that secreted antigens and antigens released by default in host cell cytoplasm will potentially be presented by the class I and II Major Histocompatibility Complex (MHC) and elicit B- and T-cell responses (Garg et al., 1997). It was inferred that during the process of replication and/or differentiation, *T. cruzi* releases plasma membrane proteins and secretory proteins in the host cell cytoplasm where they are degraded by proteosome enzymes. The resulting peptides transported to endoplasmic reticulum are associated with MHC class I molecules and displayed on the surface of infected cells, where they can be recognized by circulating $CD8^{+}$ T cells. On extracellular trypomastigotes and amastigotes, these same proteins expressed in a membrane-associated form are engulfed and processed by phagocytic cells, displayed in association with MHC class II molecules and can be recognized by $CD4^+$ T cells that provide help for the activation and proliferation of $CD8^+$ T and B cells. Armed with data on protective immune mechanisms and the features of potential antigenic targets, investigators directed their research efforts towards identifying effective antigens and antigen-delivery systems to elicit potent immune responses for control of *T. cruzi*. We, herein, update the information on various candidate antigens tested, and the efforts made to enhance the protective efficacy of vaccines by co-delivery of adjuvants, use of alternative routes of antigen delivery and increasing the amount or the number of doses.

6.5.1. Subunit vaccines

Initial studies examined the vaccine potential of purified *T. cruzi* proteins. These included GP90, GP82, GP56, cruzipain (Cz), paraflagellar rod (PFRs), TC52, complement-regulatory protein (CRP) and ASP2-purified (native) proteins, among others, some of which were then also tested as recombinant proteins (Table 6.1). Many of these antigens exhibited a number of attractive properties as vaccine candidates, including those abundantly expressed in the infective and intracellular stages of *T. cruzi* and highly immunogenic in natural infection. These studies, designed to estimate the protective efficacy of putative vaccine candidates based upon survival following a lethal challenge infection, soon made it clear that protein vaccines were more suitable for inducing antibody responses and were not efficient in eliciting the cell-mediated immunity that is essential for controlling the intracellular stage of a pathogen. It was generally accepted that the use of a vaccination approach that delivers the antigen to class I and class II pathways of antigen presentation and elicits an antigen-specific antibody response and Cytotoxic T lymphocyte (CTI) activity would likely be more effective against the extracellular and intracellular stages of *T. cruzi*. Thus, the DNA immunization approach was favoured and readily adopted for its ability to elicit antibodies, Th1 cytokines and $CD8^+$ T-cell immune responses (Donnelly et al., 2005; Dumonteil, 2007; Huygen, 2005) required for control of *T. cruzi*; ease of construction and production of the vectors; stability of DNA and the capacity to enhance the immune response by the co-delivery of genes encoding cytokines. Several *T. cruzi* proteins have been tested as DNA vaccines in experimental models. These include members of the *trans*-sialidase family (e.g. TSA1, ASP1, ASP2 and TS), TSSA, KMP11, LYT1, CRP, Cz, PFRs and others). Many of these candidates were identified as targets of antibody response and $CD8^+$ T cells or cytotoxic T lymphocytes in infected mice and humans (reviewed in Bhatia and Garg, 2005; Bhatia et al., 2009). When tested as a DNA vaccine in inbred mice, these antigens

TABLE 6.1 Subunit vaccines against *T. cruzi*

Antigen	Adjuvant (if used)	Experimental model: Mice (*T. cruzi*) strain	% Survival (dpi[a])	Reference
Protein vaccine				
GP90	Saponin	CBA, Marmoset (Y)	60 (100)[c]	Scott et al. (1985)
GP82	Alum or CpG-ODN	Balb/c (CL)	Not determined[c] or 20%	Eickhoff et al. (2010) and Santori et al. (1996)
GP56	Freund adjuvant	Swiss-Webster (Y)	40 (12)	Harth et al. (1994)
Cruzipain[b]	IL-12, CpG-ODN	C3H/HeN (RA), Balb/c (Tulahuen)	67–80 (60–100)[c]	Frank et al. (2003), Laderach et al. (1996) and Schnapp et al. (2002)
PFR1, PFR2[b]	Alum, Freund, IL-12	C57BL/6, Balb/c (Peru)	83–100 (30–60)[c]	Luhrs et al. (2003), Miller et al. (1996), Wrightsman et al. (2002) and Wrightsman and Manning (2000)
TC52	Alum, *Bordtella pertusis*	Balb/c (Y)	62 (120)[c]	Ouaissi et al. (2002)
CRP	Freund adjuvant	Balb/c (Y)	10 (40)[c]	Sepulveda et al. (2000)
ASP2	Alum, CpG-ODN	A/Sn (Y)	53 (60)[d]	Araujo et al. (2005)
TS	CpG-ODN	Balb/c (Tul)	100 (84), 80 (48)[d]	Giddings et al. (2010) and Hoft et al. (2007)
TS mutant engineered	Freund's complete	Balb/c (Tul)	100 (60)[c]	Fontanella et al. (2008)
DNA vaccine				
CRP		C3H/HeJ, Balb/c (Y)	100 (40)[c]	Sepulveda et al. (2000)
TSA1[b]	IL-12 + GM-CSF	BALB/c, C3H/HeSnJ, C57BL/6 (Brazil)	60 (140)[d]	Garg and Tarleton (2002) and Wizel et al. (1998)
ASP1[b]	IL-12 + GM-CSF	C3H/HeSnJ, C57BL/6 (Brazil)	<60 (140)[d]	Garg and Tarleton (2002)

(*continued*)

TABLE 6.1 *(continued)*

Antigen	Adjuvant (if used)	Experimental model Mice (*T. cruzi*) strain	% Survival (dpi[a])	Reference
ASP2[b]	IL-12 + GM-CSF	C3H/HeSnJ, C57BL/6 (Brazil)	80 (140)[c,f]	Garg and Tarleton (2002)
ASP2		Balb/c (Y)	63 (60)[d,f]	Vasconcelos et al. (2004)
ASP9		Balb/c (Y)	100 (60)[c]	Boscardin et al. (2003)
ASP-3		A/Sn (Col)	80 (120)[c]	Silveira et al. (2008)
TSA1 CTL epitope		C57BL/6 (Tul)	60 (60)[c]	Chou et al. (2008)
TS[b]		Balb/c (Y)	100 (50)[c,f]	Costa et al. (1998)
TSSA[b]	IL-12, RANK-L, IL-15	BALB/c, C3H/HeJ, C57BL/6, B6 (Tulahuen)	80–100 (40)[c]	Katae et al. (2002) Miyahira et al. (2003) and Eickhoff et al. (2011)
KMP11	HSP-70	Balb/c (Y)	50 (70)[c]	Planelles et al. (2001)
LYT1	IL-12 + GM-CSF	C57BL/6 (Brazil)	80 (75)	Fralish and Tarleton (2003)
FCaBP	IL-12 + GM-CSF	C57BL/6 (Brazil)	0 (75)[e]	Fralish and Tarleton (2003)
TCβ3	IL-12 + GM-CSF	C57BL/6 (Brazil)	0 (75)[e]	Fralish and Tarleton (2003)
PFR2 or PFR3	HSP70	Balb/c (Y)	100 (35)[c,f]	Morell et al. (2006)
TcG1	IL-12 + GM-CSF	C57BL/6/Sylvio		Bhatia et al. (2004) and Bhatia and Garg (2008)
TcG2	IL-12 + GM-CSF	C57BL/6/Sylvio		Bhatia et al. (2004) and Bhatia and Garg (2008)
TcG4	IL-12 + GM-CSF	C57BL/6/Sylvio		Bhatia et al. (2004) and Bhatia and Garg (2008)
TcG1 + TcG2 + TcG4	IL-12 + GM-CSF	C57BL/6/Sylvio		Bhatia et al. (2004) and Bhatia and Garg (2008)
ASP2 + TSA1	None	A/Sn (Y)	86 (60)[c,f]	Vasconcelos et al. (2004)
ASP1 + ASP2 + TSA1	IL-12 + GM-CSF	C3H/HeSnJ, C57BL/6 (Brazil)	83 (140)[c]	Garg and Tarleton (2002)

TS family members	C57BL/6 (Brazil)	75 (75)	Fralish and Tarleton (2003)
Mucin family members	C57BL/6 (Brazil)	25 (75)	Fralish and Tarleton (2003)
pELI-TcT-E library	C3H/HeN (RA)	80 (50)[c]	Tekiel et al. (2009)
Recombinant virus vaccine			
Ad-TSSA/MVA-TSSA MVA-RANK-L	C57BL/6 (Tulahuen)	100 (50)[c]	Miyahira et al. (2005)
rAD-ASP2	Balb/c (Y)	80 (160)[c]	Machado et al. (2006)
rAD-TS	Balb/c (Y)	50 (160)[d]	Machado et al. (2006)
rSeV-ASP2	C57BL/6 (Tul)	90 (50)[d]	Duan et al. (2009)
rADASP2 + rAD-TS	Balb/c (Y)	100 (160)[c]	Machado et al. (2006)
Immunotherapeutic DNA vaccine			
TSA1[b]	Balb/c (H4), acute model	70 (45)[c,f]	Dumonteil et al. (2004)
TSA1	CD1 (H1), chronic model	100 (140)[f]	Dumonteil et al. (2004)
TSA1	ICR (H1) acute model	70 (50)[c,f]	Sanchez-Burgos et al. (2007) and Zapata-Estrella et al. (2006)
Tc24[b]	Balb/c, ICR (H1) acute model	100 (50)[c,f]	Dumonteil et al. (2004) and Sanchez-Burgos et al. (2007)
TS	ICR (H1) acute model	50 (50)[c]	Sanchez-Burgos et al. (2007)
Tc52	ICR (H1) acute model	75 (50)[c]	Sanchez-Burgos et al. (2007)
ASP9		50 (50)[c]	Sanchez-Burgos et al. (2007)
TSA1 + Tc24	C57BL/6, Balb/c, ICR (H1)	80 (180)[c]	Limon-Flores et al. (2010)
SA85-1.1	C57BL/6 (CL)	Sublethal dose (90)[d,f]	Duthie et al. (2007)

[a] Experimental animals were observed for survival for *n* days post-infection.
[b] These antigens were shown to provide variable degree of protection in different mouse strains (data presented are from the animal model that exhibited best protection).
[c–e] Upon challenge infection, immunized animals exhibited very low ($\leq$10%)[c], moderate ($\sim$50%)[d] or similar[e] parasitaemia as detected in unimmunized/infected animals (data presented are from the animal model that exhibited best protection).
[f] Immunization with these antigens was effective in decreasing the severity of chronic disease, evaluated by histopathological analysis of cardiac tissue biopsies.

elicited varying levels of Th1 cytokines, CD8$^+$ CTL activity and antibody responses that correlated with the extent of parasitaemia control and survival from lethal challenge infection (Table 6.1). Considering that complete genes were incorporated into the DNA vectors, epitopes capable of being presented by many MHC alleles were expected to be present. Accordingly, several of the tested genes (e.g. *ASP-2*, *TSA-1*, *TSSA* and *Tc24*) afforded protective immunity in multiple, though not all, mouse strains. Some of the vaccine candidates (e.g. ASP-2, TSA-1 and TS) also arrested or decreased the skeletal and heart muscle inflammatory reactions and tissue necrosis, the hallmarks of chronic Chagas disease, in immunized mice (Table 6.1).

Not all of the antigenic targets were found to be useful as DNA vaccine candidates. For example, genes encoding FCaBP, TCβ3, Tc13, mucins and CCL4/MIP-1β failed to provide any protection from *T. cruzi* infection (Fralish and Tarleton, 2003; Garcia et al., 2008; Katae et al., 2002; Roffe et al., 2006). It is interesting that FCaBP and TCβ3 were recognized by CTLs in infected mice and elicited a cell-mediated immune response in mice when delivered as a DNA vaccine, a finding implying that the mere elicitation of CD8$^+$ T-cell responses by an antigen is not indicative of its vaccine potential. Tc13-induced immune responses were associated with pathology rather than protection (Garcia et al., 2008). Similarly, genes that did provide protection in one mouse strain were not protective in other inbred strains of mice. Examples include *ASP1*, *ASP2* and *TSA1* that were tested individually or in combination (Garg and Tarleton, 1998), *TSSA* (Katae et al., 2002) and cytoplasmic repetitive antigen CRA and flagellar repetitive antigen FRA (Pereira et al., 2005). All of these genes provided better protection in C57BL/6 mice than was afforded in Balb/c or C3H mice, a finding that may imply that host genetic restriction may also contribute to the inefficacy of vaccine candidates. Conversely, ASP-2 and TS isoforms, isolated from different parasite strains, contained cross-reactive epitopes. Yet, vaccination with ASP-2 and TS conferred only strain-specific protective immunity following challenge infection with *T. cruzi* (Claser et al., 2007; Haolla et al., 2009). These results alert the research community to be cautious in selection of genes/proteins that have strain variants and that consequently may not provide protection from diverse clinically relevant strains.

6.5.2. Adjuvants

In parallel with the efforts towards identification of vaccine candidates, adjuvants were tested to enhance or skew the immune responses towards a desirable Th1 type. Use of adjuvants to increase protective immunity against *T. cruzi* dates back to 1965 (Menezes, 1965) when saponin, a derivative from the bark of *Quillaja saponaria* (*Quil A*), was injected in mice to enhance the protective efficacy of immunogens. Co-inoculation of saponin with freeze–thaw-inactivated parasites stimulated a Th1-type immune response and slightly increased protection from a challenge infection (Johnson et al., 1963). Alum, licensed for human use, was shown to enhance the protective efficacy of PFRs and TS protein vaccines in mice (Table 6.1). Recent studies have examined the utility of cytokines (IL-12), co-stimulatory molecules (e.g. GM-CSF, CD40, HSP70) and CpG-ODN in enhancing the Th1 responses to defined antigen vaccines. GM-CSF was chosen as a genetic adjuvant because it is a potent cytokine capable of enhancing the antigen-presentation capability of antigen-presenting cells, such as dendritic cells. In addition, it facilitates B- and T-cell-mediated immunity (Warren and Weiner, 2000). IL-12 is a key cytokine involved in $CD8^+$ T-cell activation and proliferation and in directing the immune responses to type 1 (Pan et al., 1999). Similarly, other adjuvants were chosen for their ability either to enhance the innate and mucosal or systemic immunity or to skew the immune response to a protective Th1 type through different mechanisms (Singh and O'Hagan, 2002). IL-12 and GM-CSF, co-delivered as DNA adjuvants, did enhance the antibody response, CTL activity and IFN-γ secretion in mice immunized with single (LYT1) or mixed antigen-encoding plasmids (e.g. *ASP-2*, *TSA-1* and *TSA-2*) (Table 6.1). Similarly, an enhanced degree of Th1-type immune responses was achieved in mice by co-administration of RANK-L with TSSA and HSP70 with KMP11. The increase in the range and level of immune responses correlated with better protection from *T. cruzi* infection, as evidenced by the control of blood and tissue parasitaemia, increased longevity and reduced tissue inflammation (Table 6.1 and references therein).

Attempts to enhance the immunogenicity of Cz by using Freund's adjuvant or by co-delivery of IL-12 (plus neutralizing anti-IL-4 antibody) (Schnapp et al., 2002) and CpG-ODN (Frank et al., 2003) yielded enhanced, Th1-biased immune responses with specific IgG2a antibodies, activation of IL-2 and/or IFN-γ producing macrophages and a substantial resistance to *T. cruzi*, resulting in a >80% survival from acute infection. However, careful analysis by investigators also revealed that Cz immunization generated varying degrees of cardiac tissue injury that was dependent on the types of T-helper response triggered and adjuvant used, thus making it clear that a thorough standardization of antigen-delivery strategy is necessary. Several attempts were made using *Salmonella* as a CzDNA delivery system (with or without GM-CSF adjuvant), Sa-CzDNA/purified or recombinant protein with CpG-ODN (TLR9 stimulator) or MALP-2 (TLR2/TLR4 agonist) adjuvants delivered via various routes, including oral or nasal routes, to enhance innate or Th1 responses or to trigger mucosal and systemic immunity (Cazorla et al., 2008a; Duschak and Couto, 2009). All of these approaches promoted the elicitation of an immune response that partially controlled *T. cruzi* infection, tissue parasite loads and the subsequent damage to muscle tissues. Attempts at intranasal boosting with rCz combined with the different synthetic adjuvants yielded the finding that rCz, when co-administered with MALP-2, triggered a strong systemic and mucosal Ig response, namely IFN-γ-producing cellular immunity, but provided only partial protection from lethal challenge infection and disease (Cazorla et al., 2008b).

Similar to Cz, an enzymatically active form of TS, as well as TS mutants lacking the SAPA repeats, induced a protective state against *T. cruzi*, when tested as a recombinant protein with CpG-ODN or as a DNA vaccine (Fontanella et al., 2008). The intranasal delivery of TS mixed with CpG-ODN induced both mucosal and systemic protection against *T. cruzi* (Giddings et al., 2010; Hoft et al., 2007). However, the active TS form resulted in (or failed to prevent) myocardial tissue damage at the chronic stage (Fontanella et al., 2008), indicating the need for careful consideration of the vaccine design.

6.5.3. Multi-component vaccines

Considering that an increase in the level and diversity of *T. cruzi*-specific immune responses could enhance the protective capacity of vaccines, some investigators tested immunization with multiple genes encoding members of the TS or mucin families. The ability of the mixed genes to elicit protective immune responses depended upon (i) the amount of a given plasmid sufficient to elicit protective responses and (ii) the total amount of DNA that could be injected without toxicity. Immunization with various dilutions of TS family members (e.g. *ASP1*, *ASP2* and *TSA1*) with and without IL-12 and GM-CSF cytokine adjuvants (range: 1 ng–33 μg each) showed that the level of resistance to *T. cruzi* infection correlated with the amount of DNA delivered and was enhanced by co-delivery of cytokine adjuvants. The highest tested dose of each antigen (total 150 μg DNA) produced no toxicity (Garg and Tarleton, 1998). We did not observe an inhibitory effect on the elicitation of antigen-specific immune responses when mice were immunized with the mixture of plasmids, indicating that multiple genes with or without cytokine adjuvants can be used in developing immunization strategies for control of the *T. cruzi* infection. The level of protection from *T. cruzi* infection induced in mice immunized with a mixture of TS family members was, however, not significantly better than that induced in mice immunized with individual family members (Fralish and Tarleton, 2003; Garg and Tarleton, 2002; Table 6.1). Attempts to enhance the protective efficacy of TS family members by a DNA prime–protein boost approach were also not successful (Vasconcelos et al., 2003). No protection was observed in mice immunized with a pool of genes encoding mucin family members (Fralish and Tarleton, 2003). The findings of either no or little enhancement of protective immunity with a cocktail of antigen-encoding vectors were attributed to the fact that genes of large families may express shared epitopes that do not present any protective benefits in inbred mice. It is anticipated that the potential synergistic immunologic benefit of a combination of epitopes from multiple genes would induce a higher frequency of immune effectors in heterogeneous host populations and provide effective immunity against diverse parasite strains, both of which would likely be verified in future studies.

6.5.4. Recombinant virus vaccines

Replication-deficient recombinant human viruses have an unprecedented ability to induce strong Th1-type immune responses (Rocha et al., 2004). Several studies have been performed to evaluate the ability of the recombinant viruses encoding *T. cruzi* genes in inducing a long-lasting and protective immunity against *T. cruzi* infection in experimental models. The priming of an immune response in mice with adenovirus encoding a single $CD8^+$ T-cell epitope derived from *TSSA* antigen, followed by boosting with vaccinia virus encoding the same $CD8^+$ T-cell epitope along with vaccinia virus encoding RANK-L as adjuvant provided significant protection against lethal *T. cruzi* infection (Miyahira et al., 2005). Further, recombinant adenoviruses encoding *ASP2* and *TS* antigens, alone or in combination, elicited strong antibody and T-cell responses and provided a high level of protection against lethal *T. cruzi* challenge in mice (Machado et al., 2006). A heterologous prime/boost approach using plasmid DNA followed by replication-defective recombinant adenovirus 5 enhanced the ASP-2 elicited, $CD4^+$ and $CD8^+$ T-cell-mediated protective immunity (de Alencar et al., 2009). These studies have opened another arena for enhancing the T-cell-mediated effector functions and anti-parasite immunity by using a heterologous plasmid DNA prime-replication deficient-virus boost vaccination strategy.

6.5.5. Genome-based vaccines

By using the sequence database of *T. cruzi* (El-Sayed et al., 2005), we have the potential to conduct a large-scale, unbiased screening of the *T. cruzi* genome for the identification of genes of interest. Sophisticated bioinformatic programmes are designed to evaluate gene functions on the basis of homologies to genes characterized in other organisms and the presence of motifs predictive of targeting, cellular localization, surface expression and functional characteristics of the gene product. Such programmes, thus, circumvent time-consuming, laborious experimental techniques and allow us to directly proceed from sequence information to antigenic target identification and vaccine design. Bhatia et al. (2004) have employed web-based bioinformatic tools coupled with an experimental strategy to identify the putative genes encoding glycosyl-phosphatidylinositol-anchored or secreted proteins in a *T. cruzi*-expressed sequence tag database. Molecular and biochemical characterization of eight of the sequences selected by this approach identified three candidates (e.g. TcG1, TcG2, TcG4) that were conserved in the genome of *T. cruzi* strains of clinical importance. These were expressed in different developmental stages of the parasite and immunogenic in multiple hosts. The selected candidates were recognized by lytic Abs and $CD8^+$ T cells in infected mice (Bhatia and Garg, 2008) and antibodies in dogs and humans (unpublished observations). Mice immunized with the selected antigens presented with a trypanolytic antibody response that was in agreement with the intensity of the surface expression of these proteins in infective and intracellular stages of the parasite (Bhatia et al., 2004) and the type 1 cytokine (IFN-γ > IL4) profile. This study validated the hypothesis that a *T. cruzi* sequence database committed to appropriate screening strategies would be an efficient resource for the identification of potential vaccine candidates.

Since then, we have examined the protective efficacy of TcG1, TcG2 and TcG4 (individually or in combination with and without IL-12 and GM-CSF cytokine adjuvants) in mice. Our data clearly established that co-delivery of the antigens elicited additive immunity and protection from *T. cruzi* infection than was noted with individual candidates (Bhatia and Garg, 2008, unpublished observations), and delivery of the three antigens with cytokine adjuvants as a DNA-prime/recombinant protein boost vaccine (TcVac2) (Gupta and Garg, 2010) proved to better elicit protective immunity than did DNA-prime/DNA-boost vaccine (TcVac1) (Bhatia and Garg, 2008). The IgG and Th1-biased, antigen-specific antibody (IgG2b/IgG1 ratio > 1) titres were higher in mice vaccinated with TcVac2 than that observed in TcVac1-immunized mice. Upon challenge infection, TcVac2-vaccinated mice expanded the antigen-specific IgG2b/IgG1 antibodies (TcG4 > TcG2 > TcG1) and elicited a $CD8^+$-dominant T-cell response (CD8/CD4 ratio > 3) associated with type 1 cytokines (IFN-γ and TNF-α) when compared to controls that elicited a mixed type 1/type 2 cytokine response against *T. cruzi* infection. Subsequently, TcVac2-immunized mice exhibited a 90–97% reduction in acute parasite burden in different organs, determined by sensitive Tc18SrDNA-specific real-time PCR. At the chronic stage, real-time PCR amplification of a parasite-specific Tc18SrDNA sequence detected no signal in the heart, skeletal muscle, spleen and liver tissue of TcVac2-immunized mice. Importantly, with control of parasite burden, the splenic activation of $CD8^+$ T cells and IFN-γ/TNF-α cytokines that are of pathological importance in chronic disease subsided and IL-4/IL-10 cytokines became dominant in vaccinated mice. Accordingly, the inflammatory infiltrate and tissue fibrosis were particularly absent in the heart and skeletal muscle of TcVac2-vaccinated chronic mice (Gupta and Garg, 2010). In comparison, extensive-to-moderate levels of inflammation, tissue fibrosis and persistence of parasites dominated in the heart and skeletal muscle of chronic control mice. This report, for the first time, showed a vaccine's efficacy in reducing the tissue parasite burden by first priming a polarized type 1 T-cell response and then switching to a type 2 dominance suppressing the evolution of immunopathology and tissue damage that are an outcome of consistent immune activation in chronic Chagasic disease.

6.5.6. Therapeutic vaccines

Today, >20 million people are estimated to be infected by *T. cruzi* in Latin America and developed countries. In response to the WHO call for control of *T. cruzi,* even if the national governments develop and implement very successful strategies for control of transmission by vector, oral consumption of contaminated food, blood or organ donation and congenital transmission, many more will become infected in decades to come. Thus, post-exposure immunoprophylactic or therapeutic treatment against *T. cruzi* is required to prevent the progression of chronic disease in this population. The overall basis for therapeutic vaccines is to modulate or enhance the multiple effector mechanisms against *T. cruzi* so as to clear the parasite's persistence in the infected host. Accordingly, several candidate antigens (e.g. TSA-1, Tc52, Tc24 and ASP-2) have been tested for protective efficacy in acutely or chronically infected mice. When tested in mice immediately after infection or within 2 weeks post-infection, TSA-1 and Tc24 (as a DNA vaccine) have been shown to improve the survival and preservation of cardiac structure (Dumonteil et al., 2004; Sanchez-Burgos et al., 2007) associated with a vaccine-induced rapid increase in the number of $CD4^+$ and $CD8^+$ T cells (Zapata-Estrella et al., 2006). However, these same candidates were not protective in chronically infected mice or infected dogs (reviewed in Quijano-Hernandez et al., 2008). ASP2 and TS (individually or in combination as DNA vaccine) did not limit parasitaemia or improve the survival rate in infected mice (Dumonteil, 2007; Sanchez-Burgos et al., 2007) despite their known efficacy as a prophylactic vaccine. Likewise, SA85 (member of TS family) protein vaccination of acutely infected mice was not effective in reducing the parasite burden and inflammatory pathology. The reasons for the inefficacy of the therapeutic vaccines are not clear, and it may be that therapeutic vaccines failed to modulate the existing host response to protective Th1. Indeed, a careful dosage of TSA1/Tc24 DNA vaccine redirected the immune response to a Th1 type as evidenced by the activation of IFN-γ-producing $CD4^+$ and $CD8^+$ T cells and decreased parasitaemia in acutely infected mice (Limon-Flores et al., 2010). However, the observation of increased myocarditis in infected mice inoculated with TSA1 DNA vaccine indicates that the level of activation of CD4/CD8T cells (Zapata-Estrella et al., 2006) by vaccine needs to be regulated so as to not exacerbate the disease state.

We have shown that benznidazole treatment given to infected rats at 45 dpi, that is, after immune control of acute parasitaemia, was beneficial in controlling parasite persistence and inflammatory pathology; however, this treatment failed to avert cardiac remodelling and deterioration of ventricular contractility. Instead, maximal benefits were obtained when infected rats were treated, in conjunction with benznidazole, with PBN antioxidant to prevent free radical-mediated oxidative insult and mitochondrial deficiencies, resulting in the preservation of metabolic (mitochondrial) and contractile activity in chagasic hearts (Wen et al., 2010). We propose that therapeutic vaccines targeted to achieve a rapid, short-lived stimulation of type 1 cellular immunity to attack the persistent parasites, but prevent cellular injury, along with adjunct therapies capable of controlling the onset of oxidative insult and mitochondrial deficiencies, would prove to be maximally beneficial in preserving cardiac structure and function in Chagas disease.

6.6. FUTURE PROSPECTS

Taken together, studies in experimental models have delineated the effector mechanisms that are essential in providing resistance to *T. cruzi* infection. Several defined vaccine candidates are known to elicit partially protective immunity against *T. cruzi*. A systemic approach to vaccine development against *T. cruzi* in future studies would require further characterization of protective immune responses, development of efficient antigen-delivery systems and use of adjuvants and vaccination regimens to enhance the protective responses to known vaccine candidates. Testing and optimization of the genes or gene-mixes consisting of protective candidates that synergize in their antigenic activity would facilitate the formulation of vaccines capable of providing maximally protective immunity against multiple *T. cruzi* strains in different hosts. Further development of animal models (e.g. dogs) would be essential for conducting the field studies and adequately assessing the protective efficacy of vaccines in providing short- and long-term immunity before a clinical trial in humans can be envisioned.

DNA vaccines have demonstrated efficacy in mice; however, the results of DNA vaccination in humans have so far been disappointing. Thus, a shift to heterologous prime/boost approaches that appear to be better than the DNA or protein-based vaccines in eliciting protective immunity against *T. cruzi* is not surprising. However, a careful analysis of cost–benefit ratio will be required to justify the higher cost of producing and delivering heterologous prime/boost vaccines.

To date, vaccines have focused on eliciting type 1 T-cell-adaptive immunity. Yet, the role of $CD4^+$ and $CD8^+$ T cells or of the non-conventional T cell subsets (e.g. NK or $\gamma\delta$ T cells) in eliciting memory responses that can provide effective helper and cytotoxic functions needs to be addressed to support studies of whether vaccines elicit memory response and if vaccine-induced memory responses are expanded and effectively eliminate the parasite.

Accordingly, future efforts should address the role of different components of innate responses in controlling *T. cruzi* as well as the design of strategies to enhance these effectors to effectively eliminate parasites during acute infection and provide sterile immunity. Innate responses also contribute to the evolution of adaptive cellular immune responses that remain largely unresolved. For example, recent studies indicate that *T. cruzi*-derived components are recognized by TLR2 (GPI-anchor and Tc52), TLR4 (GIPL) and TLR9 (genomic DNA), and that the TLR-mediated activation of MyD88- and TRIF-dependent innate signalling pathways in macrophages and dendritic cells modulates the activation and expression of pro-inflammatory cytokines (e.g. IL-12) and Th1 cell development that provide resistance to *T. cruzi* infection (Kayama and Takeda, 2010). A novel TLR-independent, host–parasite interaction system mediated by Ca^{2+} is also postulated (Kayama and Takeda, 2010). Thus, an understanding of the complex nature of the innate immune responses and their role in development of protective, long-term immunity will be necessary for the development of adjuvants to enhance the efficacy of existing vaccine candidates against *T. cruzi* and Chagas disease.

ACKNOWLEDGEMENTS

The work in N. J. G.'s laboratory has been supported in part by grants from the American Heart Association, John Sealy Memorial Endowment Fund for Biomedical Research, American Health Assistance Foundation and National Institutes of Health. The work in J. C. V.-C.'s laboratory has been supported by the National Institute of Allergy and Infection Diseases and the Secretaria de Investigacion y Estudios Avanzados de la Universidad Autónoma del Estado de México. S. G. is an awardee of a postdoctoral fellowship from the Sealy Center of Vaccine Development. Our thanks are due to Ms. Mardelle Susman for proofreading and editing the chapter.

REFERENCES

Abrahamsohn, I.A., Coffman, R.L., 1996. *Trypanosoma cruzi*: IL-10, TNF, IFN-gamma, and IL-12 regulate innate and acquired immunity to infection. Exp. Parasitol. 84, 231–244.

Aliberti, J.C., Souto, J.T., Marino, A.P., Lannes-Vieira, J., Teixeira, M.M., Farber, J., et al., 2001. Modulation of chemokine production and inflammatory responses in interferon-gamma- and tumor necrosis factor-R1-deficient mice during *Trypanosoma cruzi* infection. Am. J. Pathol. 158, 1433–1440.

Almeida, I.C., Gazzinelli, R.T., 2001. Proinflammatory activity of glycosylphosphatidylinositol anchors derived from *Trypanosoma cruzi*: structural and functional analyses. J. Leukoc. Biol. 70, 467–477.

Almeida, I.C., Camargo, M.M., Procopio, D.O., Silva, L.S., Mehlert, A., Travassos, L.R., et al., 2000. Highly purified glycosylphosphatidylinositols from *Trypanosoma cruzi* are potent proinflammatory agents. EMBO J. 19, 1476–1485.

Araujo, A.F., de Alencar, B.C., Vasconcelos, J.R., Hiyane, M.I., Marinho, C.R., Penido, M.L., et al., 2005. CD8+-T-cell-dependent control of *Trypanosoma cruzi* infection in a highly susceptible mouse strain after immunization with recombinant proteins based on amastigote surface protein 2. Infect. Immun. 73, 6017–6025.

Ba, X., Gupta, S., Davidson, M., Garg, N.J., 2010. *Trypanosoma cruzi* induces ROS-PARP-1-RelA pathway for up regulation of cytokine expression in cardiomyocytes. J. Biol. Chem. 285, 11596–11606.

Bern, C., Montgomery, S.P., 2009. An estimate of the burden of Chagas disease in the United States. Clin. Infect. Dis. 49, e52–e54.

Bhatia, V., Garg, N., 2005. Current status and future prospects for a vaccine against American trypanosomiasis. Expert Rev. Vaccines 4, 867–880.

Bhatia, V., Garg, N.J., 2008. Previously unrecognized vaccine candidates control *Trypanosoma cruzi* infection and immunopathology in mice. Clin. Vaccine Immunol. 15, 1158–1164.

Bhatia, V., Sinha, M., Luxon, B., Garg, N., 2004. Utility of *Trypanosoma cruzi* sequence database for the identification of potential vaccine candidates: in silico and in vitro screening. Infect. Immun. 72, 6245–6254.

Bhatia, V., Wen, J.-J., Zacks, M.A., Garg, N.J., 2009. American trypanosomiasis and perspectives on vaccine development. In: Stanberry, L.R., Barrett, A.D. (Eds.), Vaccines for Biodefense and Emerging and Neglected Diseases. Academic Press, New York.

Bonney, K.M., Engman, D.M., 2008. Chagas heart disease pathogenesis: one mechanism or many? Curr. Mol. Med. 8, 510–518.

Boscardin, S.B., Kinoshita, S.S., Fujimura, A.E., Rodrigues, M.M., 2003. Immunization with cDNA expressed by amastigotes of *Trypanosoma cruzi* elicits protective immune response against experimental infection. Infect. Immun. 71, 2744–2757.

Brener, Z., Gazzinelli, R.T., 1997. Immunological control of *Trypanosoma cruzi* infection and pathogenesis of Chagas' disease. Int. Arch. Allergy Immunol. 114, 103–110.

Campos, S.V., Strabelli, T.M., Amato Neto, V., Silva, C.P., Bacal, F., Bocchi, E.A., et al., 2008. Risk factors for Chagas' disease reactivation after heart transplantation. J. Heart Lung Transplant. 27, 597–602.

Cardoni, R.L., Antunez, M.I., Morales, C., Nantes, I.R., 1997. Release of reactive oxygen species by phagocytic cells in response to live parasites in mice infected with *Trypanosoma cruzi*. Am. J. Trop. Med. Hyg. 56, 329–334.

Cazorla, S.I., Becker, P.D., Frank, F.M., Ebensen, T., Sartori, M.J., Corral, R.S., et al., 2008a. Oral vaccination with Salmonella enterica as a cruzipain-DNA delivery system confers protective immunity against *Trypanosoma cruzi*. Infect. Immun. 76, 324–333.

Cazorla, S.I., Frank, F.M., Becker, P.D., Corral, R.S., Guzman, C.A., Malchiodi, E.L., 2008b. Prime-boost immunization with cruzipain co-administered with MALP-2 triggers a protective immune response able to decrease parasite burden and tissue injury in an experimental *Trypanosoma cruzi* infection model. Vaccine 26, 1999–2009.

CDC, 2006. Chagas disease after organ transplantation—Los Angeles, California, 2006. MMWR Morb. Mortal. Wkly. Rep. 55, 798–800.

CDC, 2007. Blood donor screening for Chagas disease—United States, 2006–2007. MMWR Morb. Mortal. Wkly. Rep. 56, 141–143.

Chou, B., Hisaeda, H., Shen, J., Duan, X., Imai, T., Tu, L., et al., 2008. Critical contribution of immunoproteasomes in the induction of protective immunity against *Trypanosoma cruzi*

in mice vaccinated with a plasmid encoding a CTL epitope fused to green fluorescence protein. Microbes Infect. 10, 241–250.
Claser, C., Espindola, N.M., Sasso, G., Vaz, A.J., Boscardin, S.B., Rodrigues, M.M., 2007. Immunologically relevant strain polymorphism in the Amastigote Surface Protein 2 of *Trypanosoma cruzi*. Microbes Infect. 9, 1011–1019.
Cordova, E., Boschi, A., Ambrosioni, J., Cudos, C., Corti, M., 2008. Reactivation of Chagas disease with central nervous system involvement in HIV-infected patients in Argentina, 1992–2007. Int. J. Infect. Dis. 12, 587–592.
Costa, F., Franchin, G., Pereira-Chioccola, V.L., Ribeirao, M., Schenkman, S., Rodrigues, M. M., 1998. Immunization with a plasmid DNA containing the gene of trans-sialidase reduces *Trypanosoma cruzi* infection in mice. Vaccine 16, 768–774.
Coura, J.R., 1996. Current prospects of specific treatment of Chagas' disease. Bol. Chil. Parasitol. 51, 69–75.
D'Almeida, P., Keitel, E., Bittar, A., Goldani, J., Santos, A., Neumann, J., et al., 1996. Long-term evaluation of kidney donors. Transplant. Proc. 28, 93–94.
de Alencar, B.C., Persechini, P.M., Haolla, F.A., de Oliveira, G., Silverio, J.C., Lannes-Vieira, J., et al., 2009. Perforin and gamma interferon expression are required for CD4+ and CD8+ T-cell-dependent protective immunity against a human parasite, *Trypanosoma cruzi*, elicited by heterologous plasmid DNA prime-recombinant adenovirus 5 boost vaccination. Infect. Immun. 77, 4383–4395.
de Andrade, A.L., Zicker, F., de Oliveira, R.M., Almeida Silva, S., Luquetti, A., Travassos, L.R., et al., 1996. Randomised trial of efficacy of benznidazole in treatment of early *Trypanosoma cruzi* infection [see comments]. Lancet 348, 1407–1413.
de Oliveira, T.B., Pedrosa, R.C., Filho, D.W., 2007. Oxidative stress in chronic cardiopathy associated with Chagas disease. Int. J. Cardiol. 116, 357–363.
Dhiman, M., Nakayasu, E.S., Madaiah, Y.H., Reynolds, B.K., Wen, J.J., Almeida, I.C., et al., 2008. Enhanced nitrosative stress during *Trypanosoma cruzi* infection causes nitrotyrosine modification of host proteins: implications in Chagas' disease. Am. J. Pathol. 173, 728–740.
Dhiman, M., Estrada-Franco, J.G., Pando, J., Ramirez-Aguilar, F., Spratt, H., Vasquez-Corzo, S., et al., 2009. Increased myeloperoxidase activity and protein nitration are indicators of inflammation in chagasic patients. Clin. Vaccine Immunol. 16, 660–666.
Donnelly, J.J., Wahren, B., Liu, M.A., 2005. DNA vaccines: progress and challenges. J. Immunol. 175, 633–639.
DosReis, G.A., 1997. Cell-mediated immunity in experimental *Trypanosoma cruzi* infection. Parasitol. Today 13, 335–342.
Duan, X., Yonemitsu, Y., Chou, B., Yoshida, K., Tanaka, S., Hasegawa, M., et al., 2009. Efficient protective immunity against *Trypanosoma cruzi* infection after nasal vaccination with recombinant Sendai virus vector expressing amastigote surface protein-2. Vaccine 27, 6154–6159.
Dubner, S., Schapachnik, E., Riera, A.R., Valero, E., 2008. Chagas disease: state-of-the-art of diagnosis and management. Cardiol. J. 15, 493–504.
Dumonteil, E., 2007. DNA vaccines against protozoan parasites: advances and challenges. J. Biomed. Biotechnol. 2007, 90520.
Dumonteil, E., Escobedo-Ortegon, J., Reyes-Rodriguez, N., Arjona-Torres, A., Ramirez-Sierra, M.J., 2004. Immunotherapy of *Trypanosoma cruzi* infection with DNA vaccines in mice. Infect. Immun. 72, 46–53.
Duschak, V.G., Couto, A.S., 2007. An insight on targets and patented drugs for chemotherapy of Chagas disease. Recent Pat. Antiinfect. Drug Discov. 2, 19–51.
Duschak, V.G., Couto, A.S., 2009. Cruzipain, the major cysteine protease of *Trypanosoma cruzi*: a sulfated glycoprotein antigen as relevant candidate for vaccine development and drug target. A review. Curr. Med. Chem. 16, 3174–3202.

Duthie, M.S., Kahn, S.J., 2005. NK cell activation and protection occur independently of natural killer T cells during *Trypanosoma cruzi* infection. Int. Immunol. 17, 607–613.
Duthie, M.S., Kahn, S.J., 2006. During acute *Trypanosoma cruzi* infection highly susceptible mice deficient in natural killer cells are protected by a single alpha-galactosylceramide treatment. Immunology 119, 355–361.
Duthie, M.S., Khan, M., Zakayan, A., White, M., Kahn, S.J., Kahn, S.J., 2007. Parasite-induced chronic inflammation is not exacerbated by immunotherapy before or during *Trypanosoma cruzi* infection. Clin. Vaccine Immunol. 14, 1005–1012.
Eickhoff, C.S., Giddings, O.K., Yoshida, N., Hoft, D.F., 2010. Immune responses to gp82 provide protection against mucosal *Trypanosoma cruzi* infection. Mem. Inst. Oswaldo Cruz 105, 687–691.
Eickhoff, C.S., Vasconcelos, J.R., Sullivan, N.L., Blazevic, A., Bruna-Romero, O., Rodrigues, M.M., Hoft, D.F., 2011. Co-administration of a plasmid DNA encoding IL-15 improves long term protection of a genetic vaccine against Trypanosoma cruzi. PLoS Negl. Trop. Dis. 5 (3), e983.
El-Sayed, N.M., Myler, P.J., Bartholomeu, D.C., Nilsson, D., Aggarwal, G., Tran, A.N., et al., 2005. The genome sequence of *Trypanosoma cruzi*, etiologic agent of Chagas disease. Science 309, 409–415.
Fontanella, G.H., De Vusser, K., Laroy, W., Daurelio, L., Nocito, A.L., Revelli, S., et al., 2008. Immunization with an engineered mutant trans-sialidase highly protects mice from experimental *Trypanosoma cruzi* infection: a vaccine candidate. Vaccine 26, 2322–2334.
Fralish, B.H., Tarleton, R.L., 2003. Genetic immunization with LYT1 or a pool of trans-sialidase genes protects mice from lethal *Trypanosoma cruzi* infection. Vaccine 21, 3070–3080.
Frank, F.M., Petray, P.B., Cazorla, S.I., Munoz, M.C., Corral, R.S., Malchiodi, E.L., 2003. Use of a purified *Trypanosoma cruzi* antigen and CpG oligodeoxynucleotides for immunoprotection against a lethal challenge with trypomastigotes. Vaccine 22, 77–86.
Garcia, G.A., Arnaiz, M.R., Esteva, M.I., Laucella, S.A., Garavaglia, P.A., Ibarra, S.E., et al., 2008. Evaluation of immune responses raised against Tc13 antigens of *Trypanosoma cruzi* in the outcome of murine experimental infection. Parasitology 135, 347–357.
Garg, N., 2005. Mitochondrial disorders in chagasic cardiomyopathy. Front. Biosci. 10, 1341–1354.
Garg, N., Tarleton, R.L., 1998. Elicitation of protective cellular and humoral immune responses to *Trypanosoma cruzi* infection using DNA vaccines can be augmented with cytokines. New Delhi, India, Proceedings 10th International Congress of Immunology.
Garg, N., Tarleton, R.L., 2002. Genetic immunization elicits antigen-specific protective immune responses and decreases disease severity in *Trypanosoma cruzi* infection. Infect. Immun. 70, 5547–5555.
Garg, N., Nunes, M.P., Tarleton, R.L., 1997. Delivery by *Trypanosoma cruzi* of proteins into the MHC class I antigen processing and presentation pathway. J. Immunol. 158, 3293–3302.
Garraud, O., Andreu, G., Elghouzzi, M.H., Laperche, S., Lefrere, J.J., 2007. Measures to prevent transfusion-associated protozoal infections in non-endemic countries. Travel Med. Infect. Dis. 5, 110–112.
Giddings, O.K., Eickhoff, C.S., Sullivan, N.L., Hoft, D.F., 2010. Intranasal vaccinations with the trans-sialidase antigen plus CpG adjuvant induce mucosal immunity protective against conjunctival *Trypanosoma cruzi* challenges. Infect. Immun. 78, 1333–1338.
Gupta, S., Garg, N.J., 2010. Prophylactic efficacy of TcVac2 against *Trypanosoma cruzi* in mice. PLoS Negl. Trop. Dis. 4 (8), e797.
Gupta, S., Bhatia, V., Wen, J.J., Wu, Y., Huang, M.H., Garg, N.J., 2009a. *Trypanosoma cruzi* infection disturbs mitochondrial membrane potential and ROS production rate in cardiomyocytes. Free Radic. Biol. Med. 47, 1414–1421.
Gupta, S., Wen, J.J., Garg, N.J., 2009b. Oxidative stress in Chagas disease. Interdiscip. Perspect. Infect. Dis. 2009, 1–8.

Gutierrez, F.R., Guedes, P.M., Gazzinelli, R.T., Silva, J.S., 2009. The role of parasite persistence in pathogenesis of Chagas heart disease. Parasite Immunol. 31, 673–685.

Haolla, F.A., Claser, C., de Alencar, B.C., Tzelepis, F., de Vasconcelos, J.R., de Oliveira, G., et al., 2009. Strain-specific protective immunity following vaccination against experimental *Trypanosoma cruzi* infection. Vaccine 27, 5644–5653.

Harth, G., Mills, A.A., Lin, T., Araujo, F.G., 1994. *Trypanosoma cruzi* glycoprotein of M(r). 56,000 characterization and assessment of its potential to protect against fatal parasite infections. Mol. Microbiol. 11, 261–271.

Hoft, D.F., Eickhoff, C.S., Giddings, O.K., Vasconcelos, J.R., Rodrigues, M.M., 2007. Trans-sialidase recombinant protein mixed with CpG motif-containing oligodeoxynucleotide induces protective mucosal and systemic *Trypanosoma cruzi* immunity involving $CD8^+$ CTL and B cell-mediated cross-priming. J. Immunol. 179, 6889–6900.

Huygen, K., 2005. Plasmid DNA vaccination. Microbes Infect. 7, 932–938.

Johnson, P., Neal, R.A., Gall, D., 1963. Protective effect of killed *Trypanosome* vaccines with incorporated adjuvants. Nature 200, 83.

Katae, M., Miyahira, Y., Takeda, K., Matsuda, H., Yagita, H., Okumura, K., et al., 2002. Coadministration of an interleukin-12 gene and a *Trypanosoma cruzi* gene improves vaccine efficacy. Infect. Immun. 70, 4833–4840.

Kayama, H., Takeda, K., 2010. The innate immune response to *Trypanosoma cruzi* infection. Microbes Infect. 12, 511–517.

Krautz, G.M., Kissinger, J.C., Krettli, A.U., 2000. The targets of the lytic antibody response against *Trypanosoma cruzi*. Parasitol. Today 16, 31–34.

Laderach, D., Cerban, F., Motran, C., Vottero de Cima, E., Gea, S., 1996. *Trypanosoma cruzi*: the major cysteinyl proteinase (cruzipain) is a relevant immunogen of parasite acidic antigens (FIII). Int. J. Parasitol. 26, 1249–1254.

Leiby, D.A., Rentas, F.J., Nelson, K.E., Stambolis, V.A., Ness, P.M., Parnis, C., et al., 2000. Evidence of *Trypanosoma cruzi* infection (Chagas' disease) among patients undergoing cardiac surgery. Circulation 102, 2978–2982.

Leiby, D.A., Herron, R.M., Jr., Read, E.J., Lenes, B.A., Stumpf, R.J., 2002. Trypanosoma cruzi in Los Angeles and Miami blood donors: impact of evolving donor demographics on seroprevalence and implications for transfusion transmission. Transfusion 42, 549–555.

Leon, J.S., Engman, D.M., 2003. The significance of autoimmunity in the pathogenesis of Chagas heart disease. Front. Biosci. 8, e315–e322.

Limon-Flores, A.Y., Cervera-Cetina, R., Tzec-Arjona, J.L., Ek-Macias, L., Sanchez-Burgos, G., Ramirez-Sierra, M.J., et al., 2010. Effect of a combination DNA vaccine for the prevention and therapy of *Trypanosoma cruzi* infection in mice: role of $CD4^+$ and $CD8^+$ T cells. Vaccine 28, 7414–7419.

Luhrs, K.A., Fouts, D.L., Manning, J.E., 2003. Immunization with recombinant paraflagellar rod protein induces protective immunity against *Trypanosoma cruzi* infection. Vaccine 21, 3058–3069.

Macao, L.B., Filho, D.W., Pedrosa, R.C., Pereira, A., Backes, P., Torres, M.A., et al., 2007. Antioxidant therapy attenuates oxidative stress in chronic cardiopathy associated with Chagas' disease. Int. J. Cardiol. PMID: 17328977, [Epub ahead of print].

Machado, A.V., Cardoso, J.E., Claser, C., Rodrigues, M.M., Gazzinelli, R.T., Bruna-Romero, O., 2006. Long-term protective immunity induced against *Trypanosoma cruzi* infection after vaccination with recombinant adenoviruses encoding amastigote surface protein-2 and trans-sialidase. Hum. Gene Ther. 17, 898–908.

Marin-Neto, J.A., Cunha-Neto, E., Maciel, B.C., Simoes, M.V., 2007. Pathogenesis of chronic Chagas heart disease. Circulation 115, 1109–1123.

Martins, G.A., Cardoso, M.A., Aliberti, J.C., Silva, J.S., 1998. Nitric oxide-induced apoptotic cell death in the acute phase of *Trypanosoma cruzi* infection in mice. Immunol. Lett. 63, 113–120.

Melo, R.C., Fabrino, D.L., D'Avila, H., Teixeira, H.C., Ferreira, A.P., 2003. Production of hydrogen peroxide by peripheral blood monocytes and specific macrophages during experimental infection with *Trypanosoma cruzi* in vivo. Cell Biol. Int. 27, 853–861.

Menezes, H., 1965. The use of adjuvants in the vaccination of mice with lyophilized "*Trypanosoma cruzi*" Hospital (Rio J.) 68, 1341–1346.

Miller, M.J., Wrightsman, R.A., Manning, J.E., 1996. *Trypanosoma cruzi*: protective immunity in mice immunized with paraflagellar rod proteins is associated with a T-helper type 1 response. Exp. Parasitol. 84, 156–167.

Miyahira, Y., 2008. *Trypanosoma cruzi* infection from the view of CD8+ T cell immunity—an infection model for developing T cell vaccine. Parasitol. Int. 57, 38–48.

Miyahira, Y., Akiba, H., Katae, M., Kubota, K., Kobayashi, S., Takeuchi, T., et al., 2003. Cutting edge: a potent adjuvant effect of ligand to receptor activator of NF-kappa B gene for inducing antigen-specific $CD8^+$ T cell response by DNA and viral vector vaccination. J. Immunol. 171, 6344–6348.

Miyahira, Y., Takashima, Y., Kobayashi, S., Matsumoto, Y., Takeuchi, T., Ohyanagi-Hara, M., et al., 2005. Immune responses against a single $CD8^+$-T-cell epitope induced by virus vector vaccination can successfully control *Trypanosoma cruzi* infection. Infect. Immun. 73, 7356–7365.

Morell, M., Thomas, M.C., Caballero, T., Alonso, C., Lopez, M.C., 2006. The genetic immunization with paraflagellar rod protein-2 fused to the HSP70 confers protection against late *Trypanosoma cruzi* infection. Vaccine 24, 7046–7055.

Munoz-Fernandez, M.A., Fernandez, M.A., Fresno, M., 1992a. Activation of human macrophages for the killing of intracellular *Trypanosoma cruzi* by TNF-alpha and IFN-gamma through a nitric oxide-dependent mechanism. Immunol. Lett. 33, 35–40.

Munoz-Fernandez, M.A., Fernandez, M.A., Fresno, M., 1992b. Synergism between tumor necrosis factor-alpha and interferon-gamma on macrophage activation for the killing of intracellular *Trypanosoma cruzi* through a nitric oxide-dependent mechanism. Eur. J. Immunol. 22, 301–307.

Oliveira, I., Torrico, F., Munoz, J., Gascon, J., 2010. Congenital transmission of Chagas disease: a clinical approach. Expert Rev. Anti Infect. Ther. 8, 945–956.

Ouaissi, A., Guilvard, E., Delneste, Y., Caron, G., Magistrelli, G., Herbault, N., et al., 2002. The *Trypanosoma cruzi* Tc52-released protein induces human dendritic cell maturation, signals via Toll-like receptor 2, and confers protection against lethal infection. J. Immunol. 168, 6366–6374.

Padilla, A.M., Bustamante, J.M., Tarleton, R.L., 2009. $CD8^+$ T cells in *Trypanosoma cruzi* infection. Curr. Opin. Immunol. 21, 385–390.

Pan, C.H., Chen, H.W., Tao, M.H., 1999. Modulation of immune responses to DNA vaccines by codelivery of cytokine genes. J. Formos. Med. Assoc. 98, 722–729.

Pereira, V.R., Lorena, V.M., Nakazawa, M., Luna, C.F., Silva, E.D., Ferreira, A.G., et al., 2005. Humoral and cellular immune responses in BALB/c and C57BL/6 mice immunized with cytoplasmic (CRA) and flagellar (FRA) recombinant repetitive antigens, in acute experimental *Trypanosoma cruzi* infection. Parasitol. Res. 96, 154–161.

Perez-Fuentes, R., Guegan, J.F., Barnabe, C., Lopez-Colombo, A., Salgado-Rosas, H., Torres-Rasgado, E., et al., 2003. Severity of chronic Chagas disease is associated with cytokine/antioxidant imbalance in chronically infected individuals. Int. J. Parasitol. 33, 293–299.

Planelles, L., Thomas, M.C., Alonso, C., Lopez, M.C., 2001. DNA immunization with *Trypanosoma cruzi* HSP70 fused to the KMP11 protein elicits a cytotoxic and humoral immune response against the antigen and leads to protection. Infect. Immun. 69, 6558–6563.

Quijano-Hernandez, I.A., Bolio-Gonzalez, M.E., Rodriguez-Buenfil, J.C., Ramirez-Sierra, M. J., Dumonteil, E., 2008. Therapeutic DNA vaccine against *Trypanosoma cruzi* infection in dogs. Ann. N. Y. Acad. Sci. 1149, 343–346.

Rassi, A., Jr., Rassi, A., Marin-Neto, J.A., 2010. Chagas disease. Lancet 375, 1388–1402.

Ribeiro, I., Sevcsik, A.M., Alves, F., Diap, G., Don, R., Harhay, M.O., et al., 2009. New, improved treatments for Chagas disease: from the R&D pipeline to the patients. PLoS Negl. Trop. Dis. 3, e484.

Ribeiro, C.M., Budni, P., Pedrosa, R.C., Farias, M.S., Parisotto, E.B., Dalmarco, E.M., et al., 2010. Antioxidant therapy attenuates oxidative insult caused by benzonidazole in chronic Chagas' heart disease. Int. J. Cardiol. 145, 27–33.

Rocha, M.O., Ribeiro, A.L., Teixeira, M.M., 2003. Clinical management of chronic Chagas cardiomyopathy. Front. Biosci. 8, e44–e54.

Rocha, C.D., Caetano, B.C., Machado, A.V., Bruna-Romero, O., 2004. Recombinant viruses as tools to induce protective cellular immunity against infectious diseases. Int. Microbiol. 7, 83–94.

Rodriques-Coura, J., de Castro, S.L., 2002. A critical review on Chagas disease chemotherapy. Mem. Inst. Oswaldo Cruz 97, 3–24.

Roffe, E., Souza, A.L., Caetano, B.C., Machado, P.P., Barcelos, L.S., Russo, R.C., et al., 2006. A DNA vaccine encoding CCL4/MIP-1beta enhances myocarditis in experimental *Trypanosoma cruzi* infection in rats. Microbes Infect. 8, 2745–2755.

Sanchez-Burgos, G., Mezquita-Vega, R.G., Escobedo-Ortegon, J., Ramirez-Sierra, M.J., Arjona-Torres, A., Ouaissi, A., et al., 2007. Comparative evaluation of therapeutic DNA vaccines against *Trypanosoma cruzi* in mice. FEMS Immunol. Med. Microbiol. 50, 333–341.

Santori, F.R., Paranhos-Bacalla, G.S., Franco, D.A.S.J., Yamauchi, L.M., Araya, J.E., Yoshida, N., 1996. A recombinant protein based on the *Trypanosoma cruzi* metacyclic trypomastigote 82-kilodalton antigen that induces and effective immune response to acute infection. Infect. Immun. 64, 1093–1099.

Sartori, A.M., Lopes, M.H., Caramelli, B., Duarte, M.I., Pinto, P.L., Neto, V., et al., 1995. Simultaneous occurrence of acute myocarditis and reactivated Chagas' disease in a patient with AIDS. Clin. Infect. Dis. 21, 1297–1299.

Schmunis, G.A., Cruz, J.R., 2005. Safety of the blood supply in Latin America. Clin. Microbiol. Rev. 18, 12–29.

Schnapp, A.R., Eickhoff, C.S., Sizemore, D., Curtiss, R., Hoft, D.F., 2002. Cruzipain induces both mucosal and systemic protection against *Trypanosoma cruzi* in mice. Infect. Immun. 70, 5065–5074.

Schofield, C.J., Jannin, J., Salvatella, R., 2006. The future of Chagas disease control. Trends Parasitol. 22, 583–588.

Scott, M.T., Neal, R.A., Woods, N.C., 1985. Immunization of marmosets with *Trypanosoma cruzi* cell surface glycoprotein (GP90). Trans. R. Soc. Trop. Med. Hyg. 79, 451–454.

Sepulveda, P., Hontebeyrie, M., Liegeard, P., Mascilli, A., Norris, K.A., 2000. DNA-Based immunization with *Trypanosoma cruzi* complement regulatory protein elicits complement lytic antibodies and confers protection against *Trypanosoma cruzi* infection. Infect. Immun. 68, 4986–4991.

Silveira, E.L.V., Claser, C., Haolla, F.A.B., Zanella, L.G., Rodrigues, M.M., 2008. Novel protective antigens expressed by *Trypanosoma cruzi* amastigotes provide immunity to mice highly susceptible to Chagas' disease. Clin. Vaccine Immunol. 15, 1292–1300.

Singh, M., O'Hagan, D.T., 2002. Recent advances in vaccine adjuvants. Pharm. Res. 19, 715–728.

Tanowitz, H.B., Machado, F.S., Jelicks, L.A., Shirani, J., de Carvalho, A.C., Spray, D.C., et al., 2009. Perspectives on *Trypanosoma cruzi*-induced heart disease (Chagas disease). Prog. Cardiovasc. Dis. 51, 524–539.

Tarleton, R.L., Grusby, M.J., Postan, M., Glimcher, L.H., 1996. *Trypanosoma cruzi* infection in MHC-deficient mice: further evidence for the role of both class I- and class II-restricted T cells in immune resistance and disease. Int. Immunol. 8, 13–22.

Tekiel, V., Alba-Soto, C.D., González Cappa, S.M., Postan, M., Sánchez, D.O., 2009. Identification of novel vaccine candidates for Chagas' disease by immunization with sequential fractions of a trypomastigote cDNA expression library. Vaccine 27, 1323–1332.

Vallejo, G.A., Guhl, F., Schaub, G.A., 2009. Triatominae-*Trypanosoma cruzi/T. rangeli*: vector-parasite interactions. Acta Trop. 110, 137–147.
Vasconcelos, J.R., Boscardin, S.B., Hiyane, M.I., Kinoshita, S.S., Fujimura, A.E., Rodrigues, M. M., 2003. A DNA-priming protein-boosting regimen significantly improves type 1 immune response but not protective immunity to *Trypanosoma cruzi* infection in a highly susceptible mouse strain. Immunol. Cell Biol. 81, 121–129.
Vasconcelos, J.R., Hiyane, M.I., Marinho, C.R., Claser, C., Machado, A.M., Gazzinelli, R.T., et al., 2004. Protective immunity against *Trypanosoma cruzi* infection in a highly susceptible mouse strain after vaccination with genes encoding the amastigote surface protein-2 and trans-sialidase. Hum. Gene Ther. 15, 878–886.
Warren, T.L., Weiner, G.J., 2000. Uses of granulocyte-macrophage colony-stimulating factor in vaccine development. Curr. Opin. Hematol. 7, 168–173.
Wen, J.-J., Vyatkina, G., Garg, N., 2004. Oxidative damage during chagasic cardiomyopathy development: role of mitochondrial oxidant release and inefficient antioxidant defense. Free Radic. Biol. Med. 37, 1821–1833.
Wen, J.-J., Bhatia, V., Popov, V.L., Garg, N.J., 2006a. Phenyl-alpha-tert-butyl nitrone reverses mitochondrial decay in acute Chagas disease. Am. J. Pathol. 169, 1953–1964.
Wen, J.J., Yachelini, P.C., Sembaj, A., Manzur, R.E., Garg, N., 2006b. Increased oxidative stress is correlated with mitochondrial dysfunction in chagasic patients. Free Radic. Biol. Med. 41, 270–276.
Wen, J.J., Dhiman, M., Whorton, E.B., Garg, N.J., 2008. Tissue-specific oxidative imbalance and mitochondrial dysfunction during *Trypanosoma cruzi* infection in mice. Microbes Infect. 10, 1201–1209.
Wen, J.-J., Gupta, S., Guan, Z., Dhiman, M., Condon, D., Lui, C.Y., et al., 2010. Phenyl-alpha-tert-butyl-nitrone and benzonidazole treatment controlled the mitochondrial oxidative stress and evolution of cardiomyopathy in chronic chagasic rats. J. Am. Coll. Cardiol. 55, 2499–2508.
Wizel, B., Garg, N., Tarleton, R.L., 1998. Vaccination with trypomastigote surface antigen 1-encoding plasmid DNA confers protection against lethal *Trypanosoma cruzi* infection. Infect. Immun. 66, 5073–5081.
World Health Organization, 2006. Report of the Scientific Working Group on Chagas Disease. Buenos Aires, Argentina UNDP/World Bank/WHO, http://www.who.int/tdr/diseases/chagas/swg_chagas.pdf.
World Health Organization, 2010. Chagas disease: control and elimination. Report of the Secretariat. WHO, Geneva. UNDP/World Bank/WHO, http://apps.who.int/gb/ebwha/pdf_files/WHA63/A63_17-en.pdf.
Wrightsman, R.A., Manning, J.E., 2000. Paraflagellar rod proteins administered with alum and IL-12 or recombinant adenovirus expressing IL-12 generates antigen-specific responses and protective immunity in mice against *Trypanosoma cruzi*. Vaccine 18, 1419–1427.
Wrightsman, R.A., Luhrs, K.A., Fouts, D., Manning, J.E., 2002. Paraflagellar rod protein-specific CD8+ cytotoxic T lymphocytes target *Trypanosoma cruzi*-infected host cells. Parasite Immunol. 24, 401–412.
Zacks, M.A., Wen, J.J., Vyatkina, G., Bhatia, V., Garg, N., 2005. An overview of chagasic cardiomyopathy: pathogenic importance of oxidative stress. An. Acad. Bras. Cienc. 77, 695–715.
Zapata-Estrella, H., Hummel-Newell, C., Sanchez-Burgos, G., Escobedo-Ortegon, J., Ramirez-Sierra, M.J., Arjona-Torres, A., et al., 2006. Control of *Trypanosoma cruzi* infection and changes in T-cell populations induced by a therapeutic DNA vaccine in mice. Immunol. Lett. 103, 186–191.
Zingales, B., Andrade, S.G., Briones, M.R., Campbell, D.A., Chiari, E., Fernandes, O., et al., 2009. A new consensus for *Trypanosoma cruzi* intraspecific nomenclature: second revision meeting recommends TcI to TcVI. Mem. Inst. Oswaldo Cruz 104, 1051–1054.

CHAPTER 7

Genetic Epidemiology of Chagas Disease

Sarah Williams-Blangero,* **John L. VandeBerg,*,†** **John Blangero,*** and **Rodrigo Corrêa-Oliveira‡,§**

Contents

Abstract Genetic epidemiological approaches hold great promise for improving the understanding of the determinants of susceptibility to infection with *Trypanosoma cruzi* and the causes of differential disease outcome in *T. cruzi*-infected individuals. To date, a variety of

* Department of Genetics, Texas Biomedical Research Institute, San Antonio, Texas, USA
† Southwest National Primate Research Center, San Antonio, Texas, USA
‡ Centro de Pesquisas Rene Rachou, FIOCRUZ, Belo Horizonte, Minas Gerais, Brazil
§ Instituto Nacional de Ciencia e Tecnologia em Doenças Tropicais—INCTDT, Belo Horizonte, Minas Gerais, Brazil

Advances in Parasitology, Volume 75
ISSN 0065-308X, DOI: 10.1016/B978-0-12-385863-4.00007-1

approaches have been used to understand the role of genetic factors in Chagas disease. Quantitative genetic techniques have been used to estimate the heritabilities for seropositivity for *T. cruzi* infection and traits that are associated with disease progression in chronic *T. cruzi* infection. These studies have demonstrated that a significant proportion of the variation in seropositivity and a number of traits related to Chagas disease progression is attributable to genetic factors. Candidate gene studies have provided intriguing evidence for the roles of numerous individual genes in determining cardiac outcomes in chronically infected individuals. Recent results from a long-term study of Chagas disease in a rural area of Brazil have documented that over 60% of the variation in seropositivity status is attributable to genetic factors in that population. Additionally, there are significant genetic effects on a number of electrocardiographic measures and other Chagas disease-related traits. The application of genome-wide approaches will yield new evidence for the roles of specific genes in Chagas disease.

7.1. INTRODUCTION

Over 100 years after the parasitic cause of Chagas disease, or American trypanosomiasis, was elucidated, *Trypanosoma cruzi* infection and chronic Chagas disease persist as major public health problems throughout South and Central America (WHO, 2010). Chagas disease is still one of the leading causes of cardiac disease in Latin America. It is estimated that 8–10 million people are infected with *T. cruzi* and that tens of millions more are at risk for infection (Dutra et al., 2005; Rassi et al., 2010; Sanchez-Sancho et al., 2010; WHO, 2010).

Despite the success of vector control programmes in some geographic regions, active transmission occurs in many areas of Latin America (e.g. Borges et al., 2006; Coll-Cardenas et al., 2004; Grijalva et al., 2003; Gurtler et al., 2005; Pinto et al., 2004; Rizzo et al., 2003). The disease is emerging in new geographic areas both in Latin America and elsewhere in the world (e.g. Aguilar et al., 2007; Briceño-Leon, 2007; Calzada et al., 2010; Norman et al., 2010). The disease is also increasing in importance as a public health concern in the United States and is now a reportable disease in two states (Beard et al., 2003; Bern and Montgomery, 2009; Busch et al., 2003; Leiby et al., 2002; McCarthy, 2003; Sarkar et al., 2010).

Chagas disease generally occurs in two phases. First, there is an acute phase lasting 2–3 months following infection with *T. cruzi* (Kirchhoff, 1999). Many individuals are asymptomatic throughout the acute phase of the illness, although between 5% and 10% of individuals experience severe, sometimes fatal, disease during this period (Kirchhoff, 1999). About 40% of those infected who survive the acute phase remain seropositive but never experience disease progression. In the remaining 60% of cases, the disease enters a quiescent phase lasting as long as 30 years. Out of this population, it is estimated that 2% will enter the chronic phase of the disease each year. The chronic phase is characterized by progressive cardiomyopathy, or by a digestive form of the disease associated with mega-colon and/or mega-oesophagus.

The cardiac form of chronic Chagas disease is evident in data generated from electrocardiograms (ECGs). The characteristics associated with Chagas disease include bradyarrhythmias, premature ventricular contractions, atrioventricular blocks and right bundle branch blocks (Biolo et al., 2010; Goldbaum et al., 2004; Jorge et al., 2003; Kirchhoff, 1999; Maguire et al., 1987; Prata, 2001; Rangel-Flores et al., 2001; Sosa-Hurado et al., 2003; Williams-Blangero et al., 2007; Yacoub et al., 2003). Some ECG characteristics such as an elongated QT interval have been suggested to predict mortality in chagasic patients (Salles et al., 2003, 2004).

There are no drugs that can be taken to prevent infection with *T. cruzi* (Garg and Bhatia, 2005; Urbina and Docampo, 2003). Two drugs have been used for the treatment of acute *T. cruzi* infection: nifurtimox and benznidazole. Although these drugs are effective in decreasing early parasitemia during the acute phase of disease, the evidence for their efficacy during the chronic phase of Chagas disease is inconclusive (Castro et al., 2006; Lescure et al., 2010; Rodriguez Coura and de Castro, 2002; Tanowitz et al., 2009). Both drugs are carcinogenic in a variety of animal models (Castro et al., 2006; Garcia-Zapata and Marsden, 1986; Teixeira et al., 1990a,b), and they have a broad range of side effects which make them difficult to tolerate for the 1–3 months of treatment routinely administered (Castro et al., 2006; Lescure et al., 2010; Tanowitz et al., 2009). As a result, there is no consensus on their use in treatment of the chronic phase of the disease in adults (Tanowitz et al., 2009).

The lack of a generally accepted pharmacological intervention for chronic Chagas disease highlights the value of genetic studies for this disease. Modern genetic approaches can facilitate the detection of potential novel drug targets based on genetic analysis of differential disease progression in *T. cruzi*-infected individuals. The identification of genes influencing Chagas disease can suggest novel biological pathways to be targeted in drug development efforts (Ohlstein et al., 2000; Schadt et al., 2003). In addition, the novel pathways identified by genetic analysis may be treatable with existing pharmaceutical drugs. Application of existing compounds to novel pathways in the disease could lead to relatively rapid availability of new treatments for Chagas disease.

7.2. GENETIC EPIDEMIOLOGICAL APPROACHES TO CHAGAS DISEASE

Genetic epidemiological approaches can be informative for improving our understanding of the determinants of differential susceptibility to *T. cruzi* infection and differential disease outcome in individuals who are chronically infected with *T. cruzi*. Because uninfected individuals are found in all populations which experience high rates of Chagas disease, the question of whether or not there is differential susceptibility to *T. cruzi* infection naturally arises. There is familial clustering of seronegativity for *T. cruzi* infection, and genetic epidemiological studies may be designed to assess whether or not there is a genetic component to differential susceptibility to infection, assuming universal exposure to risk of infection in the population.

Among seropositive individuals, there is significant variation in disease progression. Some individuals remain asymptomatic throughout their lives, while others experience varying degrees of cardiac involvement. The question of whether or not there is a genetic component to disease progression in infected individuals is also an interesting one, which can be addressed using genetic epidemiological approaches. Disease progression can be measured in a multitude of ways. Immunological correlates of Chagas disease and ECG variables provide measures of progression of cardiac Chagas disease that can be subjected to genetic analysis using a variety of approaches.

Depending upon the type of genetic epidemiological methods used, one can determine the percent of variation in the Chagas disease-related trait attributable to genetic factors, the chromosomal location of genetic effects on the traits, the specific genes involved in determination of the traits and the individual genetic variants responsible for observed patterns of variation in disease-related traits. The knowledge of specific genes involved in disease-related traits potentially may facilitate the development of powerful tools for improving public health. Genetic information may identify novel pathways to target in drug development efforts. It may also identify pathways that may be modulated by existing drugs already on the market for other purposes. Finally, genetic information may provide a means for developing predictive tests to assess likelihood of disease progression.

There is great value to being able to reliably predict disease progression in seropositive individuals. As noted above, the available treatments for Chagas disease are generally toxic and poorly tolerated. Development of a reliable prognostic test capable of identifying those individuals who will progress to disease will allow targeting of available treatments to the individuals most likely to develop disease.

Besides the potential role of host genetic factors, genetic variation within the pathogen may also play a role in susceptibility. Substantial effort has been devoted towards documenting the genetic variation among *T. cruzi* organisms (reviewed by Campbell et al., 2004; Macedo et al., 2004; Manoel-Caetano and Silva, 2007; Miles et al., 2009). Genetic variation in the parasitic organism *T. cruzi* has been implicated in differential disease outcome, but the importance of that impact remains to be fully elucidated (Buscaglia and Di Noia, 2003; Macedo et al., 2004; Sturm et al., 2003). Severe cardiac outcomes have been observed in infections with both Type I and Type II lineages of *T. cruzi* (e.g. Añez et al., 2004). Differences in disease epidemiology between major geographic areas, such as the lack of the digestive form of Chagas disease in Venezuela, have been hypothesized to be due to variation in the parasite. However, it is acknowledged that environmental, nutritional and host immunological factors may also account for this variation (Macedo et al., 2004). While parasite genetic factors are likely to play a role in determining differential outcome in Chagas disease, the precise nature of this role remains to be determined. Much work remains to be done before the role of parasite genetics in Chagas disease is fully understood (Sturm et al., 2003).

Tibayrenc (1998, 2007, 2010) has emphasized the importance of considering genetic variation both in parasites and in hosts in the study of Chagas disease. He has recommended developing an integrated genetic epidemiological model for infectious disease that incorporates consideration of genetic variation present in the parasite, the vector and the host when working to understand the population biology of a disease such as Chagas disease.

7.2.1. Epidemiological observations of familial clustering

Before an expensive search for individual genes influencing any disease is launched, there must be documented evidence of the involvement of genes in the disease. Familial clustering of a disease is one of the most basic pieces of evidence that genetic factors are involved in the determination of a disease. The clustering of Chagas disease in familial households has long been reported (e.g. Mott et al., 1976; Tibayrenc, 1998, 1999; Zicker et al., 1990). Most frequently, this clustering is attributed to environmental factors that correlate with household and that are thought to influence exposure to the vector. However, in one examination of familial clustering of seropositivity for *T. cruzi* infection and cardiac outcomes of Chagas disease in a population from Brazil, the possibility of genetic influences was explicitly considered (Silva-Grecco et al., 2010). In this study of 41 families ranging in size from 5 to 80 individuals, there was significant evidence for familial factors influencing both seropositivity and cardiac outcome traits, although no explicit statistical evidence for the role of a major gene with large effect in determining variation was found (Silva-Grecco et al., 2010).

7.2.2. Analyses of the heritability of Chagas disease-related traits

The heritability of a disease-related trait provides an overall estimate of the importance of genetic factors in determining that trait. For example, a heritability of 0.7 for a given trait indicates that approximately 70% of the variation in that trait is attributable to genetic factors within the sample examined.

There have been few quantitative genetic assessments of Chagas disease or Chagas disease-related traits. One of the first such studies assessed the biological and cultural correlates of immunoglobulin levels in an endemic Brazil population (Barbosa et al., 1981). This study utilized a path analysis approach to estimate the heritabilities of approximately 30% for both IgA and IgG and of approximately 10% for IgM (Barbosa et al., 1981). The pedigrees, which included a total of 390 individuals, for this study were built around 40-year-old patients who were in the chronic phase of Chagas disease.

For our own quantitative genetic studies of Chagas disease and related phenotypes, we generated pedigrees for families in the Posse region of Goiás through house-to-house surveys following the approach outlined in Williams-Blangero and Blangero (2006). Our study of the heritability of seropositivity for *T. cruzi* infection included a total of 525 individuals who belonged to a total of 146 pedigrees ranging in size from 2 to 103 individuals. In addition, we included 179 independent individuals to improve parameter estimation (Williams-Blangero et al., 1997). Analysing the dichotomous trait of seropositivity on an assumed underlying continuous distribution of liability, we determined the heritability of seropositivity for *T. cruzi* infection to be 0.56 indicating that over half of the variation in seropositivity for *T. cruzi* infection is attributable to genetic factors. These results strongly suggest a genetic component to susceptibility to infection with *T. cruzi*.

7.2.3. Candidate gene studies of Chagas disease

Given that family studies support the likelihood of genetic factors playing a role in Chagas disease susceptibility and response, one approach to causal gene discovery is to focus directly on known candidate genes on the basis of our cumulative biological knowledge regarding the underlying pathways involved in the disease. Once a candidate gene is chosen, it can be examined closely for potential variation that influences quantitative variation in the focal risk factors. The central difficulty with the classical candidate gene approach is the low prior probability of picking a functional gene, given our relatively incomplete knowledge about the biological processes underlying disease. Additionally, the classical candidate gene approach is limited to incremental progress, as much has to be already known about the gene to nominate it as a candidate. Novel discoveries are thus minimized using the classical candidate gene approach.

Ramasawmy and colleagues of the Heart Institute at the University of São Paulo School of Medicine in Brazil have conducted a number of candidate gene studies assessing the genetic effects of candidate genes on risk for development of chronic Chagas cardiomyopathy in individuals seropositive for *T. cruzi* infection (Ramasawmy et al., 2006, 2007, 2008, 2009). By assessing variation in specific genes in infected individuals with Chagas-related cardiomyopathy and asymptomatic individuals who are seropositive for *T. cruzi* infection, Ramaswamy and colleagues have provided intriguing, although relatively statistically weak, evidence of genes that may be involved in disease progression in infected individuals. Variation in the monocyte chemoattractant protein-1 gene (*CCL2/MCP-1*) is associated with development of cardiomyopathy in individuals with *T. cruzi* infection (Ramasawmy et al., 2006). Polymorphisms in the gene for lymphotoxin-alpha, which is a proinflammatory cytokine, have been demonstrated to be weakly ($p = 0.035$) associated with risk for cardiomyopathy in *T. cruzi*-positive individuals (Ramasawmy et al., 2007). Similarly, variation in the inhibitory KappaB-like gene or a gene very close to it has been implicated in differential susceptibility to cardiomyopathy in individuals with chronic Chagas disease (Ramasawmy et al., 2008). A further study demonstrated an association ($p = 0.0084$) between heterozygosity for a variant of *MAL/TIRAP* gene and a lowered risk of developing cardiomyopathy in *T. cruzi* infection (Ramasawmy et al., 2009).

The associations between genes encoding for several interleukins (IL1A, IL1B and IL1RN) in the interleukin-1 gene cluster and disease progression in Chagas disease were examined using a case–control design in symptomatic and asymptomatic seropositive Colombian patients (Flórez et al., 2006). They found haplotype differences between affected and unaffected seropositive individuals that suggest that variation in the IL-1 gene cluster may influence differential susceptibility to the cardiac form of chronic Chagas disease. A similar study conducted in Mexico demonstrated an association between an *IL1RN* polymorphism and development of cardiac disease in individuals seropositive for *T. cruzi* infection (Cruz-Robles et al., 2009).

The inflammatory cytokine tumour necrosis factor-α (TNF-α) is known to be elevated in individuals with the cardiac form of chronic Chagas disease. In studies of a Brazilian population, Drigo and colleagues determined that a specific TNF genotype was associated with risk of death in

Chagas patients (Drigo et al., 2006) but did not find *TNFA* polymorphisms to be associated with severity of cardiac disease in another study (Drigo et al., 2007).

The importance of variation in the interferon-gamma gene (*IFNγ*) for Chagas disease was examined in a Colombian population (Torres et al., 2010). While they found no association between variation in *IFNγ* and differential disease progression in seropositive cases compared to controls, Torres et al. (2010) did find an association between seropositivity for *T. cruzi* infection and *IFNγ* suggesting that variation in the gene may influence differential susceptibility to infection with *T. cruzi*.

Classical markers in the human leukocyte antigen (HLA) system are frequently the focus of candidate gene studies in infectious disease (see review by Blackwell et al., 2009). Many studies have documented associations between HLA haplotypes and *T. cruzi* infection or development of Chagas disease in infected individuals (Colorado et al., 2000; Cruz-Robles et al., 2004; Fernandez-Mestre et al., 1998; García Borras et al., 2009; Layrisse et al., 2000; Llop et al., 1991; Moreno et al., 2004; Nieto et al., 2000).

Despite the intriguing nature of these studies of candidate gene associations with various aspects of Chagas disease, most of these studies are based on relatively small samples including at most several hundred individuals. Few of these studies have rigorously controlled for the number of associations tested, thus increasing the chance of observing false-positive associations. Additionally, the results may be confounded by differential admixture in the study participants. Many populations in Latin America have high rates of admixture involving European, African and Amerindian ancestry. It is critical to control for the underlying population stratification in association study designs, including candidate gene assessments. False-positive associations generated by simple population differences that are mirrored in neutral genetic variation are a likely outcome of candidate gene studies that fail to appropriately account for underlying population stratification.

7.2.4. Genome-wide assessments of Chagas disease-related traits

In the post-genomic era, our approach to understanding the genetic architecture of a complex phenotype has generally followed a specific route. First, an underlying quantitative trait locus (QTL) is localized by a genomic scan to a potentially larger chromosomal region. Until the past 5 years, this localization was usually accomplished by linkage analysis using data on the co-segregation of phenotypes and genetic markers in families. Such linkage mapping relies on information provided by the identity-by-descent status of chromosomal regions evaluated within families. It is able to potentially pick up the signals derived from both common and rare functional genetic variation. Linkage mapping will generally identify a relatively large chromosomal region (10–15 Mb) as having the likelihood of harbouring a disease-related QTL.

The second main approach to causal gene localization involves the utilization of an association mapping paradigm. Genome scanning using an association approach is dependent upon local linkage disequilibrium (LD) and is capable of finer resolution (generally pinpointing a chromosomal region of ~500 kb) than that of linkage-based localization. Genome-wide association analysis has become a popular approach to localize complex disease-related genes. This approach can be performed in unrelated samples of cases and controls or in families. It requires evaluation of a large number (typically more than 500,000) of Single Nucleotide Polymorphisms (SNPs) to adequately cover the genome. Unfortunately, this approach is only relevant for detecting the effects of common functional genetic variation. In cases where common genetic variants (with minor allele frequencies generally greater than 10%) underlie disease risk, genome-wide association may be more powerful than linkage for identifying genes or smaller chromosomal regions involved in a disease. Such an association-based discovery paradigm can also be performed in families as a safeguard against hidden stratification effects.

Following initial localization of potential QTLs influencing the risk of the phenotype under investigation, we can attempt to refine the chromosomal location by saturating the positional candidate region with additional genetic markers and simultaneously exploiting information on both linkage and linkage disequilibrium (whose effective signal spans a much smaller region than a linkage signal does). However, with the marker density afforded by new genome-wide genotyping technologies, this second phase of LD mapping is largely unnecessary. Instead, identification can proceed with comprehensive resequencing of those genes showing the most prior evidence for association. This resequencing step is no longer limited to the examination of common genetic variants but will also include rare functional variants that are segregating in families. Genome scanning approaches hold great promise for Chagas disease. These approaches can be used to identify the specific genes influencing risk for *T. cruzi* infection and risk for cardiac outcomes in Chagas disease

7.3. EXPLORING THE GENETIC ARCHITECTURE OF CHAGAS DISEASE

7.3.1. Quantitative genetic methods

Quantitative genetic approaches were used to examine multiple traits associated with *T. cruzi* infection and Chagas disease progression. For these genetic analyses, we employed SOLAR (Almasy and Blangero,

1998), a general computer package for statistical genetic analyses. These analyses permit the estimation of the heritabilities of the traits being examined. The variance component approach implemented in SOLAR can be used for both quantitative traits such as QRS intervals determined from ECGs and discrete traits such as the presence or absence of a right bundle branch block (Williams et al., 1999). At the heart of SOLAR lies a general variance component engine that makes it possible to analyse family-based quantitative data for pedigrees of any size and complexity. Quantitative genetic analysis partitions the observed covariance among related individuals into genetic versus environmental components. Covariates such as sex, age and their interactions were routinely included in the genetic models.

These analyses can be extended to the joint analysis of multiple traits to allow for the genetic decomposition of the observed correlations. Using the information contained in the kinship coefficients among family members and maximum likelihood variance decomposition techniques, the phenotypic correlations between any two traits can be partitioned into additive genetic and random environmental components. For example, one could examine the genetic correlation between right bundle branch block and the QT interval. The additive genetic correlation ranges between -1 and 1 and is a measure of the shared genetic basis of two traits. An absolute additive genetic correlation of 1.0 indicates complete pleiotropy (i.e. the same genes are affecting the two traits). Alternatively, a genetic correlation whose absolute value is less than 1 shows incomplete pleiotropy indicating that the two traits are influenced to some extent by the same genes but that each trait also has a genetic basis unique from the other. Similarly, the random environmental correlation serves as a measure of the strength of the correlated response of the traits to non-genetic factors. In this maximum likelihood framework, the likelihood of models that constrain the genetic correlation (or environmental correlation) between traits to zero will be compared to the likelihood of models that allow the genetic correlation (or environmental correlation) between the traits to be estimated. In this manner, pairs of Chagas disease-related traits were screened for those that were significantly genetically (and/or environmentally) correlated with one another.

We also explicitly tested for evidence of a heritable basis of the phenotypic response to infection using the quantitative genetic approach to the general examination of genotype-by-environment interaction developed by Blangero (1993). Seropositivity status can be considered an environment to which Chagas-related traits respond. Optimal detection of genotype-by-environment interaction is obtained when individuals can be experimentally manipulated to be examined in both possible environments. For the case of Chagas infection, this is clearly impossible. However, because the uninfected individuals are related to the infected individuals in our large extended pedigrees, and therefore represent the same genes exposed to two different environments, it is possible to specifically test for the genetic factors involved in differential response to seropositivity status. For this case, it is still possible to estimate the genetic variance in response to infection, although it is not possible to directly estimate the total heritability due to the absence of a statistically identifiable environmental variance due to our inability to measure any single individual prior to both infection and post-infection in a standard population-based study.

7.3.2. Quantitative genetics of Chagas disease-related traits: An example

As an example of genetic analyses related to Chagas disease, data obtained from a pedigree-based study in Brazil were analysed. These data were collected in Posse, a rural region of the state of Goiás located approximately 350 km from Brasilia in 1995. Over the past 15 years, we have collected and documented pedigree information for over 1300 individuals who have been characterized for some aspect of Chagas disease. This ongoing longitudinal study is the first large-scale genetic epidemiological study of Chagas disease.

7.3.2.1. Heritability of Chagas disease-related traits

The detailed pedigree information available for the families participating in our studies of Chagas disease in Posse permits the estimation of the heritabilities for a broad range of Chagas disease-related traits. Individuals born in 1975 or earlier (i.e. at least 10 years before the vector control insecticide spraying programme was initiated in the area) are all assumed to have been at risk of infection with *T. cruzi*. As noted earlier, the heritability of a trait provides an estimate of the proportion of variation in the trait attributable to genetic factors. The results of the quantitative genetic analyses of Chagas disease-related traits are provided in Table 7.1, along with the sample sizes for each of the traits.

ECGs were collected from participants with a portable Marquette MAC5000 System (GE Medical Systems Information Technologies, Milwaukee, WI). Seropositivity assessments were determined using three standardized tests (enzyme-linked immunosorbent assay, hemagglutination and immunofluorescence) by the Laboratory of Cellular and Molecular Immunology at the Rene Rachou Research Center, FIOCRUZ. Individuals were considered positive if two or more of these standardized tests were positive.

Seropositivity is a discrete dichotomous trait but is analysed assuming a continuous underlying distribution of liability. Seropositivity for *T. cruzi* infection is significantly heritable. The observed prevalence of

TABLE 7.1 Heritabilities for *T. cruzi* seropositivity, cardiovascular phenotypes and the effects on infection

Trait	*N*	h^2	$p\ (h^2)$	Δ Infection (SDU)	*p* (infect)
T. cruzi seropositivity	1350	0.636	2.2×10^{-15}	–	–
QRS (ms)	1190	0.250	9.0×10^{-7}	0.344	3.5×10^{-8}
QT (ms)	1199	0.411	3.5×10^{-20}	0.417	5.2×10^{-12}
PR (ms)	1168	0.458	5.7×10^{-17}	0.095	0.136
Ventricular rate (bpm)	1190	0.386	3.9×10^{-17}	−0.244	1.2×10^{-4}
Diastolic BP (mmHg)	1104	0.414	2.1×10^{-15}	−0.250	1.1×10^{-4}
Systolic BP (mmHg)	1104	0.365	5.2×10^{-13}	−0.272	1.6×10^{-5}
Right bundle branch block	1190	0.536	4.1×10^{-4}	1.301	7.5×10^{-12}
Abnormal ECG	1190	0.377	5.6×10^{-5}	0.577	5.1×10^{-10}

seropositivity is approximately 60% among adults in the community of Posse. The heritability of seropositivity for *T. cruzi* infection in this sample of 1350 individuals born in 1975 or earlier is 0.636, indicating that approximately 64% of the observed variation in seropositivity status is attributable to genetic factors. This highly significant estimate ($p = 2.2 \times 10^{-15}$) is somewhat higher than our initial estimate of 0.56 that we calculated for a smaller ($n = 525$) set of individuals (Williams-Blangero et al., 1997).

We also examined several quantitative traits determined from ECG readings. The procedures used for the collection of the ECGs from study participants are outlined in Williams-Blangero et al. (2007). Table 7.1 provides evidence that most of these phenotypes are influenced by seropositivity status as reflected in the mean difference between seropositives and seronegatives (provided by the column Δ Infection which is given in standard deviation units). As also can be seen in Table 7.1, there are significant genetic components to all of the cardiovascular-related quantitative traits determined from ECG measures. The QRS interval is significantly heritable, with approximately 25% of the variation in the trait attributable to genetic factors. The QT interval shows evidence for significant genetic effects, with approximately 41% of the variation in the trait attributable to genetic factors. The PR interval is similarly heritable, with approximately 46% of the variation due to genetic effects.

We also measured blood pressure in the participants of our Chagas disease study in Posse. The blood pressure traits were also significantly heritable with about 40% of the variation in diastolic blood pressure and systolic blood pressure being attributable to genetic factors. The heritability of diastolic blood pressure was 0.414 and the heritability of systolic blood pressure was 0.365.

We also considered the potential genetic determinants of right bundle branch block, the cardiac abnormality most closely associated with Chagas disease. The presence of a right bundle branch block is significantly heritable in the Posse population, with about 54% of the variation in the trait being attributable to genetic factors.

Finally, we treated the presence of an abnormal ECG due to any reason as a phenotype in our analyses. The variation among individuals in presence of an abnormal ECG was also heritable with 38% of the variation in the trait attributable to genetic factors. The heritability of this trait was highly significant, indicating that genes do play a role in the development of cardiac outcomes in this population which is endemic for Chagas disease.

7.3.2.2. Shared genetic effects among Chagas disease-related traits

The question of whether or not the genes that influence seropositivity for *T. cruzi* infection and the genes which influence the cardiac-related traits overlap can be addressed by testing for the presence of pleiotropy, that is, genes having effects on multiple traits. There is no strong evidence for direct pleiotropy of genes jointly influencing seropositivity for *T. cruzi* infection and cardiovascular-related phenotypes, meaning that the genes which influence seropositivity status are distinct from those which determine cardiac outcomes in chronic Chagas disease. Bivariate genetic analyses were used to estimate the genetic correlation between seropositivity for *T. cruzi* infection status and each of the cardiovascular phenotypes. While all of them were in the expected direction as given by the differential mean effects shown in Table 7.1, none of these genetic correlations were significantly different from zero. However, both diastolic and systolic blood pressure showed negative genetic correlations (-0.156 and -0.161) which both reached suggestive levels ($p < 0.10$) of significance indicating that there may be some overlap of genetic effects on the blood pressure-related traits and the seropositivity status trait, but that a larger sample will be necessary to have sufficient power to determine this unambiguously.

These same questions of pleiotropy or genetic overlap can be addressed regarding the source of the phenotypic relationships among the cardiovascular-related traits. Table 7.2 shows the results of the bivariate quantitative genetic analyses of the quantitative cardiovascular phenotypes with the significant p values indicated by italics. The results indicate not only substantial pleiotropy across some of the traits but also that there are clearly trait-specific genes acting on these phenotypes. The overall strongest evidence for the pleiotropic effects of genes is seen for

TABLE 7.2 Genetic correlations between quantitative cardiovascular phenotypes

Trait	Trait	ρ_G	$p\ (\rho_G = 0)$
QT	QRS	*0.59*	3.1×10^{-6}
QT	PR	0.21	0.0757
QT	Ventricular rate	*−0.93*	3.0×10^{-17}
QT	Diastolic BP	*−0.28*	*0.0169*
QT	Systolic BP	−0.14	0.2623
QRS	PR	0.28	0.0534
QRS	Ventricular rate	*−0.48*	*0.0013*
QRS	Diastolic BP	0.21	0.1609
QRS	Systolic BP	0.24	0.1294
PR	Ventricular rate	−0.22	0.0808
PR	Diastolic BP	0.17	0.1687
PR	Systolic BP	0.22	0.0804
Ventricular rate	Diastolic BP	*0.44*	*0.0004*
Ventricular rate	Systolic BP	0.25	0.0521
Diastolic BP	Systolic BP	*0.80*	4.2×10^{-10}

the QT interval and ventricular rate which exhibit a very substantial negative genetic correlation of −0.93 ($p = 3.0 \times 10^{-17}$). Thus, about 86% ($-0.93^2 \times 100$) of the genetic variation is due to shared genetic effects between these two traits. Similarly, as expected, diastolic and systolic blood pressure exhibit a high positive genetic correlation of 0.80 ($p = 4.2 \times 10^{-10}$), suggesting that 64% of the observed genetic variation is due to the effects of pleiotropic genes.

7.3.2.3. Genotype-by-infection interaction

Table 7.3 presents the results of quantitative genetic tests for genotype-by-environment interaction where infection status is the environment. This statistical approach requires the availability of relatives in each of the two environments. In the present case, the environments are (1) the state of being seropositive for *T. cruzi* infection and (2) the state of not being seropositive for infection. Our large pedigrees allow such contrasts to be made. As described by Blangero (1993), a significant genotype-by-environment interaction is evidence for a heritable response to the environment. There are two possible tests for such interaction. The first is a test for differences in the additive genetic variance for the trait as expressed in each environment. When there is a difference in genetic variance, there is obligate evidence for the heritability of the response to the environment.

Table 7.3 shows that three of the cardiovascular traits (the QRS interval, systolic blood pressure and ventricular rate) show significant evidence for different additive genetic variances in individuals

TABLE 7.3 Tests of genotype-by-infection interaction suggesting a genetic basis of response to infection

Trait	Observed genetic variance	p (equal σ_G^2)	ρ_G	p ($\rho_G = 1$)
QRS	Seropos > seroneg	0.050	0.50	0.081
QT	Seropos = seroneg	0.369	0.99	0.493
PR	Seropos = seroneg	0.391	1	0.500
Ventricular rate	Seropos > seroneg	0.035	0.93	0.338
Diastolic BP	Seropos = Seroneg	0.748	1	0.500
Systolic BP	Seropos > Seroneg	0.042	1	0.500
Right bundle branch block	Seropos = Seroneg	0.799	0.42	0.338
Abnormal ECG	Seropos = Seroneg	0.856	0.36	0.044

seropositive for *T. cruzi* infection as compared to seronegative individuals. For both the QRS interval and the ventricular rate, seropositive individuals express larger amounts of genetic variance than do seronegatives. However, for systolic blood pressure, this is reversed. The second test for genotype-by-environment interaction examines whether the additive genetic correlation (ρ_G) between the trait's expression levels in the two environments is different from 1. When $\rho_G \neq |1|$, there is evidence for different genes influencing the expression of the trait in the two environments which again induces obligate heritability for the response to the environment. In Table 7.3, one important trait, the presence or absence of an abnormal ECG, provides significant evidence for such Genotype × Infection interaction with an estimated genetic correlation of 0.36 between the environments. This suggests that there are different genes acting on the risk of abnormal ECG in infected individuals versus uninfected individuals. The QRS interval provides suggestive evidence for such interaction ($\rho_G = 0.50, p = 0.081$).

Overall, our quantitative genetic analyses provide evidence that the cardiovascular response to seropositivity for *T. cruzi* infection is heritable for at least four traits (QRS interval, systolic blood pressure, ventricular rate and abnormal ECG). Because such tests provide lower power than a direct longitudinal assessment of change in these characters, the absence of such an interaction should not be counted as evidence against a genetic basis of the response to infection. Our ongoing mixed longitudinal collection of cardiovascular phenotypes in infected individuals will ultimately provide a more powerful basis for the formal test of the role of genetic factors in the cardiovascular response to *T. cruzi* infection.

7.4. MAPPING THE FUTURE OF GENETIC EPIDEMIOLOGICAL STUDIES OF CHAGAS DISEASE

We have presented an overview of past and ongoing assessments of host genetic factors in Chagas disease. To date, the focus has been on the demonstration that host factors in both susceptibility to *T. cruzi* infection and cardiovascular response to infection have heritable components. The task of localization of the underlying QTLs has just begun. In our study in Brazil, we are currently completing a genome-wide high-density SNP screen with over 1 M SNPs. Because we are studying very large pedigrees, we will be able to jointly utilize both linkage and association information in order to cover the complete functional allelic spectrum from rare to common. However, this joint linkage/association approach will also be limited to the genomic localization of the underlying QTLs. Actual gene identification will require a deep-sequencing approach in which all of the sequence variation is evaluated in the regions of localization and intensive genetic work performed to identify both causal variants and causal genes. The advent of high-throughput next-generation sequencing should make gene identification feasible. Indeed, we are soon approaching the day when we will be able to economically obtain whole genome sequence data on our subjects. This should allow a direct search for the functional variants involved in both susceptibility to Chagas disease and the cardiovascular response to infection. Large pedigrees will be particularly useful if the underlying variation is rare. Such pedigrees allow for the examination of multiple copies of even private founder variants. Therefore, founder lineage size should be maximized in order to be able to examine the effects of both common and rare variants. Additionally, as seen in our analyses above, tests for genotype-by-environment interaction are also optimal in large families, as relatives can often be observed in both environments.

ACKNOWLEDGEMENTS

This work was supported by a grants (R01 HL089849, R01 HL066480, C06 RR017515) from the National Institutes of Health. Statistical genetics support was provided by R01 MH059490. We thank Antonio R.L. Teixeira for his contributions to initiating the research effort in Posse. We are also grateful to the people of Posse for their generous cooperation with this study.

REFERENCES

Aguilar, H.M., Abad-Franch, F., Pinto Dias, J.C., Junqueira, A.C.V., Coura, J.R., 2007. Chagas disease in the Amazon region. Mem. Inst. Oswaldo Cruz 102, 47–55.

Almasy, L.A., Blangero, J., 1998. Multipoint quantitative-trait linkage analysis in general pedigrees. Am. J. Hum. Genet. 62, 1198–1211.

Añez, N., Crisante, G., Maia da Silva, F., Rojas, A., Carrasco, H., Umezawa, W.S., et al., 2004. Predominance of lineage I among *Trypanosoma cruzi* isolates from Venezuelan patients with different clinical profiles of acute Chagas disease. Trop. Med. Int. Health 9, 1319–1326.

Barbosa, C.A.A., Morton, N.E., Rao, D.C., Krieger, H., 1981. Biological and cultural determinants of immunoglobulin levels in a Brazilian population with Chagas' disease. Hum. Genet. 59, 161–163.

Beard, C.B., Pye, G., Steurer, F.J., Rodrigues, R., Campman, R., Peterson, A.T., et al., 2003. Chagas disease in a domestic transmission cycle, southern Texas, USA. Emerg. Infect. Dis. 9, 103–105.

Bern, C., Montgomery, S.P., 2009. An estimate of the burden of Chagas disease in the United States. Clin. Infect. Dis. 49, e52–e254.

Biolo, A., Ribeiro, A.L., Clausell, N., 2010. Chagas cardiomyopathy—where do we stand after a hundred years? Prog. Cardiovasc. Dis. 52, 300–316.

Blackwell, J.M., Jamieson, S.E., Burgner, D., 2009. HLA and infectious diseases. Clin. Microbiol. Rev. 22, 370–385.

Blangero, J., 1993. Statistical genetic approaches to human adaptability. Hum. Biol. 65, 941–946.

Borges, J.S., Machada de Assis, G.F., Gomes, L.V., Dias, J.C.P., Pinto, I.D.M., Martins-Filho, O.A., et al., 2006. Seroprevalence of Chagas disease in school children from two municipalities of Jequitinhonha Valley, Minas Gerais, Brazil: six years following the onset of epidemiological surveillance. Rev. Inst. Med. Trop. Sao Paulo 48, 81–86.

Briceño-Leon, R., 2007. Chagas disease and globalization of the Amazon. Cad. Saúde Pública 23 (Suppl. 1), S33–S40.

Busch, M.P., Kleinman, S.H., Nemo, G.J., 2003. Current and emerging infectious risks of blood transfusions. J. Am. Med. Assoc. 289, 959–961.

Buscaglia, C.A., Di Noia, J.M., 2003. Trypanosoma cruzi clonal diversity and the epidemiology of Chagas disease. Microbes Infect. 5, 419–427.

Calzada, J.E., Pineda, V., Garisto, J.D., Samudio, F., Santamaria, A.M., Saldaña, A., 2010. Human trypanosomiasis in the eastern region of the Panama province: new endemic areas for Chagas disease. Am. J. Trop. Med. Hyg. 82, 580–582.

Campbell, D.A., Westenberger, S.J., Strum, N.R., 2004. The determinants of Chagas disease: connecting parasite and host genetics. Curr. Mol. Med. 4, 549–562.

Castro, J.A., de Mecca, M.M., Bartel, L.C., 2006. Toxic side effects of drugs used to treat Chagas' disease (American trypanosomiasis). Hum. Exp. Toxicol. 25, 471–479.

Coll Cardenas, R., Espinoza-Gomez, F., Maldonado-Rodriguez, A., Reyes-Lopez, P.A., Huerta-Viera, M., Rojas-Larios, F., 2004. Active transmission of human Chagas disease in Colima Mexico. Mem. Inst. Oswaldo Cruz 99, 363–368.

Colorado, I.A., Acquatella, H., Catalioti, F., Fernandez, M.T., Layrisse, Z., 2000. HLA class II DRB1, DPB1 polymorphisms and cardiomyopathy due to *Trypanosoma cruzi* chronic infection. Hum. Immunol. 61, 320–325.

Cruz-Robles, D., Reyes, P.A., Monteon-Padilla, V.M., Ortiz-Muniz, A.R., Varga-Alarcon, G., 2004. MHC class I and class II genes in Mexican patients with Chagas disease. Hum. Immunol. 65, 60–65.

Cruz-Robles, D., Chávez-Gonzáles, J.P., Cavazos-Quero, M.M., Pérez-Méndez, O., Reyes, P.A., Vargas-Alarcón, G., 2009. Association between IL-1B and IL-1RN gene polymorphisms and Chagas' disease development susceptibility. Immunol. Invest. 38, 231–239.

Drigo, S.A., Cunha-Neto, E., Ianni, B., Cardosa, M.R., Braga, P.E., Fae, F.C., et al., 2006. TNF gene polymorphisms are associated with reduced survival in severe Chagas disease cardiomyopathy patients. Microbes Infect. 8, 598–603.

Drigo, S.A., Cunha-Neto, E., Ianni, B., Mady, C., Faé, K.C., Buck, P., et al., 2007. Lack of association of tumor necrosis factor-α polymorphisms with Chagas disease in Brazilian patients. Immunol. Lett. 108, 109–111.

Dutra, W.O., Rocha, M.O.C., Teixeira, M.M., 2005. The clinical immunology of Chagas disease. Trends Parasitol. 21, 581–587.

Fernandez-Mestre, M.T., Layrisse, Z., Mantagnani, S., Acquatella, H., Cataloiti, F., Matos, M., et al., 1998. Influence of HLA class II polymorphism in chronic Chagas disease. Parasite Immunol. 20, 197–203.

Flórez, O., Zafra, G., Morillo, C., Martín, J., González, C.I., 2006. Interleukin-1 gene cluster polymorphism in Chagas disease in a Colombian case-control study. Hum. Immunol. 67, 741–748.

García Borras, S., Racca, L., Cotorruelo, C., Biondi, C., Beloscar, J., Racca, A., 2009. Distribution of HLA-DRB1 alleles in Argentinean patients with Chagas disease cardiomyopathy. Immunol. Invest. 38, 268–275.

Garcia-Zapata, M.T.A., Marsden, P.D., 1986. Chagas disease. Clin. Trop. Med. Commun. Dis. 1, 557–585.

Garg, N., Bhatia, V., 2005. Current status and future prospects for a vaccine against American trypanosomiasis. Exp. Rev. Vaccines 4, 867–880.

Goldbaum, M., Ajimura, F.Y., Litvoc, J., Alves de Carvalho, S., Eluf-Neto, J., 2004. American trypanosomiasis and electrocardiographic alterations among industrial works in São Paulo Brazil. Rev. Inst. Med. Trop. Sao Paulo 46, 299–302.

Grijalva, M.J., Escalante, L., Paredes, R.A., Costales, J.A., Padilla, A., Rowland, E.C., et al., 2003. Seroprevalence and risk factors for *Trypanosoma cruzi* infection in the Amazon region of Ecuador. Am. J. Trop. Med. Hyg. 69, 380–385.

Gurtler, R.E., Cecere, M.C., Lauricella, M.A., Petersen, R.M., Chuit, R., Segura, E.L., Cohen, J. E., 2005. Incidence of *Trypanosoma cruzi* infection among children following domestic reinfection after insecticide spraying in rural northwestern Argentina. Am. J. Trop. Med. Hyg. 73, 95–103.

Jorge, M.T., Macedo, T.A., Janones, R.S., Carizzi, D.P., Heredia, R.A., Acha, R.E., 2003. Types of arrhythmia among cases of American trypanosomiasis compared with those in other cardiology patients. Ann. Trop. Med. Parasitol. 97, 139–148.

Kirchhoff, L.V., 1999. American trypanosomiasis (Chagas' disease). In: Guerrant, R.L., Walker, D.H., Weller, P.F. (Eds.), Tropical Infectious Diseases: Principles, Pathogens, and Practice. Churchill Livingstone, New York, pp. 785–796.

Layrisse, Z., Fernandez, M.T., Montagnani, D., Matos, M., Balbas, O., Herrera, F., et al., 2000. HLA-C(*)03 is a risk factor for cardiomyopathy in Chagas disease. Hum. Immunol. 61, 925–929.

Leiby, D.A., Herron, R.M., Read, E.J., Lenes, B.A., Stumpf, R.J., 2002. *Trypanosoma cruzi* in Los Angeles and Miami blood donors: impact of evolving donor demographics on seroprevalence and implications for transfusion transmission. Transfusion 42, 549–555.

Lescure, F.X., LeCoup, G., Ferilij, H., Develoux, M., Paris, L., Brutus, L., et al., 2010. Chagas disease: changes in knowledge and management. Lancet Infect. Dis. 10, 556–570.

Llop, E.R., Rothhammer, F., Acuña, M., Apt, W., Arribada, A., 1991. Antigenos HLA en cariopatas chagasicos: nueva evidence basada en un analisis de casos y controles. Rev. Med. Chile 119, 633–636.

Macedo, A.M., Machado, C.R., Oliveira, R.P., Pena, S.D.J., 2004. *Trypanosoma cruzi*: genetic structure of populations and relevance of genetic variability to the pathogenesis of Chagas disease. Mem. Inst. Oswaldo Cruz 99, 1–12.

Maguire, J.H., Hoff, R., Sherlock, I., Guimaraes, A.C., Sleigh, A.C., Ramos, N.B., et al., 1987. Cardiac morbidity and mortality due to Chagas disease: prospective electrocardiographic study of a Brazilian community. Circulation 75, 1140–1145.

Manoel-Caetano, F.S., Silva, A.E., 2007. Implications of genetic variability of *Trypanosoma cruzi* for the pathogenesis of Chagas disease. Cad. Saude Publica Rio de Janeiro 23, 2263–2274.

McCarthy, M., 2003. American Red Cross to screen blood for Chagas disease. Lancet 362, 1988.

Miles, M.A., Llewellyn, M.S., Lewis, M.D., Yeo, M., Baleela, R., Fitzpatrick, S., et al., 2009. The molecular epidemiology and phylogeography of *Trypanosoma cruzi* and parallel research on *Leishmania*: looking back and to the future. Parasitology 136, 1509–1528.

Moreno, M., Silva, E.L., Ramirez, L.E., Palacio, L.G., Rivera, D., Arcos-Burgos, M., 2004. Chagas disease susceptibility/resistance: linkage disequilibrium suggests epistasis between major histocompatibility complex and interleukin 10. Tissue Antigens 64, 18–24.

Mott, K.E., Lehman, J.S., Jr., Hoff, R., Morrow, R.H., Muniz, T.M., Sherlock, I., et al., 1976. The epidemiology and household distribution of seroreactivity to *Trypanosoma cruzi* in a rural community in northeast Brazil. Am. J. Trop. Med. Hyg. 25, 552–562.

Nieto, A., Beraun, Y., Collado, M.D., Caballero, A., Alonso, A., Gonzalez, A., et al., 2000. HLA haplotypes are associated with differential susceptibility to *Trypanosoma cruzi* infection. Tissue Antigens 55, 195–198.

Norman, F.F., Pérez de Ayala, A., Pérez-Molina, J.A., Monge-Maillo, B., Zamarrón, P., López-Vélez, R., 2010. Neglected tropical diseases outside the tropics. PLoS Negl. Trop. Dis. 4, e762.

Ohlstein, W.H., Ruffolo, R.R., Jr., Elliott, J.D., 2000. Drug discovery in the next millennium. Ann. Rev. Pharmacol. Toxicol. 40, 177–191.

Pinto, A.Y.N., Valente, S.A.S., Valente, V.C., 2004. Emerging acute Chagas disease in Amazonian Brazil: case reports with serious cardiac involvement. Braz. J. Infect. Dis. 8, 454–460.

Prata, A., 2001. Clinical and epidemiological aspects of Chagas' disease. Lancet Infect. Dis. 1, 92–100.

Ramasawmy, R., Cunha-Neto, E., Fae, K.C., Martello, F.G., Müller, N.G., Cavalcanti, V.L., et al., 2006. The monocyte chemoattractant protein-1 gene polymorphism is associated with cardiomyopathy in human Chagas disease. Clin. Infect. Dis. 43, 305–311.

Ramasawmy, R., Fae, K.C., Cunha-Neto, E., Müller, N.G., Cavalcanti, V.L., Ferreira, R.C., et al., 2007. Polymorphisms in the gene for lymphotoxin-alpha predispose to chronic Chagas cardiomyopathy. J. Infect. Dis. 196, 1836–1843.

Ramasawmy, R., Fae, K.C., Cunha-Neto, E., Borba, S.C., Ianni, B., Mady, C., et al., 2008. Variants in the promoter region of IKBL/NFKBIL1 gene may mark susceptibility to the development of chronic Chagas' cardiomyopathy among *Trypanosoma cruzi*-infected individuals. Mol. Immunol. 45, 283–288.

Ramasawmy, R., Cunha-Neto, E., Fae, K.C., Borba, S.C.P., Teixeira, P.C., Ferreira, S.C.P., et al., 2009. Heterozygosity for the A180L variant of *MAL/TIRAP*, a gene expressing an adaptor protein in the toll-like receptor pathway, is associated with lower risk of developing chronic Chagas cardiomyopathy. J. Infect. Dis. 199, 1838–1845.

Rangel-Flores, H., Sánchez, B., Mendoza-Duarte, J., Barnabé, C., Brenière, F.S., Ramos, C., et al., 2001. Serologic and parasitologic demonstration of *Trypanosoma cruzi* infections in an urban area of central Mexico: correlation with electrocardiographic alterations. Am. J. Trop. Med. Hyg. 65, 887–895.

Rassi, A., Jr., Rassi, A., Marin-Neto, J.A., 2010. Chagas disease. Lancet 375, 1388–1402.

Rizzo, N.R., Arana, B.A., Diaz, A., Cordon-Rosales, C., Klein, R.W., Powell, M.R., 2003. Seroprevalence of *Trypanosoma cruzi* infection among school-age children in the endemic area of Guatamala. Am. J. Trop. Med. Hyg. 68, 678–682.

Rodriguez Coura, J., de Castro, S.L., 2002. A critical review on Chagas disease chemotherapy. Mem. Inst. Oswaldo Cruz 97, 3–24.

Salles, G., Xavier, S., Sousa, A., Hasslocher-Moreno, A., Cardosa, C., 2003. Prognostic value of QT interval parameters for mortality risk stratification in Chagas disease: results of a long-term follow-up study. Circulation 108, 305–312.

Salles, G., Xavier, S., Sousa, A., Hasslocher-Moreno, A., Cardosa, C., 2004. T-wave axis deviation as an independent predictor of mortality in chronic Chagas disease. Am. J. Cardiol. 93, 1136–1140.

Sanchez-Sancho, F., Campillo, N.E., Páez, J.A., 2010. Chagas disease: progress and new perspectives. Curr. Med. Chem. 17, 423–452.

Sarkar, S., Strutz, S.E., Frank, D.M., Rivaldi, C.L., Sissel, N., Sanchez-Cordero, V., 2010. Chagas disease risk in Texas. PLoS Negl. Trop. Dis. 4, e836.

Schadt, E.E., Monks, S.A., Friend, S.H., 2003. A new paradigm for drug discovery: integrating clinical, genetic, genomic, and molecular phenotype data to identify drug targets. Drug Discov. Des. 31, 437–443.

Silva-Grecco, R.L., Balarin, M.A., Correia, D., Prata, A., Rodrigues, V., Jr., 2010. Familial analysis of seropositivity to *Trypanosoma cruzi* and of clinical forms of Chagas disease. Am. J. Trop. Med. Hyg. 82, 45–48.

Sosa-Hurado, F., Mazariego-Aranda, M., Hernandez-Becerril, N., Garza-Murillo, V., Cardenas, M., Reyes, P.A., et al., 2003. Electrocardiographic findings in Mexican chagasic subjects living in high and low endemic regions of *Trypanosoma cruzi* infection. Mem. Inst. Oswaldo Cruz 98, 605–610.

Sturm, N.R., Vargas, N.S., Westenberger, S.J., Zingales, B., Campbell, D.A., 2003. Evidence for multiple hybrid groups in *Trypanosoma cruzi*. Int. J. Parasitol. 33, 269–279.

Tanowitz, H.B., Machado, F.S., Jelicks, L.A., Shirani, J., Campos de Carvalho, A.C., Spray, D.C., et al., 2009. Perspectives on *Trypanosoma cruzi*-induced heart disease (Chagas disease). Prog. Cardiovasc. Dis. 51, 524–539.

Teixeira, A.R.L., Cordoba, J.C., Maior, I.S., Solorzano, E., 1990a. Chagas disease: lymphoma growth in rabbits treated with benznidazole. Am. J. Trop. Med. Hyg. 43, 146–158.

Teixeira, A.R.L., Silva, R., Neto, E.C., Santano, J.M., Rizzo, L.V., 1990b. Malignant, non-Hodgkin's lymphoma in *Trypanosoma cruzi* infected rabbits treated with nitroarenes. J. Comp. Pathol. 103, 37–48.

Tibayrenc, M., 1998. Integrated genetic epidemiology of infectious diseases: the Chagas model. Mem. Inst. Oswaldo Cruz 93, 577–580.

Tibayrenc, M., 1999. Toward an integrated genetic epidemiology of parasitic protozoa and other pathogens. Ann. Rev. Genet. 33, 449–477.

Tibayrenc, M., 2007. Human genetic diversity and the epidemiology of parasitic and other transmissible diseases. Adv. Parasitol. 64, 377–422.

Tibayrenc, M., 2010. Modelling the transmission of *Trypanosoma cruzi*: the need for an integrated genetic epidemiological and population genomics approach. Adv. Exp. Med. Biol. 673, 200–211.

Torres, O.A., Calzada, J.E., Beraún, Y., Morillo, C.A., González, A., González, C.I., et al., 2010. Role of the IFNG +874T/A polymorphism in Chagas disease in a Columbian population. Infect. Genet. Evol. 10, 682–685.

Urbina, J.A., Docampo, R., 2003. Specific chemotherapy of Chagas disease: controversies and advances. Trends Parasitol. 19, 495–501.

WHO, 2010. Chagas (American trypanosomiasis) fact sheet (revise June 2010). Weekly Epidemiol. Rec. 85 (34), 334–336.

Williams, J.T., Van Eerdewegh, P., Almasy, L., Blangero, J., 1999. Joint multipoint linkage analysis of multivariate qualitative and quantitative traits. I. Likelihood formulation and simulation results. Am. J. Hum. Genet. 65, 1134–1147.

Williams-Blangero, S., Blangero, J., 2006. Collection of pedigree data for genetic analysis in isolate populations. Hum. Biol. 78, 89–101.

Williams-Blangero, S., VandeBerg, J.L., Blangero, J., Teixeira, A.R., 1997. Genetic epidemiology of seropositivity for *Trypanosoma cruzi* infection in rural Goias, Brazil. Am. J. Trop. Med. Hyg. 57, 538–543.
Williams-Blangero, S., Magalhaes, T., Rainwater, E., Blangero, J., Corrêa-Oliveira, R., VandeBerg, J.L., 2007. Electrocardiographic characteristics in a population with high rates of seropositivity for *Trypanosoma cruzi* infection. Am. J. Trop. Med. Hyg. 77, 495–499.
Yacoub, S., Birks, E.J., Slavik, Z., Henein, M., 2003. Early detection of myocardial dysfunction in Chagas disease using novel echocardiographic indices. Trans. R. Soc. Trop. Med. Hyg. 97, 528–534.
Zicker, F., Smith, P.G., Netto, J.C., Oliveira, R.M., Zicker, E.M., 1990. Physical activity, opportunity for reinfection, and sibling history of heart disease as risk factors for Chagas cardiopathy. Am. J. Trop. Med. Hyg. 43, 498–505.

CHAPTER 8

Kissing Bugs. The Vectors of Chagas

Lori Stevens,* Patricia L. Dorn,† Justin O. Schmidt,‡ John H. Klotz,§ David Lucero,* and **Stephen A. Klotz¶**

Contents

* Department of Biology, University of Vermont, Burlington, Vermont, USA
† Department of Biological Sciences, Loyola University of New Orleans, New Orleans, Los Angeles, USA
‡ Southwestern Biological Institute, Tucson, Arizona, USA
§ Department of Entomology, University of California Riverside, Riverside, California, USA
¶ Section of Infectious Diseases, University of Arizona, Tucson, Arizona, USA

Advances in Parasitology, Volume 75
ISSN 0065-308X, DOI: 10.1016/B978-0-12-385863-4.00008-3

Abstract

A complete picture of Chagas disease requires an appreciation of the many species of kissing bugs and their role in transmitting this disease to humans and other mammals. This chapter provides an overview of the taxonomy of the major species of kissing bugs and their evolution. Knowledge of systematics and biological kinship of these insects may contribute to novel and useful measures to control the bugs. The biology of kissing bugs, their life cycle, method of feeding and other behaviours contributing to the transmission of *Trypanosoma cruzi* are explained. We close with a discussion of vector control measures and the allergic complications of kissing bug bites, a feature of particular importance in the United States.

8.1. INTRODUCTION

Vectors of Chagas disease are remarkable in being the only true bugs capable of transmitting disease to people. These bugs in the order Hemiptera differ from most other blood-feeding vectors by developing from egg to adult via nymphs that appear similar to adults but lack a pupal stage. All stages live in the same locations and exhibit nearly identical lifestyles. Most other insect vectors (lice are an exception) exhibit complete development including a pupal stage, thereby having dramatically different life stages and ecologies that can be targeted for control. All vectors of *Trypanosoma cruzi* are in the subfamily Triatominae, in the family Reduviidae, known as assassin bugs, so named because the majority of insects in this group are predators that hunt other arthropods and feed by digesting and sucking out their prey's bodily juices. These predators were presumed to have arisen from earlier plant feeding "sap suckers" (Carcavallo et al., 2000). The Triatominae are known as kissing bugs. Except for a group transported to seaports worldwide, Triatominae are restricted geographically to the American continents and probably emerged as a separate lineage coincident with the formation of the American continents.

Blood feeding evolved less than a dozen times in insects. Three groups of insects with a nymphal stage (bed bugs, lice and Triatominae) and another three groups with a pupal stage (fleas, flies and a butterfly) became hematophagous (Benoit and Denlinger, 2010). Most groups of blood-feeding insects are monophyletic (Yoshizawa and Johnson, 2010). However, in Diptera (flies), blood feeding is thought to have evolved at least five times (Yuval, 2006). Triatomines are unusual arthropod vectors because they may harbour two trypanosome parasites with different modes of transmission, that is, faecal contamination for *T. cruzi* and salivary transmission for *Trypanosoma rangeli* (Gaunt and Miles, 2000).

The Triatominae contain an estimated 140 species; however, biological species are not always precisely defined (Knowles and Carstens, 2007) and some of the recognized groups likely contain multiple lineages, subspecies or morphological variants (Dorn et al., 2009). The family is subdivided into five tribes: Triatomini with nine genera and ~110 species; Rhodniini with ~20 species in two genera; Alberproseniini (one genus with two species), Bolboderini (four genera with 14 species) and Carvernicolini (two species in a single genus).

Although most Chagas transmission is vector-mediated via parasite-contaminated faeces, other routes include blood transfusion and organ transplant, and vertical transmission (i.e. mother to child) such that 2–10% of infants born to infected mothers are infected. Because the parasite cannot penetrate the skin, horizontal transmission from insect vector to mammalian host requires penetration of mucosal membranes (around the eye or mouth) or through the bite wound by parasites contained in faeces deposited while the vector is taking a blood meal. A second mode of horizontal transmission, thought to be rare in humans but perhaps common for other mammals, occurs when parasites penetrate the mucosa of the digestive system following ingestion of an infected vector (Diaz-Suarez, 2009).

8.2. VECTOR GENERA AND SPECIES

The relative importance of the various triatomine species as human disease vectors depends on behavioural and biological factors, especially the preferred vector ecotope with adaptation to domestic and peridomestic structures (corrals, chicken coops, wood piles, etc.) as well as the sylvatic habitat. Other important traits include degree of anthropophily and host preference, feeding time, dispersal capabilities and time span between blood meal and defecation (Lent and Wygodzinsky, 1979). The epidemiologically important vectors vary among geographic regions. Only about a dozen species appear to have strictly domestic populations over at least a part of their geographic range, while another two dozen or so species are described as secondary vectors because they seasonally or opportunistically invade houses from peridomestic and sylvatic habitats (Vallejo et al., 2009). The two most epidemiologically significant tribes include the Rhodniini and the Triatomini. Within the Triatomini, many taxa in the genus *Triatoma* have been organized into species groups called complexes.

8.2.1. North American taxa

Of the ~40 species found in North America, 8 are shared between Mexico and the United States, 4 are found only in the U.S. and 28 only in Mexico (some of these are also present in Central America) (Ibarra-Cerdena et al., 2009). Temperature is thought to limit the northern range to the lower approximately two-thirds of the United States. In Mexico, the species included in the phyllosoma complex are responsible for the majority of Chagas transmission (Ibarra-Cerdena et al., 2009; Martinez-Ibarra et al., 2008). These species are found associated with human dwellings in central and southern Mexico and include *Triatoma pallidipennis*, *T. longipennis*, *T. barberi*, *T. mazzotti*, *T. phyllosoma*, *T. picturata* and *T. mexicana.*

In the United States, transmission from insect vector to human host is rare and the major concern is anaphylactic reactions to their bites (Klotz et al., 2010). In Texas, *T. gerstaeckeri*, the principle vector of zoonotic *T. cruzi*, is associated with the southern plains woodrat, *Neotoma micropus* (Kjos et al., 2009). Other *Triatoma* species in Texas include *T. protracta*, *T. indictiva*, *T. rubida* and *T. neotomae.* In Arizona and California, *T. protracta* and *T. rubida* are commonly found, whereas *T. recurva* is rare. In the southeastern United States, *T. sanguisuga* has been found in large numbers around human dwellings and is associated with raccoons and opossums from Florida to Texas (de la Rua et al., 2010; Ponce, 2007).

8.2.2. Central American taxa

In Mesoamerica (roughly, central Mexico to Costa Rica), anti-Chagas campaigns have dramatically reduced the numbers of the introduced, domestic vector *R. prolixus* in most localities leaving the indigenous and widespread *Triatoma dimidiata* as the predominant vector except in Panama, where *R. pallescens* predominates. Additional minor species that may cause infection in humans include *T. nitida* and *T. ryckmani* (Ponce, 2007; Zeledón et al., 2007).

8.2.3. South American taxa

Chagas disease vectors in South America can be divided into three ecological groups, Andean, Amazonian and Southern Cone. The most significant domestic vectors in the Andes region, which includes part of five countries, Bolivia, Colombia, Ecuador, Peru and Venezuela, are *R. prolixus*, *T. dimidiata* and *Triatoma infestans.* Secondary vectors in this region are *T. maculata*, *R. ecuadoriensis*, *R. pallescens*, *T. venosa*, *T. carrioni*, *P. herreri*, *P. chinai*, *P. geniculatus* and *P. rufotuberculatus* (Guhl, 2007). It is in this region that *T. infestans* is thought to have originated in the Andean highlands and desert regions of Bolivia and Argentina (Giordano et al., 2005).

Deforestation and human settlement in the Amazon region have increased contact between humans and vectors. No species is reported to live year round strictly in human dwellings; however, several species are routinely associated with human dwellings including *T. maculata, P. geniculatus, R. neglectus* and *R. stali*. Humans also routinely have contact with several sylvatic species including *R. robustus, R. pictipes* and *R. brethesi* (Aguilar et al., 2007).

The Southern Cone region includes parts of Argentina, Bolivia, Brazil, Chile, Paraguay and Uruguay, and the major vector is *T. infestans*. Occasionally, *Panstrongylus megistus, T. brasiliensis, T. sordida, T. pseudomaculata* and *R. nasutus* are found (Dias, 2007).

8.2.4. The important human disease vectors

The most important human disease vector *is T. infestans*, followed by *R. prolixus*, and *T. dimidiata*. Different vector genera appear to be adapted to different niches with the result that the major subgroups of *T. cruzi* are associated with particular vectors and mammalian hosts (Gaunt and Miles, 2000). The major human disease vectors represent recent expansion into domestic and peridomestic habitats by only a few species. The habitat preferences of *Rhodnius* and *Triatoma* are reflected in their distribution within infested houses: *R. prolixus* is found in palm roofs and *T. infestans* in mud-walled houses or tiled roofs (Gaunt and Miles, 2000; Pizarro et al., 2008).

T. infestans occurs over a wide geographic range. Human dwellings and peridomestic structures are its preferred ecotope. Based on Zeledón's "defecation index", *T. infestans* adults are not quite as efficient as *R. prolixus* at defecating during feeding; however, both defecate within 10 min of feeding and this is thought to be the critical threshold for efficient *T. cruzi* transmission (Zeledón et al., 1977).

In the Andean highlands, *T. infestans* is found in rocky habitats in association with rodent burrows including wild guinea pigs (Pizarro et al., 2008). *T. cruzi* II appears to have evolved with *T. infestans* in rocky habitats or burrows associated with edentates or possibly ground dwelling marsupials (Gaunt and Miles, 2000).

R. prolixus is exclusively domestic in Central America. In northern South America, it occurs in domestic and sylvatic habitats, primarily palm trees (Lent and Wygodzinsky, 1979) where it feeds on opossums as well as birds. These bugs are well adapted to climbing on the smooth stems and trunks of palms. *T. cruzi* I predominates in domestic and sylvatic habitats in the regions north of the Amazon (Gaunt and Miles, 2000), and the sylvatic vectors are associated with opossums (Carrasco et al., 1996; Povoa et al., 1984).

Studies examining local adaptation between vector and parasite strains are relatively few, but experimental studies have shown that not all *T. cruzi* strains can be transmitted by all species of Triatominae (Garcia and Azambuja, 1991). The insect vectors have a complex association with symbiotic intestinal bacteria, which may affect the numbers of the trypanosomatid parasites including *T. cruzi*, *T. rangelli* and *Blastocrithidia triatomae* (Azambuja et al., 2005; Eichler and Schaub, 2002).

8.3. EVOLUTION OF THE TRIATOMINES

The main evolutionary questions regarding Triatominae are as follows: Is this a monophyletic group, or alternatively, is it a polyphyletic group, having arisen from more than one predator ancestor? Did the Triatominae arise only in the New World or in both the New and Old Worlds? And finally, which species definition reveals the true taxonomic subdivisions? Answers to these questions give scientists the ability to infer shared characteristics, some of which, such as preference for human habitations and blood meals, are epidemiologically important.

8.3.1. Monophyly of Triatominae

Lent and Wygodzinsky (1979) concluded that the Triatominae subfamily are a monophyletic group possessing the following shared, derived characters: they are hematophagous, with a generally painless bite and have a membranous connection between the second and third rostral segments that allows them to bend the rostrum up during feeding.

The monophyly theory has been challenged based on several lines of evidence including biogeography and morphology, salivary proteins, cuticular hydrocarbons and DNA sequence differences between the Triatomini and the Rhodniini tribes (Dujardin and Schofield, 2004; Schofield and Galvao, 2009). When an insufficient number of shared characters or outgroups are used, the classification of monophyly or polyphyly suffers (Gorla et al., 1997; Schofield, 1988). So morphology, especially with a limited set of characters, may overestimate the differences among groups.

The differences in salivary proteins between Triatomini and Rhodniini are often cited as evidence for polyphyly (Ribeiro et al., 1998); however, other studies show that the anticoagulant mechanism utilized by the genus *Panstronglyus*, which is clearly within the Triatomini tribe (de Paula et al., 2005), is similar to that of *Rhodnius* and different from *Triatoma* (Pereira et al., 1996). Further, the differences in epicuticular hydrocarbons represent relatively primitive characters that differ quantitatively and not qualitatively (Juarez et al., 2002).

Results from many studies utilizing allozyme analyses and morphometry (Dujardin et al., 1999) and DNA sequence (Marcilla et al., 2001; Monteiro et al., 2000; Stothard et al., 1998) clearly show the separation of Triatomini from Rhodniini (Dujardin and Schofield, 2004). These studies used a single outgroup and showed the sister taxa relationship between the two tribes; however, with an insufficient number of outgroups, they cannot be used to prove or disprove mono- or polyphyly of the subfamily (Schaefer, 2003).

Cladistic analysis, with a large number (162) of morphological characters (Weirauch, 2008) or DNA sequences and a large number of outgroups (Weirauch and Munro, 2009), reveals the monophyly of the Triatominae subfamily. In addition, the power of this approach is that out of the 162 characters examined, Weirauch (2008) identified 12 shared characteristics that define the Triatominae subfamily. The best approach seems to be an evolutionary species concept using cladistic analysis with many characters, molecular as well as phenotypic and a sufficient number of outgroups to elucidate the phylogenic relationships among taxa.

The evolution of the Triatominae from the Reduviidae ancestor appears to be fairly recent and originated in the Americas. This is supported by the lack of autochthonous species in Africa, the fact that the vast majority of species occur in the Western hemisphere (Dujardin and Schofield, 2004) and those found in Asia likely originated in the Americas (Hypsa et al., 2002). Dujardin and Schofield (2004) speculate they evolved "well after the mid-Tertiary period", perhaps even later than the Quaternary period.

8.3.2. Evolution within the subfamily Triatominae

Among the epidemiologically important taxa are the previously mentioned sister taxa: Triatomini and Rhodniini. This division is well documented by phenotypic, morphometric and molecular (allozymes, DNA sequence, etc.) comparisons. The number of autosomes or sex chromosomes is not helpful in distinguishing the tribes, as the autosomal complement is nearly uniform (only three species have other than 20 autosomes). Genome size varies, and in general, Rhodniini has a smaller genome size correlating with smaller chromosomes rather than differences in the amount of heterochromatin (Panzera et al., 2010). The other three tribes of Alberproseniini, Bolboderini and Carvernicolini have never been included in a formal cladistic analysis (Weirauch and Munro, 2009), and molecular genetic analysis to date has been limited to DNA regions coding for mitochondrial and nuclear ribosomal RNA (Patterson and Gaunt, 2010; Weirauch and Munro, 2009) and mitochondrial genes involved in electron transport (Patterson and Gaunt, 2010).

Within the Triatomini tribe, the *Triatoma* genus comprises ~80 species (Schofield and Galvao, 2009) that further subdivide into two clades found north and south of the Amazon region based on mtDNA (Lyman et al., 1999) and nuclear DNA sequence (Marcilla et al., 2001). More recently, a third clade has been added consisting of the dispar complex, located west of the Amazon region (Bargues et al., 2010). Cytogenetics is useful in distinguishing the two clades as all *Triatoma* in the "northern" clade, with one exception, show multiple sex chromosomes (fragmented X chromosomes), whereas most, but not all, "southern" clade *Triatoma* have the XY system (Panzera et al., 2010). The *Rhodnius* genus includes 16 species (Schofield and Galvao, 2009) that are divided into three clades based on mtDNA sequence (Lyman et al., 1999), allozyme analysis and morphometry (Dujardin et al., 1999), and they also are geographically localized.

Most workers have concentrated on understanding the evolution of *T. infestans*. The finding of wild foci of *T. infestans* in the Andean valleys of Cochabamba, Bolivia (Torrico, 1946) led to the hypothesis that this was the site of origin of the species (Schofield, 1988) and the vectors became domesticated as they moved from wild guinea pig burrows to quite similar microhabitats in human dwellings (Usinger et al., 1966). As might be expected from remnants of a founding population, results from early studies showed that although overall genetic diversity in *T. infestans* is low, these Andean *T. infestans* populations from Bolivia were more diverse than those found in Peru (Dujardin and Tibayrenc, 1985). Interestingly, some Argentinean populations show higher genetic diversity than is found in Bolivia (De Rosas et al., 2007; Garcia et al., 1995), presumably for reasons other than originating in Argentina, possibly from pesticide pressures (De Rosas et al., 2007). Chromosomal make-up is informative about the origin and dispersal of *T. infestans* as "Andean". The putative ancestral form shows ~30% more DNA due to ~50% more heterochromatin than the "non-Andean" (Panzera et al., 2004). *T. infestans* appears to have lost heterochromatin as it spreads out across South America. Sequence of the internal transcribed spacer regions of the rDNA supports a northern/southern split in *T. infestans* populations (Bargues et al., 2006), and intermediate chromosomal forms have been detected in the overlapping area (Noireau, 2009; Panzera et al., 2007).

The interfertility of many species of the Phyllosoma (Mazzotti and Osorio, 1942) and Infestans complexes (Usinger et al., 1966) violates the traditional species definition of reproductive isolation (Mayr, 1970). Therefore, an ecological species concept (van Valen, 1976) of spatial or temporal division has been invoked for the separation of *T. infestans* and *T. platensis* that have some natural hybrids (Abalos, 1948) even though they occupy different niches, *T. infestans* in the domestic environment and *T. plantensis* in bird nests (Carcavallo et al., 2000). With the increasing availability of DNA sequence data, quantitative differences in DNA sequence (genetic distance) measures may be useful in constructing taxonomic subdivisions (Monteiro et al., 2004; Pfeiler et al., 2006).

8.4. BIOLOGY OF THE BUGS

The Triatominae are a nearly obligatory hematophagous subfamily, although some species feed on the hemolymph of arthropods in addition to vertebrate blood and appear to represent the ancestral trait of the subfamily (Sandoval et al., 2010). They are relatively large bugs with adults ranging in length from about 12 to 36 mm and having five immature instars, morphologically similar to adults, except lacking wings. Both sexes and all five instars feed on blood of vertebrates, starting with the first instars which take a blood meal as soon as 2–3 days after hatching from the egg. All instars are also capable of transmitting *T. cruzi*, though first instars probably rarely transmit the parasite as they must acquire the parasites from an initial blood meal and often moult to second instars before feeding again.

The life cycle of kissing bugs can be completed in several months in tropical areas where temperatures are warm and when food is readily available. In temperate higher latitude regions having extended cooler periods of the year, the bugs typically have only one generation per year. In these environments, bugs seek refuge in cavities, rodent burrows, caves or similar locations with moderate temperatures and pass the unfavourable times in various nymphal stages. Adults live several months, occasionally a year or more (Gorla et al., 2010) and feed throughout their lives. In captivity, adults of *T. rubida*, *T. protracta*, and *T. recurva* live 4–5 months on average (J. Schmidt, unpublished data). Mating is of short duration relative to many other hemipterans, lasting only about 10 min. Females readily mate with multiple males and can lay several hundred eggs during their lifetime, but numbers vary widely depending on conditions including density of bugs in the immediate environment, presence of preferred hosts, continuous availability of hosts and time of season the bug matured (Gorla et al., 2010). Dispersal is achieved both actively by crawling immatures and flying adults (Schofield, 2000) and passively in some species either by transport of attached eggs to new locations or by human transport of materials harbouring eggs or free-living stages. A classic example of human passive transport is the species *T. rubrofasciata* which has been inadvertently transported via commerce to many seaports around the world (Schofield, 2000). Active dispersal of immatures appears to be in response to a shortage of food sources leading to bugs crawling towards locations potentially having new hosts. Adults typically disperse by flight during optimal seasons, often just before or during the rainy season. Hunger is a powerful driver of dispersal (Lehane et al., 1992). Another is the reproductive strategy in which gravid females retain a portion of their eggs for deposition after flight (Klotz et al., 2010; McEwen and Lehane, 1994). Mate seeking is apparently not a cause of dispersal as evidenced by nearly equal numbers of males and females being captured at lights and the captured females rapidly ovipositing fertile eggs (Klotz et al., 2010; McEwen and Lehane, 1994).

Triatomine bugs can inhabit a variety of ecological environments from highly specialized to generalized, including human domestic environments. Within these habitats, they can range from specialists feeding on a limited number of hosts or to opportunists feeding on a variety of host species. Specialists include *Cavernicola pilosa*, which feed on bats, the members of *Psammolestes* living in twig constructed nests of birds, and *Rhodnius* spp. living in palm trees where they feed on birds and mammals. Living in somewhat more general areas are *T. rubrofasciata* and members of the *T. protracta* complex that prefer feeding on rodents. *T. infestans*, *T. dimidiata* and *R. prolixus* are inhabitants of human domestic environments (Lehane et al., 1992). Most species, irrespective of their preferred habitat, can be opportunistic and feed on available species when encountered. Species that are generally opportunists can also be facultative specialists that prefer to feed mainly on one group of hosts if given the opportunity (de la Fuente et al., 2008; Gurtler et al., 2009; Pizarro and Stevens, 2008). The *Triatoma* living in Arizona are all non-domestic species that often feed on pack rats (*Neotoma* spp.), yet they readily feed on a variety of encountered vertebrate hosts including humans (L. Stevens et al., unpublished data). In Tucson, the Arizona-Sonora Desert Museum, an educational living zoo of regional animals, supports large populations of *T. rubida* and *T. protracta* which plague many of the captive animals. Their extensive feeding is considered the cause of anaemia in several reptiles and the death of a rare protected mountain rattlesnake (James L. Jarchow, DVM, personal communication).

Exactly how and when some species of triatomines became specialists on humans is unclear. Human beings are relatively recent inhabitants of the New World, with exact arrival dates debated, but arrival around 14,000–20,000 years ago is reasonable. Thus, the shifts in some triatomine species to specializing on our species are evolutionarily recent events and might well explain some of our vulnerability to the *T. cruzi* parasites the bugs transmit to us.

8.4.1. Feeding behaviour

Triatomine bugs rely on a multitude of sensory modalities to locate hosts. These include carbon dioxide (CO_2) gradients, odours, moisture, heat and air flow (Guerenstein and Lazzari, 2009). They are exquisitely sensitive to

CO_2, being able to detect 75 ppm above the background air levels of 350 ppm when a trace of lactic acid, another attractant, is present. Exothermic hosts such as resting reptiles generate very low levels of CO_2; nevertheless, triatomines use many other host-generated chemical cues including short-chained aliphatic amines and acids, 7- to 9-carbon aldehydes and alcohols and lactic acid to locate these hosts. Triatomines also detect very low infrared radiation enabling them to orient towards endothermic hosts from several metres. Finally, they follow air currents impregnated with host odours to the host (Guerenstein and Lazzari, 2009).

Feeding by bugs in human domiciles usually takes place at night, with bugs secreting themselves during the day in cracks and crevices away from the feeding areas. Much less is known about feeding times for sylvatic species. Likely, they adjust their daily activity periods to match the inactive periods of their host, thereby minimizing danger and interference from hosts. *T. rubida* and *T. protracta* do not hesitate to approach and feed on rodents during bright daylight (Klotz et al., 2010), a behaviour that might well be adaptive for bugs that often feed on rodents in their burrows while they are sleeping or quiescent during the day.

Once a host is located, a hungry bug extends its proboscis and inserts it into the skin of the host. Often a host detects the minor sensation caused by a bug's probing and moves or shifts position, causing the bug to retract before returning to continue probing one or several more times until feeding is complete. Uninterrupted feeding is relatively rapid—considering that the bug often imbibes more blood than its own weight (Klotz et al., 2010) and feeds on average 22 min for *T. protracta*, 28 min for *T. rubida* and between 11 and 28 min for *T. infestans*, *T. dimidiata* and *R. prolixus* (Klotz et al., 2009b; Zeledón et al., 1977). To rid their bodies of the excess fluids from their blood meals, bugs often defecate during feeding, at completion of feeding, or after leaving the feeding site. Some species, especially those domestic species that are major vectors of Chagas disease, defecate rapidly, frequently, often near or on the host (Zeledón et al., 1977). Others not considered important vectors tend to defecate less rapidly and frequently, and often at a distance from the host (Klotz et al., 2009b). Frequency and proximity of defecation to the host are considered factors in transmitting *T. cruzi* to humans.

8.5. URBANIZATION OF THE BUGS

Many species of bugs like *T. dimidiata* occupy multiple ecotopes including sylvan, peridomestic and domestic environments providing reservoirs to readily occupy treated houses. For example, *T. mexicana* of central Mexico and *T. dimidiata* of the Yucatan, Mexico and Belize do not colonize homes but seasonally migrate from sylvan and peridomestic ecotopes and infest homes (Ramirez-Sierra et al., 2009). Thus, the efficacy of insecticide programmes is greatly reduced as new populations of triatomines infest homes annually. Molecular markers have been used to determine the source of bugs in houses after treatment and whether they are survivors of ineffective pesticide applications (the usual case) or are immigrants from a particular ecotope. A number of studies of vector-borne infectious diseases demonstrate that their resurgence is due to human expansion into forested areas and Chagas disease in Latin America follows this paradigm. For example, the diversity of *T. dimidiata* niches defies public health initiatives because of continued reinfestation from sylvatic habitats posing a greater threat than *R. prolixus* even though *R. prolixus* is more efficient at transmitting disease (Ponce, 1999). Other examples include niche expansion into houses in a forested community in Bolivia and homes in Calilegua National Park, Argentina where light attracts *P. rufotuberculatus* (Salomon et al., 1999).

8.6. CONTROL OF VECTORS

8.6.1. Multinational efforts

Vector transmission of Chagas disease accounts for more than 80% of disease transmission (Yamagata and Nakagawa, 2006). Over the past two decades, several regional initiatives in Latin America have made tremendous strides in reducing and in some cases, interrupting vector transmission of the disease. The Southern Cone Initiative was launched first (1991) and focused on blood screening and insecticide-based elimination of *T. infestans*, a primarily domestic species that is the main disease vector in the southern cone region of South America. Success, although considerable, was measured mainly by the significant reduction of *T. infestans* in Uruguay by 1997, Chile by 1999, Brazil by 2000, Argentina by 2001 and Paraguay by 2002. Bolivia was the only country that did not see a significant reduction of the primary vector, *T. infestans*.

The Central American Initiative followed (1997) with the goal of eliminating *R. prolixus*, a South American species with only domestic populations in Central America and reducing household infestations of *T. dimidiata*, a native domestic, peridomestic and sylvatic species (Ponce, 2007). Other regional initiatives were launched in the Andean Region (1997), Mexico (2003) and Amazon (2004). To date, Brazil, Chile, Uruguay and Guatemala have been declared free of Chagas disease transmission by their main vectors, as well as some areas in Argentina and Paraguay (Gorla et al., 2010).

Large-scale initiatives like these face formidable challenges. The operational logistics of controlling vectors over vast geographic areas should be designed to maximize efficacy and minimize costs (Levy et al., 2010). The sustainability of these programmes relies on political and economic commitments that may change quickly in developing countries, and the decentralization of health care services across Latin America during the 1980s places the burden of responsibility on vector control and surveillance on the local community (Gürtler et al., 2007; Tarleton et al., 2007). Although there exists technical expertise in management strategies, there is always room for improvement and yet applied research in vector control lags far behind basic research on triatomines (Abad-Franch et al., 2010). Finally, a successful control campaign can often be its own worst enemy if complacency sets in and vector control and surveillance programmes are not maintained (Gorla et al., 2010).

8.6.2. Housing improvement

Vector control programmes for triatomines generally include three components that should be carried out by trained personnel (Schofield, 2000): (1) geographical reconnaissance to locate infestation foci, which entails inspections of homes and peridomestic environments in areas suspected of infestation; (2) application of residual insecticide sprays in and around infested structures and (3) long-term surveillance to monitor treated homes and peridomestic environments for reinfestation and retreatments when necessary. Homeowners should also be educated on the vector control programme and encouraged to report any triatomines that they find.

8.6.3. Chemical control

Insecticide spraying has been the cornerstone of vector control of triatomines ever, since the advent of organic insecticides in the late 1940s made effective control possible. The organochlorines such as dieldrin and lindane were the first line of defense in the 1950s, followed by organopho sphates and carbamates in the 1960s and 1970s, and pyrethroids since the 1980s, such as cypermethrin, cyfluthrin, deltamethrin and lambda-cyhalothrin, particularly wettable powder and soluble concentrate formulations (Gorla et al., 2010; Toloza et al., 2008). Ideally, chemical control measures should be tailored to the biology of the targeted species, as for example, with *T. dimidiata* in the Yucatán Peninsula, by spraying at the beginning of April, right before the start of their seasonal infestation period (Barbu et al., 2009).

Chemical failures due to pyrethroid resistance have been reported in areas of Argentina and Bolivia in controlling *T. infestans* including evidence of resistance in eggs to the pyrethroids deltamethrin and lambda-cyhalothrin (Toloza et al., 2008). Resistance may be slowed by rotating or mixing carbamates or organophosphates with pyrethroids (Lardeux et al., 2010). Other chemical control strategies include pyrethroid-impregnated curtains (Ferral et al., 2010) and bed nets (Kroeger et al., 2003), and xenointoxication, as for example, using pyrethroid-treated dog collars (Reithinger et al., 2006). Because young children spend much of their time in and around their household, efforts need to consider the effect of insecticide sprayings in domestic settings (Chaudhuri, 2004).

8.6.4. Non-chemical measures

Chagas disease is considered one of the neglected tropical diseases that have primarily impacted the poorest people living in Latin America (Hotez et al., 2008). Early on, Carlos Chagas recognized the potential benefits of improved housing in the prevention of triatomine infestation (Dias, 2007). According to Zeledon and Rabinovich (1981), some of the risk factors associated with triatomine infestations include "palm thatched roofs or walls" for *R. prolixus*, "cracks in mud and cane walls" for *T. infestans*, and "wooden or mud houses with earthen floors or under houses built on stilts" for *T. dimidiata*. Replacing thatched roofs with metal sheets (Bustamante et al., 2007) and plastering walls (Monroy et al., 2009) removes potential harbourage sites for triatomines, as well as physical modifications in the peridomestic environment such as replacing piled brushwood with wire fencing for animal enclosures (Gürtler et al., 2007).

Investigations of potential biological control agents have been undertaken in order to provide alternative strategies to chemical control measures and/or management of pyrethroid-resistant populations of triatomines (Pedrini et al., 2009). The entomopathogenic fungus, *Beauveria bassiana*, has been isolated from field populations of *T. infestans* in Argentina. Pathogenicity tests of these isolates in the laboratory yielded 100% mortality of bugs 15 days after infection (Marti et al., 2005). Field tests of traps infected with *B. bassiana* were conducted in rural village homes infested with pyrethroid-resistant bugs, and their mortality was estimated at $>50\%$ (1). Other pathogens isolated from *T. infestans* include a picorna-like virus (Muscio et al., 1988). Ryckman and Blankenship compiled a list of a number of potential parasites and predators of the Triatominae. How practical and where in the life cycle of the kissing bugs these biological agents could be used remains to be established (Ryckman and Blankenship, 1984).

BOX Non-chemical measures to reduce risk of household infestation

Sanitation measures

- Maintaining good hygiene and reducing clutter inside houses (Monroy et al., 2009)
- Eliminating junk, wood or rock piles, trash, and other objects in peridomestic environments (Ferral et al., 2010)
- Managing surrounding vegetation and conserving local fauna (Teixeira et al., 2009)
- Home improvement
- Installing insect screens (Guzman-Tapia et al., 2007)
- Replacing outside white lights with yellow lights (Gouge et al., 2010)
- Sealing structural cracks and crevices (Gouge et al., 2010)

8.7. NON-INFECTIOUS CONSEQUENCES OF A TRIATOMINE BITE

The major importance of kissing bugs from a medical perspective is their ability to transmit *T. cruzi* to humans and other animals, including pets. The transmission of *T. cruzi* remains an ongoing problem in Mexico, Central and South America. An unappreciated health-related association important in the United States is allergic responses to kissing bug bites. The allergic reactions can be trivial to life-threatening (Klotz et al., 2010). For example, anaphylaxis caused by a *Triatoma* bite led to the death of an adult woman in Phoenix, Arizona (Lo Vecchio and Tran, 2004). *Triatoma* bites are the leading cause of anaphylaxis due to insect bites in the United States (Hoffman, 1987).

Kissing bugs rarely transmit Chagas in the United States. Why this is so is unknown and is an active area of interest. To date, only six autochthonous cases of Chagas are documented in the United States (Dorn et al., 2007). Lack of domestication of sylvatic species is likely the most important factor (Zeledón, 1974). Observers have further postulated that because Triatominae in the United States do not defecate at the time of feeding there is little or no transmission of *T. cruzi* (Edwards and Lynch, 1984). The latter speculation is borne out by direct observations of *T. sanguisuga* (Shields and Walsh, 1956) feeding on humans and *T. rubida* and *T. protracta* feeding on rodents (Klotz et al., 2009b; Wood, 1951). It is interesting to note that victims of kissing bug bites in the United States do not report faecal drops or smears on their bed sheets (Shields and Walsh, 1956) yet defecation while feeding or shortly after the insect is replete is very characteristic of other Triatominae.

8.7.1. Nature of the bite

There is considerable misinformation concerning kissing bug bites, in particular, whether the bite is painful or not. Early accounts of bites of *T. sanguisuga* stated the bite is "...very painful and often even dangerous" (Kimball, 1893–1894) and "...a most painful wound" often confused with a spider bite (Le Conte, 1854–1855). From the standpoint of successful hematophagous insects, it is helpful that the host remains unaware of the presence of the insect; hence, the act of biting is often painless. Patients presenting to emergency rooms with anaphylaxis due to kissing bugs bites are rarely aware of a preceding bite—they awaken with intense itching over the body and difficulty breathing (Shields and Walsh, 1956). Shields and Walsh carefully observed *T. sanguisuga* feeding on humans and concluded that the bite is painless (Nichols and Green, 1963).

The typical kissing bug bite leads to a small raised skin lesion with a central punctum and an inflammatory infiltrate in the subcutaneous tissue (Shields and Walsh, 1956). Swelling of tissue at the bite site over several days may lead to nodular, urticarial lesions associated with pain and may last up to 7 days (Lynch and Pinnas, 1978). Some severe reactions may last for up to a month and include lesions at the bite site. Lymphadenitis and vasculitic rashes such as erythema multiforme may occur as well (Shields and Walsh, 1956). These delayed allergic responses are uncomfortable or painful and undoubtedly account for the many claims that the bite itself "hurts". Romana's sign (unilateral eyelid oedema), found in patients in endemic areas of Chagas, is held to be pathognomonic of acute disease, but when seen in the United States is likely to be an allergic manifestation of the bite (Klotz et al., 2010).

Allergic reactions to bites of many species including the epidemiologically important vectors of Chagas disease (*T. infestans, R. prolixus, P. megistus* and *T. dimidiata*) are documented (Mott et al., 1980). The use of xenodiagnosis has been limited as a result of allergic skin reactions occurring after bites—patients experienced accelerated allergic reactions such as wheals and hives (i.e. IgE-mediated responses; Costa et al., 1981).

8.7.2. Triatomine saliva and its antigenic components

Whole bug extracts of *T. infestans* are capable of eliciting IgE and IgG antibodies in atopic patients, and the allergens may be similar to those of the American cockroach, *Periplaneta americana* (Alonso et al., 2004). However, mere contact of kissing bugs with human skin has not been reported to cause allergic reactions such as are seen with, for example, the urticating hairs of some caterpillars (Klotz et al., 2009a).

Allergic host responses to kissing bug bites are due to allergens present in the saliva of the bugs. In kissing bug endemic areas in the United

States, allergies are common. About 7% of the inhabitants of one community in California had evidence of IgE allergy to *T. protracta* (Marshall et al., 1986b). Bioassays of salivary gland extracts have demonstrated the presence of allergens capable of eliciting IgE antibody in patients and are highly species specific, that is, there is no cross-reactivity of extracts, for example, between *T. rubida* and *T. protracta* or extracts from *R. prolixus*, *T. rubrofasciata* or *T. cavernicola* (Marshall et al., 1986a). The allergens appear to be low molecular weight proteins (Marshall et al., 1986a). Procalin, a 20-kDa protein, was identified from *T. protracta* (Paddock et al., 2001). This protein, or one very similar, accounted for ~90% of the allergenic activity of the saliva (Chapman et al., 1986).

In the classical description of anaphylaxis by Richet and Portier, two steps were required: exposure to an allergen (which "primed" or "set the stage") followed by repeat exposure to the same allergen *after* sufficient time (usually weeks) for lymphocytes to produce IgE antibody to the foreign antigen and thus elicit the allergic cascade known as a type I hypersensitivity reaction (Klotz et al., 2009a). This reaction is the most extreme of allergic reactions mediated by IgE antibody. During the reaction, antibodies bind to mast cells located throughout the body and cause the release of histamine which in turn leads to swelling of the mucosa especially in the airways and larynx that can impair breathing, syncope, hypotension and shock, urticaria (hives), intense itching, diarrhoea and even uterine bleeding (Nichols and Green, 1963; Pinnas et al., 1986). IgG antibodies may result in a similar, but not identical response known as an anaphylactoid reaction, but this has not been reported with kissing bug bites and usually follows some form of envenomation (Klotz et al., 2009a). Anaphylaxis has been reported following bites with important Chagas vectors including as *R. prolixus* and *T. infestans* but is apparently not common (Mott et al., 1980).

Currently, there is no effective preventive therapy for anaphylaxis due to kissing bug bites. Moffitt et al. (2003) compiled the data regarding immunotherapy and its use and success in patients with a history of anaphylaxis, but this is an intensive procedure and without standardized allergens it is unlikely to be of much widespread benefit.

8.8. CONCLUSION

Extensive research on the primary vectors of Chagas has provided scientists with a wealth of knowledge regarding the origin and expansion of domesticated triatomines and has led to many successful control programmes. However, secondary vectors that are often cryptic in nature and enjoy a relatively large niche in forests and burrows readily move into vacated ecotopes and pose an ongoing risk for transmission of *T. cruzi*.

Consequently, kissing bugs will remain a menace to human populations for some time to come as well as a subject of intense research.

ACKNOWLEDGEMENT

Part of this material is based upon work supported by the National Science Foundation under core faculty funding from Grant No. NSF EPS-0701410 (L. S.) and NIH Grant 1R15 A1079672-01A1 (P. L. D.).

REFERENCES

Abad-Franch, F., Santos, W.S., Schofield, C.J., 2010. Research needs for Chagas disease prevention. Acta Trop. 115, 44–54.

Abalos, J.W., 1948. Sobre híbridos naturales y experimentales de Triatoma. An. Inst. Med. Region. 2, 209–223.

Aguilar, H.M., Abad-Franch, F., Dias, J.C., Junqueira, A.C., Coura, J.R., 2007. Chagas disease in the Amazon region. Mem. Inst. Oswaldo Cruz 102 (Suppl. 1), 47–56.

Alonso, A., Potenza, M., Mouchian, K., Albonico, J., Pionetti, C., 2004. Proteinase and gelatinolytic properties of a Triatoma infestans extract. Allergol. Immunopathol. (Madr.) 32, 223–227.

Azambuja, P., Garcia, E., Ratcliffe, N., 2005. Gut microbiota and parasite transmission by insect vectors. Trends Parasitol. 21, 568–572.

Barbu, C., Dumonteil, E., Gourbiere, S., 2009. Optimization of control strategies for non-domiciliated Triatoma dimidiata, Chagas disease vector in the Yucatan Peninsula, Mexico. PLoS Negl. Trop. Dis. 3, e416.

Bargues, M.D., Klisiowicz, D.R., Panzera, F., Noireau, F., Marcilla, A., Perez, R., et al., 2006. Origin and phylogeography of the Chagas disease main vector Triatoma infestans based on nuclear rDNA sequences and genome size. Infect. Genet. Evol. 6, 46–62.

Bargues, M.D., Schofield, C.J., Dujardin, J.P., 2010. Classification and phylogeny of the Triatominae. In: Telleria, J., Tibayrenc, M. (Eds.), American Trypanosomiasis Chagas Disease—100 Years of Research. Elsevier, Burlington, MA, pp. 117–147.

Benoit, J.B., Denlinger, D.L., 2010. Meeting the challenges of on-host and off-host water balance in blood-feeding arthropods. J. Insect Physiol. 56, 1366–1376.

Bustamante, D.M., Monroy, M.C., Rodas, A.G., Juarez, J.A., Malone, J.B., 2007. Environmental determinants of the distribution of Chagas disease vectors in south-eastern Guatemala. Geospat. Health 1, 199–211.

Carcavallo, R.U., Jurberg, J., Lent, H., Noireau, F., Galvao, C., 2000. Phylogeny of the Triatominae. (Hemiptera: Reduviidae). Proposals for taxonomic arrangements. Entomol. Vect. 7 (Suppl. 1), 1–99.

Carrasco, H.J., Frame, I.A., Valente, S.A., Miles, M.A., 1996. Genetic exchange as a possible source of genomic diversity in sylvatic populations of *Trypanosoma cruzi*. Am. J. Trop. Med. Hyg. 54, 418–424.

Chapman, M., Marshall, N., Saxon, A., 1986. Identification and partial purification of species-specific allergens from Triatoma protracta (Heteroptera:Reduviidae). J. Allergy Clin. Immunol. 78, 436–442.

Chaudhuri, N., 2004. Interventions to improve children's health by improving the housing environment. Rev. Environ. Health 19, 197–222.

Costa, D., Costa, M., Weber, J., Gilks, G., Castro, C., Marsden, P., 1981. Sin reactions to bug bites as a result of xenodiagnosis. Trans. R. Soc. Trop. Med. Hyg. 75, 405–408.

de la Fuente, A., Dias-Lima, A., Lopes, C., Emperaire, L., Walter, A., Ferreira, A., et al., 2008. Behavioral plasticity of Triatominae related to habitat selection in northeast Brazil. J. Med. Entomol. 45, 14–19.

de la Rua, N., Stevens, L., Wesson, D., Dorn, P.L., 2010. High genetic diversity in a single population of *Triatoma sanguisuga* (LeConte, 1855) inferred from two mitochondrial markers: cytochrome *b* and 16S ribosomal DNA. Infect. Genet. Evol. 11, 671–677.

de Paula, A.S., Diotaiuti, L., Schofield, C.J., 2005. Testing the sister-group relationship of the Rhodniini and Triatomini (Insecta: Hemiptera: Reduviidae: Triatominae). Mol. Phylogenet. Evol. 35, 712–718.

De Rosas, A.R.P., Segura, E.L., Garcia, B.A., 2007. Microsatellite analysis of genetic structure in natural Triatoma infestans (Hemiptera: Reduviidae) populations from Argentina: its implication in assessing the effectiveness of Chagas' disease vector control programmes. Mol. Ecol. 16, 1401–1412.

Dias, J.C., 2007. Southern Cone Initiative for the elimination of domestic populations of Triatoma infestans and the interruption of transfusional Chagas disease. Historical aspects, present situation, and perspectives. Mem. Inst. Oswaldo Cruz 102 (Suppl. 1), 11–18.

Diaz-Suarez, O., 2009. Chagas disease: re-emergent or neglected. Invest. Clin. 50, 415–418.

Dorn, P.L., Perniciaro, L., Yabsley, M.J., Roellig, D.D.M., Balsamo, G., Diaz, J., et al., 2007. Autochthonous transmission of Trypanosoma cruzi, Louisiana. Emerg. Infect. Dis. 13, 605–607.

Dorn, P.L., Calderon, C., Melgar, S., Moguel, B., Solorzano, E., Dumonteil, E., et al., 2009. Two distinct Triatoma dimidiata (Latreille, 1811) taxa are found in sympatry in Guatemala and Mexico. PLoS Negl. Trop. Dis. 3, e393.

Dujardin, J.P., Schofield, C.J., 2004. Triatominae: systematics, morphology, and population biology. In: Maudlin, I., Holmes, P.H., Miles, M.A. (Eds.), The Trypanosomiases. CABI Publishing, Cambridge, Part 2. Chapter 9, pp. 181–201.

Dujardin, J.P., Tibayrenc, M., 1985. Isoenzymatic studies of the principal vector of Chagas disease: Triatoma infestans (Hemiptera: Reduviidae). Ann. Soc. Belg. Med. Trop. 65 (Suppl. 1), 165–169.

Dujardin, J.P., Chavez, T., Moreno, J.M., Machane, M., Noireau, F., Schofield, C.J., 1999. Comparison of isoenzyme electrophoresis and morphometric analysis for phylogenetic reconstruction of the Rhodniini (Hemiptera: Reduviidae: Triatominae). J. Med. Entomol. 36, 653–659.

Edwards, L., Lynch, P., 1984. Anaphylactic reaction to kissing bugs. Arizona Med. 41, 159–161.

Eichler, S., Schaub, G., 2002. Development of symbionts in triatomine bugs and the effects of infections with trypanosomids. Exp. Parasitol. 100, 17–27.

Ferral, J., Chavez-Nunez, L., Euan-Garcia, M., Ramirez-Sierra, M.J., Najera-Vazquez, M.R., Dumonteil, E., 2010. Comparative field trial of alternative vector control strategies for non-domiciliated Triatoma dimidiata. Am. J. Trop. Med. Hyg. 82, 60–66.

Garcia, E.S., Azambuja, P., 1991. Development and interactions of *Trypanosoma cruzi* within the insect vector. Parasitol. Today 7, 240–244.

Garcia, B.A., Canale, D.M., Blanco, A., 1995. Genetic structure of four species of Triatoma (Hemiptera: Reduviidae) from Argentina. J. Med. Entomol. 32, 134–137.

Gaunt, M., Miles, M., 2000. The ecotopes and evolution of triatomine bugs (Triatominae) and their associated trypanosomes. Mem. Inst. Oswaldo Cruz 95, 557–565.

Giordano, R., Cortez, J.C., Paulk, S., Stevens, L., 2005. Genetic diversity of Triatoma infestans (Hemiptera: Reduviidae) in Chuquisaca, Bolivia based on the mitochondrial cytochrome *b* gene. Mem. Inst. Oswaldo Cruz 100, 753–760.

Gorla, D.E., Dujardin, J.P., Schofield, C.J., 1997. Biosystematics of Old World Triatominae. Acta Trop. 63, 127–140.

Gorla, D., Ponce, C., Dujardin, J., Schofield, C., 2010. Control strategies against Triatominae. In: Telleria, J., Tibayrenc, M. (Eds.), American Trypanosomiasis Chagas Disease One Hundred Years of Research. Elsevier, Burlington, MA, pp. 233–245.
Guerenstein, P.G., Lazzari, C.R., 2009. Host-seeking: how triatomines acquire and make use of information to find blood. Acta Trop. 110, 148–158.
Guhl, F., 2007. Chagas disease in Andean countries. Mem. Inst. Oswaldo Cruz 102 (Suppl. 1), 29–38.
Gurtler, R.E., Ceballos, L.A., Ordonez-Krasnowski, P., Lanati, L.A., Stariolo, R., Kitron, U., 2009. Strong host-feeding preferences of the vector Triatoma infestans modified by vector density: implications for the epidemiology of Chagas disease. PLoS Negl. Trop. Dis. 3, e447.
Gürtler, R.E., Kitron, U., Ceceré, M.C., Segura, E.L., Cohen, J.E., 2007. Sustainable vector control and management of Chagas disease in the Gran Chaco, Argentina. Proc. Natl. Acad. Sci. USA 104, 16194–16199.
Guzman-Tapia, Y., Ramirez-Sierra, M.J., Dumonteil, E., 2007. Urban infestation by Triatoma dimidiata in the city of Merida, Yucatan, Mexico. Vector Borne Zoonotic Dis. 7, 597–606.
Hoffman, D., 1987. Allergy to biting insects. Clin. Rev. Allergy 5, 177–190.
Hotez, P.J., Bottazzi, M.E., Franco-Paredes, C., Ault, S.K., Periago, M.R., 2008. The neglected tropical diseases of Latin America and the Caribbean: a review of disease burden and distribution and a roadmap for control and elimination. PLoS Negl. Trop. Dis. 2, e300.
Hypsa, V., Tietz, D.F., Zrzavy, J., Rego, R.O., Galvao, C., Jurberg, J., 2002. Phylogeny and biogeography of Triatominae (Hemiptera: Reduviidae): molecular evidence of a New World origin of the Asiatic clade. Mol. Phylogenet. Evol. 23, 447–457.
Ibarra-Cerdena, C.N., Sanchez-Cordero, V., Townsend Peterson, A., Ramsey, J.M., 2009. Ecology of North American Triatominae. Acta Trop. 110, 178–186.
Juarez, M.P., Carlson, D.A., Salazar Schettino, P.M., Mijailovsky, S., Rojas, G., 2002. Cuticular hydrocarbons of Chagas disease vectors in Mexico. Mem. Inst. Oswaldo Cruz 97, 819–827.
Kimball, B., 1893–18. Conorhinus sanguisugus: its habits and life history. Trans. Annu. Meetings Kansas Acad. Sci. 14, 128–131.
Kjos, S.A., Snowden, K.F., Olson, J.K., 2009. Biogeography and *Trypanosoma cruzi* infection prevalence of Chagas disease vectors in Texas, USA. Vector Borne Zoonotic Dis. 9, 41–49.
Klotz, J., Klotz, S., Pinnas, J., 2009a. Animal bites and stings with anaphylactic potential. J. Emerg. Med. 36, 148–156.
Klotz, S., Dorn, P., Klotz, J., Pinnas, J., Weirauch, C., Kurtz, J., et al., 2009b. Feeding behavior of triatomines from the southwestern United States: an update on potential risk for transmission of Chagas disease. Acta Trop. 111, 114–118.
Klotz, J., Dorn, P., Logan, J., Stevens, L., Pinnas, J., Schmidt, J., et al., 2010. "Kissing bugs": potential disease vectors and cause of anaphylaxis. Clin. Infect. Dis. 50, 1629–1634.
Knowles, L.L., Carstens, B.C., 2007. Delimiting species without monophyletic gene trees. Syst. Biol. 56, 887–895.
Kroeger, A., Villegas, E., Ordonez-Gonzalez, J., Pabon, E., Scorza, J.V., 2003. Prevention of the transmission of Chagas' disease with pyrethroid-impregnated materials. Am. J. Trop. Med. Hyg. 68, 307–311.
Lardeux, F., Depickere, S., Duchon, S., Chavez, T., 2010. Insecticide resistance of Triatoma infestans (Hemiptera, Reduviidae) vector of Chagas disease in Bolivia. Trop. Med. Int. Health 15, 1037–1048.
Le Conte, J., 1854–18. Remarks on two species of American Cimex. Proc. Acad. Nat. Sci. Philadelphia 7, 404.
Lehane, M.J., McEwen, P.K., Whitaker, C.J., Schofield, C.J., 1992. The role of temperature and nutritional status in flight initiation by Triatoma infestans. Acta Trop. 52, 27–38.

Lent, H., Wygodzinsky, P., 1979. Revision of the Triatominae (Hemiptera, Reduviidae), and their significance as vectors of Chagas' disease. Bull. AMNH 163, 127–520.

Levy, M.Z., Malaga Chavez, F.S., Cornejo Del Carpio, J.G., Vilhena, D.A., McKenzie, F.E., Plotkin, J.B., 2010. Rational spatio-temporal strategies for controlling a Chagas disease vector in urban environments. J. R. Soc. Interface 7, 1061–1070.

Lo vecchio, F., Tran, T., 2004. Allergic reactions from insect bites. Am. J. Emerg. Med. 22, 631.

Lyman, D.F., Monteiro, F.A., Escalante, A.A., Cordon-Rosales, C., Wesson, D.M., Dujardin, J.P., et al., 1999. Mitochondrial DNA sequence variation among triatomine vectors of Chagas' disease. Am. J. Trop. Med. Hyg. 60, 377–386.

Lynch, P., Pinnas, J., 1978. Kissing bug bites. Cutis 22, 585–589.

Marcilla, A., Bargues, M.D., Ramsey, J.M., Magallon-Gastelum, E., Salazar-Schettino, P.M., Abad-Franch, F., et al., 2001. The ITS-2 of the nuclear rDNA as a molecular marker for populations, species, and phylogenetic relationships in Triatominae (Hemiptera: Reduviidae), vectors of Chagas disease. Mol. Phylogenet. Evol. 18, 136–142.

Marshall, N., Chapman, M., Saxon, A., 1986a. Species-specific allergens from salivary glands of Triatominae (Heteroptera: Reduviidae). J. Allergy Clin. Immunol. 78, 430–435.

Marshall, N., Liebhaber, M., Dyer, Z., Saxon, A., 1986b. The prevalence of allergic sensitization to Triatoma protracta (Heteroptera: Reduviidae) in southern California, USA, community. J. Med. Entomol. 23, 117–124.

Marti, G.A., Scorsetti, A.C., Siri, A., Lopez Lastra, C.C., 2005. Isolation of *Beauveria bassiana* (Bals.) Buill. (Deuteromycotina: Hyphomycetes) from the Chagas diseases vector *Triatoma infestans* (Hemiptera: Reduviidae) in Argentina. Mycopathologica 159 (3), 389–391.

Martinez-Ibarra, J.A., Grant-Guillen, Y., Morales-Corona, Z.Y., Haro-Rodriguez, S., Ventura-Rodriguez, L.V., Nogueda-Torres, B., et al., 2008. Importance of species of Triatominae (Heteroptera: Reduviidae) in risk of transmission of *Trypanosoma cruzi* in western Mexico. J. Med. Entomol. 45, 476–482.

Mayr, E., 1970. Populations, Species, and Evolution. Harvard University Press, Cambridge, MA.

Mazzotti, L., Osorio, M.T., 1942. Cruzamientos experimentales entre varias especies de triatomas. Med. Rev. Mexicana 22, 215–222.

McEwen, P.K., Lehane, M.J., 1994. Relationship between flight initiation and oviposition in Triatoma infestans (Klug) (Hem., Reduviidae). J. Appl. Entomol. 117, 217–223.

Moffitt, J., Venarske, D., Goddard, J., Yates, A., DeShazo, R., 2003. Allergic reactions to Triatoma bites. Ann. Allergy Asthama Immunol. 91, 122–128.

Monroy, C., Bustamante, D.M., Pineda, S., Rodas, A., Castro, X., Ayala, V., et al., 2009. House improvements and community participation in the control of Triatoma dimidiata re-infestation in Jutiapa, Guatemala. Cad. Saude Publica 25 (Suppl. 1), S168–S178.

Monteiro, F.A., Wesson, D.M., Dotson, E.M., Schofield, C.J., Beard, C.B., 2000. Phylogeny and molecular taxonomy of the Rhodniini derived from mitochondrial and nuclear DNA sequences. Am. J. Trop. Med. Hyg. 62, 460–465.

Monteiro, F.A., Donnelly, M.J., Beard, C.B., Costa, J., 2004. Nested clade and phylogeographic analyses of the Chagas disease vector *Triatoma brasiliensis* in Northeast Brazil. Mol. Phylogenet. Evol. 32, 46–56.

Mott, K., Franca, J., Barrett, T., Hoff, R., de Oliveira, T., Sherlock, I., 1980. Cutaneous allergic reactions to *Triatoma infestans* after xenodiagnosis. Mem. Inst. Osaldo Cruz 75, 3–10.

Muscio, O.A., La Torre, J.L., Scodeller, E.A., 1988. Characterization of *Triatoma* Virus, a picorna-like virus isolated from the triatomine bug *Triatoma infestans*. J. Gen. Virol. 69 (1), 2929–2934.

Nichols, N., Green, T., 1963. Allergic reactions to "kissing bug" bites. Calif. Med. 98, 267–268.

Noireau, F., 2009. Wild *Triatoma infestans*, a potential threat that needs to be monitored. Mem. Inst. Oswaldo Cruz 104, 60–64.

Paddock, C., McKerrow, J., Hansell, E., foreman, K., Hsieh, I., Marshall, N., 2001. Identification, cloning, and recombinant expression of procalin, a major triatome allergen. J. Immunol. 167, 2694–2699.
Panzera, F., Dujardin, J.P., Nicolini, P., Caraccio, M.N., Rose, V., Tellez, T., et al., 2004. Genomic changes of Chagas disease vector, South America. Emerg. Infect. Dis. 10, 438–446.
Panzera, F., Perez, R., Lucero, C., Ferrandis, I., Ferreiro, M.J., Calleros, L., et al., 2007. Cambios genómicos en la subfamilia Triatominae, con énfasis en Triatoma infestans. In: Cortez, M.R. (Ed.), Triatominos de Bolivia y la enfermedad de Chagas. Ministerio de Salud y Deportes—Programa Nacional de Chagas, La Paz, Bolivia pp.
Panzera, F., Perez, R., Panzera, Y., Ferrandis, I., Ferreiro, M.J., Calleros, L., 2010. Cytogenetics and genome evolution in the subfamily Triatominae (Hemiptera, Reduviidae). Cytogenet. Genome Res. 128, 77–87.
Patterson, J.S., Gaunt, M.W., 2010. Phylogenetic multi-locus codon models and molecular clocks reveal the monophyly of haematophagous reduviid bugs and their evolution at the formation of South America. Mol. Phylogenet. Evol. 56, 608–621.
Pedrini, N., Mijailovsky, S.J., Girotti, J.R., Stariolo, R., Cardozo, R.M., Gentile, A., et al., 2009. Control of pyrethroid-resistant Chagas disease vectors with entomopathogenic fungi. PLoS Negl. Trop. Dis. 3, e434.
Pereira, M.H., Souza, M.E., Vargas, A.P., Martins, M.S., Penido, C.M., Diotaiuti, L., 1996. Anticoagulant activity of *Triatoma infestans* and *Panstrongylus megistus* saliva (Hemiptera/Triatominae). Acta Trop. 61, 255–261.
Pfeiler, E., Bitler, B.G., Ramsey, J.M., Palacios-Cardiel, C., Markow, T.A., 2006. Genetic variation, population structure, and phylogenetic relationships of *Triatoma rubida* and T-recurva (Hemiptera: Reduviidae: Triatominae) from the Sonoran Desert, insect vectors of the Chagas' disease parasite *Trypanosoma cruzi*. Mol. Phylogenet. Evol. 41, 209–221.
Pinnas, J., Lindberg, R., Chen, T., Meinke, G., 1986. Studies of kissing bug-sensitive patients: evidence for the lack of cross-reactivity between *Triatoma protracta* and *Triatoma rubida* salivary gland extracts. J. Allergy Clin. Immunol. 77, 364–370.
Pizarro, J.C., Stevens, L., 2008. A new method for forensic DNA analysis of the blood meal in Chagas disease vectors demonstrated using *Triatoma infestans* from Chuquisaca, Bolivia. PLoS One 3, e3585.
Pizarro, J.C., Gilligan, L.M., Stevens, L., 2008. Microsatellites reveal a high population structure in *Triatoma infestans* from Chuquisaca, Bolivia. PLoS Negl. Trop. Dis. 2, e202.
Ponce, C., 1999. Towards the elimination of the transmission of *Trypanosoma cruzi* in Honduras and Central American countries. Medicinea (Baires) 59 (Suppl. 2), 117–119.
Ponce, C., 2007. Current situation of Chagas disease in Central America. Mem. Inst. Oswaldo Cruz 102 (Suppl. 1), 41–44.
Povoa, M.M., de Souza, A.A., Naiff, R.D., Arias, J.R., Naiff, M.F., Biancardi, C.B., et al., 1984. Chagas' disease in the Amazon basin IV. Host records of *Trypanosoma cruzi* zymodemes in the states of Amazonas and Rondonia, Brazil. Ann. Trop. Med. Parasitol. 78, 479–487.
Ramirez-Sierra, M.J., Herrera-Aguilar, M., Gourbiere, S., Dumonteil, E., 2009. Patterns of house infestation dynamics by non-domiciliated *Triatoma dimidiata* reveal a spatial gradient of infestation in rural villages and potential insect manipulation by Trypanosoma cruzi. Trop. Med. Int. Health 15, 77–86.
Reithinger, R., Ceballos, L., Stariolo, R., Davies, C.R., Gurtler, R.E., 2006. Extinction of experimental Triatoma infestans populations following continuous exposure to dogs wearing deltamethrin-treated collars. Am. J. Trop. Med. Hyg. 74, 766–771.
Ribeiro, J.M.C., Schneider, M., Isaias, T., Jurberg, J., Galvao, C., Guimaraes, J.A., 1998. Role of salivary antihemostatic components in blood feeding by triatomine bugs (Heteroptera). J. Med. Entomol. 35, 599–610.

Ryckman, R.E., Blankenship, C.M., 1984. The parasites, predators and symbionts of the Triatominae (Hemiptera: Reduviidae: Triatominae). Bull. Soc. Vector Ecol. 9 (2), 84–111.
Salomon, O.D., Ripoll, C.M., Rivetti, E., Carcavallo, R.U., 1999. Presence of *Panstrongylus rufotuberculatus* (champion, 1899) (hemiptera: reduviidae: Triatominae) in artentina. Mem. Inst. Oswaldo Cruz 94, 285–288.
Sandoval, C.M., Ortiz, N., Jaimes, D., Lorosa, E., Galvao, C., Rodriguez, O., et al., 2010. Feeding behaviour of Belminus ferroae (Hemiptera: Reduviidae), a predaceous Triatominae colonizing rural houses in Norte de Santander, Colombia. Med. Vet. Entomol. 24, 124–131.
Schaefer, C.W., 2003. Triatominae (Hemiptera: Reduviidae): systematic questions and some others. Neotrop. Entomol. 32, 01–10.
Schofield, C.J., 1988. Biosystematics of the Triatominae. Biosystematics of Haematophagous Insects. Clarendon Press, Oxford, pp. 287–312.
Schofield, C.J., 2000. Biosystematics and evolution of the Triatominae. Cad. Saude Publica 16 (Suppl. 2), 89–92.
Schofield, C.J., Galvao, C., 2009. Classification, evolution, and species groups within the Triatominae. Acta Trop. 110, 88–100.
Shields, T., Walsh, E., 1956. Kissing bug bite. Arch. Dermatol. 74, 14–21.
Stothard, J.R., Yamamoto, Y., Cherchi, A., Garcia, A.L., Valente, S.A.S., Schofield, C.J., 1998. A preliminary survey of mitochondrial sequence variation within triatomine bugs (Hemiptera: Reduviidae) using polymerase chain reaction-based single strand conformational polymorphism (SSCP) analysis and direct sequencing. Bull. Entomol. Res. 88, 8.
Tarleton, R.L., Reithinger, R., Urbina, J.A., Kitron, U., Gurtler, R.E., 2007. The challenges of Chagas disease—grim outlook or glimmer of hope. PLoS Med. 4, e332.
Teixeira, A.R., Gomes, C., Lozzi, S.P., Hecht, M.M., Rosa Ade, C., Monteiro, P.S., et al., 2009. Environment, interactions between Trypanosoma cruzi and its host, and health. Cad. Saude Publica 25 (Suppl. 1), S32–S44.
Toloza, A.C., Germano, M., Cueto, G.M., Vassena, C., Zerba, E., Picollo, M.I., 2008. Differential patterns of insecticide resistance in eggs and first instars of Triatoma infestans (Hemiptera: Reduviidae) from Argentina and Bolivia. J. Med. Entomol. 45, 421–426.
Torrico, R.A., 1946. Hallazgo de Eratyrus mucronatus, infestación natural de "vinchucas" de cerro y Eutriatoma sordida en Cochabamba. An. Lab. Central 1, 19–23.
Usinger, R., Wygodzinsky, P., Ryckman, R., 1966. The biosystematics of Triatominae. Ann. Rev. Entomol. 11, 309–330.
Vallejo, G.A., Guhl, F., Schaub, G.A., 2009. Triatominae-Trypanosoma cruzi/T. rangeli: vector-parasite interactions. Acta Trop. 110, 137–147.
van Valen, L., 1976. Ecological species, multispecies, and oaks. Taxon 25, 233–239.
Weirauch, C., 2008. Cladistic analysis of Reduviidae (Heteroptera: Cimicomorpha) based on morphological characters. Syst. Entomol. 33, 229–274.
Weirauch, C., Munro, J.B., 2009. Molecular phylogeny of the assassin bugs (Hemiptera: Reduviidae), based on mitochondrial and nuclear ribosomal genes. Mol. Phylogenet. Evol. 53, 287–299.
Wood, S., 1951. Importance of feeding and defecation times of insect vectors in transmission of Chagas' disease. J. Econ. Entomol. 44, 52–54.
Yamagata, Y., Nakagawa, J., 2006. Control of Chagas disease. Adv. Parasitol. 61, 129–165.
Yoshizawa, K., Johnson, K., 2010. How stable is the "Polyphyly of Lice" hypothesis (Insecta: Psodocea)? A comparison of phylogenetic signal in multiple genes. Mol. Phylogenet. Evol. 55, 939–951.
Yuval, B., 2006. Mating systems of blood-feeding flies. Annu. Rev. Entomol. 51, 413–440.
Zeledón, R., 1974. Epidemiology, modes of transmission and reservoir hosts of Chagas' disease. In: Eliot, K., O'connor, M., Wolstenholme, G. (Eds.), Trypanosomiasis and

Leishmaniasis with Special Reference to Chagas' Disease. Associated Scientific Publishers, Amsterdam, pp. 51–85.

Zeledon, R., Rabinovich, J.E., 1981. Chagas' disease: an ecological appraisal with special emphasis on its insect vectors. Annu. Rev. Entomol. 26, 101–133.

Zeledón, R., Alvarado, R., Jiron, L.F., 1977. Observations on the feeding and defecation patterns of three triatomine species (Hemiptera: Reduviidae). Acta Trop. 34, 65–77.

Zeledón, R., Ponce, C., Mendez-Galvan, J.F., 2007. Epidemiological, social, and control determinants of Chagas disease in Central America and Mexico–group discussion. Mem. Inst. Oswaldo Cruz 102 (Suppl. 1), 45–46.

CHAPTER 9

Advances in Imaging of Animal Models of Chagas Disease

Linda A. Jelicks* and **Herbert B. Tanowitz**[†,‡]

Contents

Abstract

Since serial studies of patients are limited, researchers interested in Chagas disease have relied on animal models of *Trypanosoma cruzi* infection to explore many aspects of this important human disease. These studies have been important for evaluation of the immunology, pathology, physiology and other aspects of pathogenesis. While larger animals have been employed, mice have remained

* Department of Physiology and Biophysics, Albert Einstein College of Medicine, Bronx, New York, USA
† Department of Pathology, Albert Einstein College of Medicine, Bronx, New York, USA
‡ Department of Medicine, Albert Einstein College of Medicine, Bronx, New York, USA

Advances in Parasitology, Volume 75
ISSN 0065-308X, DOI: 10.1016/B978-0-12-385863-4.00009-5

the most favoured animal model, as they recapitulate many aspects of the human disease, are easy to manipulate genetically and are amenable to study by small animal imaging technologies. Further, developments in non-invasive imaging technologies have permitted the study of the same animal over an extended period of time by multiple imaging modalities, thus permitting the study of the transition from acute infection through the chronic stage and during therapeutic regimens.

9.1. INTRODUCTION

For several decades, researchers interested in Chagas disease have relied on animal models of *Trypanosoma cruzi* infection to explore many aspects of this important human disease. Since serial studies on humans are limited, researchers have relied on animal models to evaluate the immunology, pathology, physiology and other aspects of pathogenesis. In addition, animal models have been routinely employed to screen for novel anti-*T. cruzi* drugs (Buckner and Navabi, 2010) and for vaccine development (Gupta and Garg, 2010).

The primary animal model employed to date has been the mouse because it has been demonstrated to recapitulate many of the immunological, pathological and physiological features of human Chagas disease. However, some have argued that the mouse model is not a credible model. Interestingly, similar arguments have recently appeared in the literature questioning the relevance of the mouse model of cerebral malaria to human cerebral malaria (Taylor-Robinson, 2010). Thus, several studies have employed *T. cruzi*-infected larger animals such as rabbits, rats, guinea pigs, dogs and subhuman primates (Barbabosa-Pliego et al., 2009; Bonecini-Almeida Mda et al., 1990; Chandrasckar et al., 1998; Chen et al., 1996; Cruz-Chan et al., 2009; da Silva et al., 1996; de Almeida et al., 1992; de Meirelles Mde et al., 1990; Figueiredo et al., 1986; Guedes et al., 2002, 2009; Junqueira Junior et al., 1992; Labrador-Hernandez et al., 2008; Milei et al., 1982; Morris et al., 1991; Perez et al., 2009; Ramirez and Brener, 1987; Teixeira et al., 1983; Zabalgoitia et al., 2004).

Mice are a good model because of ease of handling, housing and cost. In addition, the use of mice allows for acquiring greater numbers of samples, whereas with larger animals, the number of animals in the study is limited by cost and ethical considerations. However, even studies involving mice have been hampered by the inability to compare studies because of variability in parasite and mouse strains employed. For example, among the strains of *T. cruzi* often used in mice experiments are CL Brener (the strain used in the *T. cruzi* genome project), the Y, SylvioX10,

Colombian, Brazil and Tulahuen strains. Each strain is a particular laboratory or country "favourite." Thus, the combination of a particular *T. cruzi* strain and mouse strain results in early death with high parasitemia and high tissue parasitism, while other combinations result in a transient parasitemia, no death in the acute phase and the development of chronic disease often manifested by a cardiomyopathy. Similarly, infection of cultured myoblasts with different strains of *T. cruzi* may result in the up- or down-regulation of different genes in the host cell (Adesse et al., 2010).

Once having selected a parasite strain, another challenge is the choice of an appropriate mouse model. Among the important mouse strains that have been used are outbred strains such as CD-1 and inbred strains such as A/J, Balb/C, C57BL/6, C3H and others. Additionally, experiments may use various null and transgenic mice. Then there are the issues involving the size of the original infecting inoculum as well as the sex (de Souza et al., 2001; McHardy, 1978) and age (Maletto et al., 1996) of the mice. Although most investigators infect mice within 6–10 weeks of age, infection of mice at other ages may result in variability in mortality, parasitemia and pathology. The temperature of the environment may also be a confounding factor (Amrein, 1967; Anderson and Kuhn, 1989; Dimock et al., 1992). All of these factors have been demonstrated to be important, and one can achieve different results depending on the combination of many of these factors.

As far back as 1978, we demonstrated that when various inbred mice available at that time were infected with a standard inocula of trypomastigotes of the Brazil strain and observed for mortality, certain mouse strains were resistant and others highly susceptible (Trischmann et al., 1978). We further observed that infection of C57BL/6 mice with 1×10^4 trypomastigotes of the Brazil strain resulted in a transient parasitemia, no mortality and the appearance of a dilated cardiomyopathy by day 90 post-infection (Jelicks et al., 1999). However, infection of the same mouse strain with 1×10^3 trypomastigotes of the Tulahuen strain resulted in high parasitemia and death by day 20–25 post-infection (Chandra et al., 2002b).

In the use of various null mice, there are variations as well. For example, when nitric oxide synthase 2 (NOS2) null mice were infected with 10^4 trypomastigotes of the Brazil strain, none of the mice died, but they displayed less right ventricular dilation than displayed by Brazil strain-infected wild-type (WT) mice. Presumably, the reason was that there was less nitric oxide (NO) to contributing to development of cardiomyopathy. Prior to these experiments, it was thought that the mice would die, as NO is required for intracellular parasite killing. The interpretation at that time was that the genetic background of the host (C57BL/6) was more important than whether the mice could produce NO. However, when NOS2 null mice were infected with the Tulahuen strain, the mortality rate was 100%. Athymic nude mice lacking T-cells have a 100% mortality that was not dependant of parasite strain used (Kierszenbaum, 1980; Trischmann et al., 1978).

9.2. LARGER ANIMAL MODELS

9.2.1. Rabbit studies

Rabbits have been evaluated as a model for Chagas disease by several laboratories (da Silva et al., 1996; Figueiredo et al., 1986; Ramirez and Brener, 1987; Teixeira et al., 1983). In 1983, Teixeira et al. reported studies of the electrocardiogram (ECG) of rabbits infected with the Ernestina or Albuquerque strains of *T. cruzi* (Teixeira et al., 1983). During latent infection, there were no detectable alterations in the ECG of the infected rabbits. However, in the chronic stage of the disease, ECG changes consistent with enlargement and overload of cardiac chambers, alterations of ventricular repolarization, S-T changes and bundle-branch blocks were frequently recorded. Autopsy substantiated these findings. Megacolon was seen in two rabbits inoculated with the Ernestina strain of the parasite. In 1986, Figueiredo et al. reported findings in young rabbits infected with the Colombia strain of *T. cruzi*. Cineventriculography in the left ventricle of the rabbits during the chronic phase disclosed regional myocardial dysfunction, with typical apical systolic bulging.

9.2.2. Dog studies

Dogs are both an important reservoir of the parasite and a good model to study the pathogenesis of *T. cruzi* infection. Cruz-Chan et al. (2009) found that three of nine *T. cruzi* seropositive stray dogs presented electrocardiographic alterations including right bundle-branch block, sinusal block and QRS complex alterations and some right-ventricle enlargement was noted. Dogs infected with a *T. cruzi* isolate from Mexico exhibited electrocardiographic alterations, left- and right-ventricle dilation and hydropericardium (Barbabosa-Pliego et al., 2009). Guedes et al. (2009) studied dogs infected with *T. cruzi* as a model to understand the immunopathogenic mechanisms involved in chronic chagasic infection. They have also used the dog model to evaluate chemotherapy (Guedes et al., 2002). Studies of the myocardial beta-adrenergic adenylate cyclase complex have also been performed in dogs (Chen et al., 1996; Morris et al., 1991).

9.2.3. Rat studies

Rats have been used to study potential therapeutic strategies (Perez et al., 2009) and to investigate the inflammatory response (Chandrasekar et al., 1998), cardiac autonomic dysfunction (Junqueira Junior et al., 1992) and mechanisms that lead to chronic chagasic cardiomyopathy (Labrador-Hernandez et al., 2008). These studies helped establish the role of immune system and involvement of the parasympathetic nervous system in the pathogenesis of chagasic cardiomyopathy.

9.2.4. Non-human primates

Non-human primates have also been explored as models for Chagas disease (Bonecini-Almeida Mda et al., 1990; de Almeida et al., 1992; de Meirelles Mde et al., 1990; Milei et al., 1982). Early studies revealed that ECG changes in infected monkeys were correlated with specific anatomic lesions (Milei et al., 1982). In later studies, *Cebus apella* sp. monkeys were infected with different strains of *T. cruzi* and were submitted to xenodiagnosis, serological testing clinical examination and electrocardiography (de Almeida et al., 1992). The ECGs were always normal for the 12 infected monkeys in the study, and at autopsy, only three of the monkeys exhibited chronic myocarditis. High parasitemia and positive serology, despite the normal ECG, lead the authors to conclude that *Cebus* monkeys were not susceptible to the development of the disease but they could be used to maintain strains and study serology in long-term infections. In another study, seropositive baboons were studied using myocardial contrast echocardiography (Zabalgoitia et al., 2004). Chagasic heart disease was present in 24% of seropositive baboons as evidenced by decreased fractional shortening, although there was no significant difference in the coronary microcirculation pattern in those animals.

9.3. MOUSE MODELS

The studies of Chagas disease in animals provide a good framework for the evaluation of novel drugs and vaccines. Here, we focus on the mouse model which has been most extensively studied.

9.3.1. Chagasic cardiomyopathy in mice

9.3.1.1. ECG studies

Although ECG studies are electrophysiological studies, they give insight into the morphological alterations in the heart. The first well-designed comprehensive ECG-based study in mice over a prolonged period after infection was that of Postan et al. (1987). These investigators infected C3H and C57Bl/6 mice with various *T. cruzi* strains. They found that there were differences in the degree of myocardial fibrosis and in ECG abnormalities. They also reported that prolongation in the P-R intervals and complete atrial–ventricular dissociation was mouse strain and parasite strain dependent. More recently, Eickhoff et al. reported an ECG study of chagasic cardiomyopathy in BALB/c, SCID, C57BL/6 and CH3 mice infected with the Tulahuen, Brazil and Sylvio-X10/4 strains of *T. cruzi* (Eickhoff et al., 2010). In this study, a prolongation of the QRS and QT intervals was consistently detected in BALB/c mice infected with the Brazil strain, and these alterations were correlated with the histopathological changes associated with chagasic cardiomyopathy. These studies over 20 years apart underscore the fact that the combination of mouse and parasite strain yields varying results.

9.3.1.2. Cardiac magnetic resonance imaging, echocardiography and positron emission tomography

In 1999, we reported the first magnetic resonance imaging (MRI) studies of mice infected with *T. cruzi* (Brazil strain; Huang et al., 1999; Jelicks et al., 1999). MRI is a non-invasive imaging modality with high resolution (~50–100 μm for small animal studies) and excellent soft tissue contrast. MRI can be used to image anatomic structures, blood flow and diffusion. For our studies, mice were anaesthetized with 1.5% of isoflurane; a set of standard, shielded, nonmagnetic electrocardiographic leads ending in silver wires were attached to the four limbs for monitoring the ECG and using the R wave to provide a cardiac gating signal to the MRI system. Infection of CD1 mice was associated with a significant increase in the right ventricular inner diameter (RVID) that was reversed in some mice by the calcium-channel blocker verapamil. We also evaluated chagasic cardiomyopathy in NOS2 null and syngeneic WT mice. Infected WT mice exhibited an increase in RVID in the acute phase that was more marked during chronic infection. Chronically infected NOS2 null mice also exhibited increased RVID; however, the increase was less than that in WT mice. The data supported the notion that the NOS2/NO pathway contributes to the pathogenesis of murine chagasic cardiomyopathy. Subsequently, we examined the cardiac structural and functional correlates of verapamil treatment in CD1 mice infected with the Brazil strain of *T. cruzi* using serial transthoracic echocardiography (Chandra et al., 2002a). That study was the first demonstration of the utility of echocardiography to study the functional and structural abnormalities in chronic murine chagasic heart disease. Ultrasound imaging has high spatial resolution (~50 μm) and contrast in soft tissue. In additional to being portable, it is a fast and economical technique and has been extensively used for echocardiography studies of small animals. Mice in the untreated-infected group compared with the mice in the infected-verapamil-treated group showed thinning of the left ventricular wall, increase in the left ventricular end-diastolic diameter and a reduction in percent fractional shortening. Verapamil is known to increase coronary blood flow and inhibit platelet aggregation. These properties of verapamil may be important in the amelioration of *T. cruzi*-induced cardiomyopathy. Other compounds, such as risedronate, a bisphosphonate, reduce mortality but have no effect on development cardiomyopathy in Brazil strain-infected CD1 mice (Bouzahzah et al., 2005). We also reported echocardiography studies of mice infected with the Tulahuen strain of *T. cruzi*, which results in an acutely fatal myocarditis with a toxic shock-like syndrome (Chandra et al., 2002b).

Endothelin-1, a 21-amino acid peptide, is a powerful vasoconstrictor synthesized by many cell types in the cardiovascular system including endothelial cells, fibroblasts and cardiac myocytes. Endothelin has been implicated in the pathogenesis of chagasic cardiomyopathy in mice (Huang et al., 2002; Petkova et al., 2001; Tanowitz et al., 2005). Employing MRI and echocardiography, we demonstrated that early treatment of *T. cruzi* infected mice with phosphoramidon, a compound that inhibits endothelin-converting enzyme at neutral endopeptidases, or verapamil, which inhibits the actions of endothelin at a post-receptor site are effective for reducing mortality and development of cardiac pathology (De Souza et al., 2004; Jelicks et al., 2002a,b; Tanowitz et al., 1999). These imaging methods were also valuable for studying the roles of interferon-gamma-inducible gene IGTP (de Souza et al., 2003), and in other studies, we validated the use of the MRI methods for measuring the right ventricular dimensions and for monitoring wall motion abnormalities (de Souza et al., 2005; Durand et al., 2006).

Recently, we used MRI to evaluate changes in the cardiac morphology of *T. cruzi*-infected mice following administration of bone marrow-derived cell therapy and selenium supplementation (Goldenberg et al., 2008; Souza et al., 2010). These studies revealed regression of the right ventricular dilatation typically observed in the chagasic mouse model with bone marrow cell therapy and prevention of right ventricular dilatation with selenium supplementation. Selenium supplementation also resulted in regression of ECG abnormalities (prolonged P wave duration) in mice with pre-existing cardiac pathology (Souza et al., 2010).

Our group performed multimodality imaging employing MRI, echocardiography and microPET imaging in a longitudinal study of Brazil strain-infected CD1 mice (Prado et al., 2009). Positron emission tomography (PET) is a highly sensitive (pM) molecular imaging technique that can be used to visualize a variety of *in vivo* biological processes. The resolution of microPET (1–2 mm) is not as high as CT or MRI but is adequate for small animal imaging. We used the molecule 2-deoxy-2-[^{18}F]-fluoro-D-glucose, which is routinely used in the clinical setting. Cardiac gating of the PET acquisition was accomplished using standard ECG leads interfaced to the microPET scanner. Figure 9.1 shows representative MRI, microPET and echocardiography data from that study. Using these three complementary imaging technologies, it was possible to non-invasively quantify cardiovascular function, morphology and metabolism from the earliest days of infection through the chronic phase.

9.3.2. Megasyndromes of the gastrointestinal tract and other organs in mice

For many years, it was difficult to establish that *T. cruzi*-infected mice could display alterations in gastrointestinal tract (GI) function. Mori et al. (1995) used X-ray methods to investigate GI tract abnormalities in *T. cruzi*-infected mice (Mori et al., 1995). In those mice, intestinal transit time was normal during acute infection, although delayed evacuation time was observed in the chronic phase. Another X-ray study of infected mice demonstrated swelling of the stomach and colon (Guillen-Pernia et al., 2001). Histological examination revealed extensive changes of the intestinal muscle layer and the loss of colonic folds and myenteric plexus. Recently, de Oliveira et al. (2008) demonstrated decreased intestinal motility in *T. cruzi* (Y strain)-infected Swiss Webster mice using charcoal.

MRI was employed to monitor alterations in the GI tract of Brazil strain-infected mice and to assess the role of NO in the development of intestinal dilation (Ny et al., 2008). In that study, infected C57BL/6 WT mice exhibited dilatation of the intestines by 30 days post-infection with the average intestine lumen diameter increased by 72%. Levels of intestinal NO synthase (NOS) isoforms, NOS2 and NOS3, were elevated in infected WT mice. Inflammation and ganglionitis were observed in all infected mice. Intestinal dilation was observed in infected WT, NOS1, NOS2 and NOS3 null mice. The data strongly suggested that NO is not the sole contributor to intestinal dysfunction resulting from this infection. In a more recent study, we employed MRI to non-invasively monitor the effect of selenium supplementation on alterations in the GI tract of *T. cruzi*-infected mice (de Souza et al., 2010). CD1 mice infected with the Brazil strain exhibited dilatation of the intestines similar to what we observed in infected C57BL/6 mice. The average intestine lumen diameter increased by 65%, and the increase was reduced to 29% in mice supplemented with 2-ppm selenium in the drinking water. When supplemented with 3-ppm selenium in chow, the lumen diameter was also

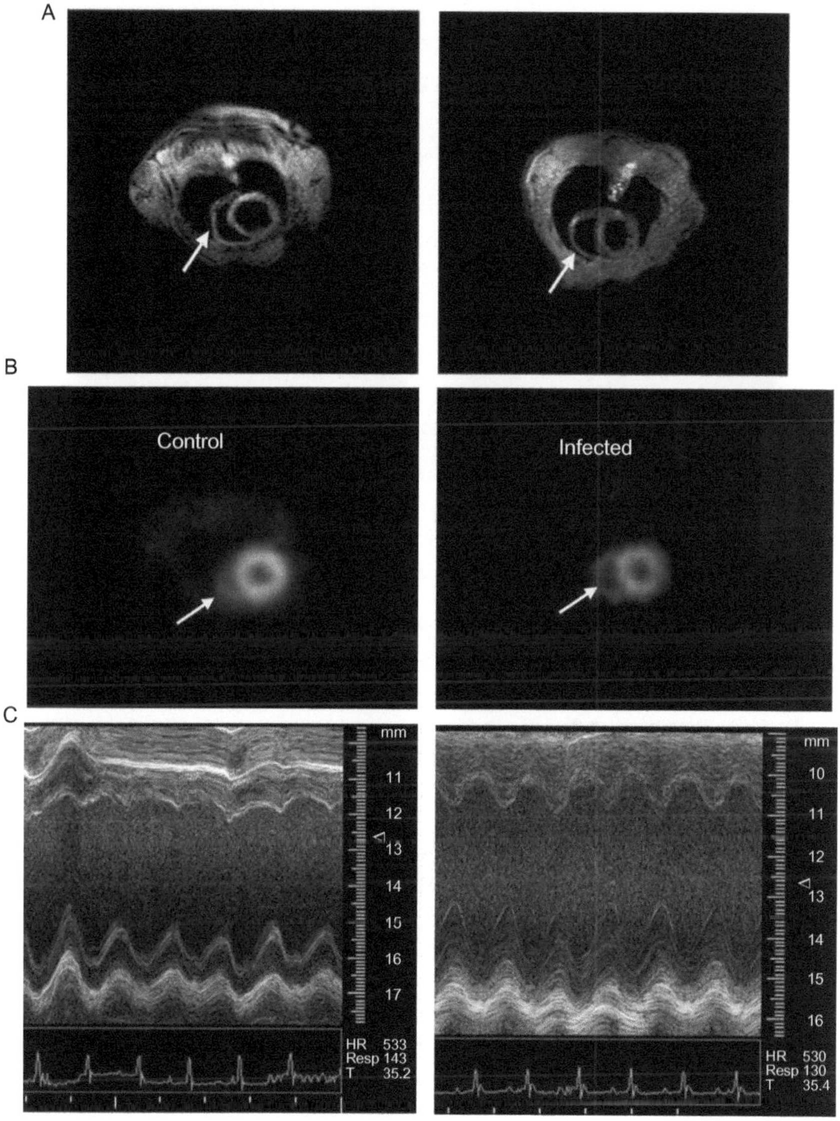

FIGURE 9.1 Representative MRI (A), microPET (B) and echocardiography M-mode data (C) for uninfected control mice (left) and CD1 mice infected with the Brazil strain of *T. cruzi* (right). Arrows indicate the right ventricle in the MRI and microPET images.

significantly reduced, although the difference between the infected and infected supplemented mice was smaller. Intestinal motility in infected mice fed with selenium-enriched chow was increased compared with infected mice fed with normal unsupplemented chow and was not

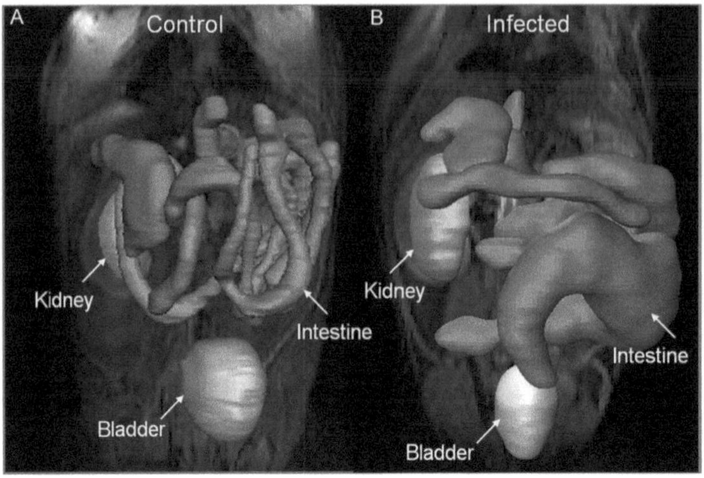

FIGURE 9.2 Representative MRI of an uninfected CD1 mouse (A) and a CD1 mouse infected with the Brazil strain of *T. cruzi* (B). One of the kidneys, the bladder and the GI tract are indicated in the 3D greyscale overlay. Note the enlargement of the intestine in the infected mouse.

significantly different from intestinal motility in uninfected mice. Figure 9.2 shows representative MRI data of mice showing intestinal dilation.

T. cruzi infection has also been shown to induce megasyndromes in other organs. We reported megabladder accompanied by fibrosis and decreased bladder compliance (Boczko et al., 2005) in mice infected with the Brazil strain. Figure 9.3 shows a comparison of the MRI of the normal bladder of a control mouse and the enlarged flaccid bladder of an infected mouse. Although there had been only rare descriptions of megaureter in humans (Koeberle, 1968), megabladder had been reported before in experimental *T. cruzi* infection in mice and dogs (Barr et al., 1991; Scremin et al., 1999). Hepatosplenomegaly has also been reported in patients with Chagas disease, and we have observed enlargement of both the spleen and the liver in mice infected with the Brazil strain of *T. cruzi*. Figure 9.4 shows representative MRI of the abdominal region of control and infected mice highlighting the enlarged spleen in the infected mouse.

9.3.3. Adipose tissue

In 2005, we reported the first detailed analysis of the consequences of *T. cruzi* (Brazil strain) infection on adipose tissue (Combs et al., 2005). Infected mice gained more weight than controls, and MRI studies revealed that total fat and abdominal fat depots were reduced in infected mice, consistent with reduced levels of leptin. Infected mice exhibiting

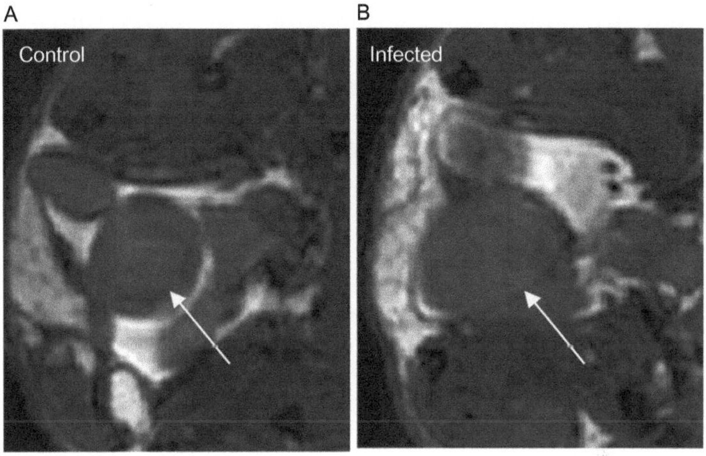

FIGURE 9.3 Zoomed region of the transverse MRI of an uninfected control CD1 mouse (A) and a CD1 mouse infected with the Brazil strain of *T. cruzi* (B) at the region of the bladder (indicated by the white arrow). Note the large irregular shape of the flaccid bladder in the infected mouse.

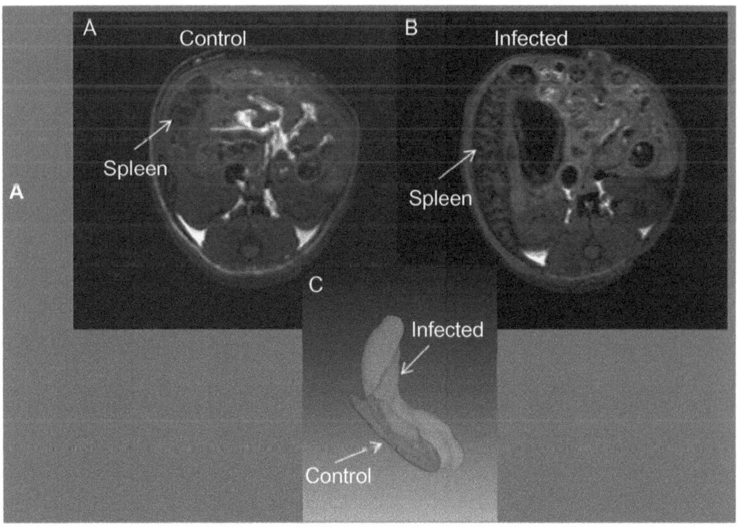

FIGURE 9.4 Representative MRI of an uninfected CD1 mouse (A) and a CD1 mouse infected with the Brazil strain of *T. cruzi* (B). The 3D reconstructions of the normal (darker grey translucent) enlarged (lighter opaque grey) spleens are shown in (C).

dilated cardiomyopathy had even further reduced fat stores and weight gain in those infected animals appeared to be related to oedema, a consequence of cardiac dysfunction in these animals.

Recently, we measured body composition in *T. cruzi*-infected mice. This was determined by magnetic relaxometry with the EchoMRI-100 System (Echo Medical Systems), which provides quantitative measurements of fat mass and fat-free mass in live mice weighing up to 130 g without anaesthesia or sedation. Daily tuning occurs through automated calibration and testing procedures with self-correcting adjustments via custom software. Saturated and unsaturated fat standards are used to calibrate the instrument immediately prior to each set of MRI scans that were performed, and at the end of the study, these were validated by analysis of the carcasses (Nagajyothi et al., 2010). Using this technique, we determined that infection resulted in reduction in fat mass, which correlates with the infection-associated decrease in leptin. This decrease in fat may be a consequence of both decreased food intake and infection-associated lipolysis.

9.4. FUTURE DIRECTIONS: MULTIMODALITY IMAGING APPROACHES

As we have shown in our studies employing MRI, echocardiography and microPET, the imaging techniques appropriate for study of small animal models of Chagas disease are complementary and may be applied in a multiple modality manner. With the advent of new integrated technologies, such as PET/CT (computed tomography), and molecular imaging probes, the co-registration of functional images from PET with CT will be easier and will permit more detailed and accurate analysis of function/metabolism (Brewer et al., 2008). Similar integrated technologies are under development for PET/MRI that will permit anatomic co-registration without the additional exposure to radiation inherent in the PET/CT systems (Judenhofer et al., 2008).

Serial imaging of animals infected with *T. cruzi* allows for detailed study of the pathogenesis of Chagas disease that cannot be obtained solely by examination of the pathology which requires the sacrifice of animals. Serial imaging allows for assessment of the efficacy of chemotherapeutic agents. Many drugs are capable of lowering or eliminating parasites from peripheral blood or tissue, but imaging of the heart or GI systems is also required to assess whether these agents also ameliorate the progression to chronic disease.

ACKNOWLEDGEMENTS

This study was supported by grants from the United States National Institutes of Health AI-062730 and CA-123334 (L. A. J.) and AI-076248 (H. B. T.).

REFERENCES

Adesse, D., Iacobas, D.A., Iacobas, S., Garzoni, L.R., Meirelles Mde, N., Tanowitz, H.B., et al., 2010. Transcriptomic signatures of alterations in a myoblast cell line infected with four distinct strains of *Trypanosoma cruzi*. Am. J. Trop. Med. Hyg. 82, 846–854.

Amrein, Y.U., 1967. Effects of environmental temperature on *Trypanosoma cruzi* infection in mice. J. Parasitol. 53, 1160.

Anderson, K.J., Kuhn, R.E., 1989. Elevated environmental temperature enhances immunity in experimental Chagas' disease. Infect. Immun. 57, 13–17.

Barbabosa-Pliego, A., Diaz-Albiter, H.M., Ochoa-Garcia, L., Aparicio-Burgos, E., Lopez-Heydeck, S.M., Velasquez-Ordonez, V., et al., 2009. *Trypanosoma cruzi* circulating in the southern region of the State of Mexico (Zumpahuacan) are pathogenic: a dog model. Am. J. Trop. Med. Hyg. 81, 390–395.

Barr, S.C., Schmidt, S.P., Brown, C.C., Klei, T.R., 1991. Pathologic features of dogs inoculated with North American *Trypanosoma cruzi* isolates. Am. J. Vet. Res. 52, 2033–2039.

Boczko, J., Tar, M., Melman, A., Jelicks, L.A., Wittner, M., Factor, S.M., et al., 2005. *Trypanosoma cruzi* infection induced changes in the innervation, structure and function of the murine bladder. J. Urol. 173, 1784–1788.

Bonecini-Almeida Mda, G., Galvao-Castro, B., Pessoa, M.H., Pirmez, C., Laranja, F., 1990. Experimental Chagas' disease in rhesus monkeys. I. Clinical, parasitological, hematological and anatomo-pathological studies in the acute and indeterminate phase of the disease. Mem. Inst. Oswaldo Cruz 85, 163–171.

Bouzahzah, B., Jelicks, L.A., Morris, S.A., Weiss, L.M., Tanowitz, H.B., 2005. Risedronate in the treatment of Murine Chagas' disease. Parasitol. Res. 96, 184–187.

Brewer, S., McPherson, M., Fujiwara, D., Turovskaya, O., Ziring, D., Chen, L., et al., 2008. Molecular imaging of murine intestinal inflammation with 2-deoxy-2-[18F]fluoro-D-glucose and positron emission tomography. Gastroenterology 135, 744–755.

Buckner, F.S., Navabi, N., 2010. Advances in Chagas disease drug development: 2009–2010. Curr. Opin. Infect. Dis. 23, 609–616.

Chandra, M., Shirani, J., Shtutin, V., Weiss, L.M., Factor, S.M., Petkova, S.B., et al., 2002a. Cardioprotective effects of verapamil on myocardial structure and function in a murine model of chronic *Trypanosoma cruzi* infection (Brazil Strain): an echocardiographic study. Int. J. Parasitol. 32, 207–215.

Chandra, M., Tanowitz, H.B., Petkova, S.B., Huang, H., Weiss, L.M., Wittner, M., et al., 2002b. Significance of inducible nitric oxide synthase in acute myocarditis caused by *Trypanosoma cruzi* (Tulahuen strain). Int. J. Parasitol. 32, 897–905.

Chandrasekar, B., Melby, P.C., Troyer, D.A., Colston, J.T., Freeman, G.L., 1998. Temporal expression of pro-inflammatory cytokines and inducible nitric oxide synthase in experimental acute Chagasic cardiomyopathy. Am. J. Pathol. 152, 925–934.

Chen, G., Barr, S., Walsh, D., Rohde, S., Brewer, A., Bilezikian, J.P., et al., 1996. Cardioprotective actions of verapamil on the beta-adrenergic receptor complex in acute canine Chagas' disease. J. Mol. Cell. Cardiol. 28, 931–941.

Combs, T.P., Nagajyothi, Mukherjee, S., de Almeida, C.J., Jelicks, L.A., Schubert, W., et al., 2005. The adipocyte as an important target cell for *Trypanosoma cruzi* infection. J. Biol. Chem. 280, 24085–24094.

Cruz-Chan, J.V., Bolio-Gonzalez, M., Colin-Flores, R., Ramirez-Sierra, M.J., Quijano-Hernandez, I., Dumonteil, E., 2009. Immunopathology of natural infection with *Trypanosoma cruzi* in dogs. Vet. Parasitol. 162, 151–155.

da Silva, A.M., Eduardo Ramirez, L., Vargas, M., Chapadeiro, E., Brener, Z., 1996. Evaluation of the rabbit as a model for Chagas disease. II. Histopathologic studies of the heart, digestive tract and skeletal muscle. Mem. Inst. Oswaldo Cruz 91, 199–206.

de Almeida, E.A., Navarro, M.R., Guariento, M.E., Carvalhal Sdos, S., 1992. The experimental infection of *Cebus apella* sp. monkeys with *Trypanosoma cruzi*. Its clinical, electrocardiographic and anatomicopathological assessment. Rev. Soc. Bras. Med. Trop. 25, 7–12.

de Meirelles Mde, N., Bonecini-Almeida Mda, G., Pessoa, M.H., Galvao-Castro, B., 1990. *Trypanosoma cruzi*: experimental Chagas' disease in rhesus monkeys. II. Ultrastructural and cytochemical studies of peroxidase and acid phosphatase activities. Mem. Inst. Oswaldo Cruz 85, 173–181.

de Oliveira, G.M., de Melo Medeiros, M., da Silva Batista, W., Santana, R., Araujo-Jorge, T.C., de Souza, A.P., 2008. Applicability of the use of charcoal for the evaluation of intestinal motility in a murine model of *Trypanosoma cruzi* infection. Parasitol. Res. 102, 747–750.

de Souza, E.M., Rivera, M.T., Araujo-Jorge, T.C., de Castro, S.L., 2001. Modulation induced by estradiol in the acute phase of *Trypanosoma cruzi* infection in mice. Parasitol. Res. 87, 513–520.

de Souza, A.P., Tang, B., Tanowitz, H.B., Factor, S.M., Shtutin, V., Shirani, J., et al., 2003. Absence of interferon-gamma-inducible gene IGTP does not significantly alter the development of chagasic cardiomyopathy in mice infected with *Trypanosoma cruzi* (Brazil strain). J. Parasitol. 89, 1237–1239.

De Souza, A.P., Tanowitz, H.B., Chandra, M., Shtutin, V., Weiss, L.M., Morris, S.A., et al., 2004. Effects of early and late verapamil administration on the development of cardiomyopathy in experimental chronic *Trypanosoma cruzi* (Brazil strain) infection. Parasitol. Res. 92, 496–501.

de Souza, A.P., Tang, B., Tanowitz, H.B., Araujo-Jorge, T.C., Jelicks, E.L., 2005. Magnetic resonance imaging in experimental Chagas disease: a brief review of the utility of the method for monitoring right ventricular chamber dilatation. Parasitol. Res. 97, 87–90.

de Souza, A.P., Sieberg, R., Li, H., Cahill, H.R., Zhao, D., Araujo-Jorge, T.C., et al., 2010. The role of selenium in intestinal motility and morphology in a murine model of *Trypanosoma cruzi infection*. Parasitol. Res. 106, 1293–1298.

Dimock, K.A., Davis, C.D., Kuhn, R.E., 1992. Changes in humoral responses to *Trypanosoma cruzi* during the course of infection in mice held at elevated temperature. J. Parasitol. 78, 687–696.

Durand, J.L., Tang, B., Gutstein, D.E., Petkova, S., Teixeira, M.M., Tanowitz, H.B., et al., 2006. Dyskinesis in Chagasic myocardium: centerline analysis of wall motion using cardiac-gated magnetic resonance images of mice. Magn. Reson. Imaging 24, 1051–1057.

Eickhoff, C.S., Lawrence, C.T., Sagartz, J.E., Bryant, L.A., Labovitz, A.J., Gala, S.S., et al., 2010. ECG detection of murine chagasic cardiomyopathy. J. Parasitol. 96, 758–764.

Figueiredo, F., Marin-Neto, J.A., Rossi, M.A., 1986. The evolution of experimental *Trypanosoma cruzi* cardiomyopathy in rabbits: further parasitological, morphological and functional studies. Int. J. Cardiol. 10, 277–290.

Goldenberg, R.C., Jelicks, L.A., Fortes, F.S., Weiss, L.M., Rocha, L.L., Zhao, D., et al., 2008. Bone marrow cell therapy ameliorates and reverses chagasic cardiomyopathy in a mouse model. J. Infect. Dis. 197, 544–547.

Guedes, P.M., Veloso, V.M., Tafuri, W.L., Galvao, L.M., Carneiro, C.M., Lana, M., et al., 2002. The dog as model for chemotherapy of the Chagas' disease. Acta Trop. 84, 9–17.

Guedes, P.M., Veloso, V.M., Afonso, L.C., Caliari, M.V., Carneiro, C.M., Diniz, L.F., et al., 2009. Development of chronic cardiomyopathy in canine Chagas disease correlates with high IFN-gamma, TNF-alpha, and low IL-10 production during the acute infection phase. Vet. Immunol. Immunopathol. 130, 43–52.

Guillen-Pernia, B., Lugo-Yarbuh, A., Moreno, E., 2001. Digestive tract dilation in mice infected with *Trypanosoma cruzi*. Invest. Clin. 42, 195–209.

Gupta, S., Garg, N.J., 2010. Prophylactic efficacy of TcVac2 against *Trypanosoma cruzi* in mice. PLoS Negl. Trop. Dis. 4, e797.

Huang, H., Chan, J., Wittner, M., Jelicks, L.A., Morris, S.A., Factor, S.M., et al., 1999. Expression of cardiac cytokines and inducible form of nitric oxide synthase (NOS2) in *Trypanosoma cruzi*-infected mice. J. Mol. Cell. Cardiol. 31, 75–88.

Huang, H., Yanagisawa, M., Kisanuki, Y.Y., Jelicks, L.A., Chandra, M., Factor, S.M., et al., 2002. Role of cardiac myocyte-derived endothelin-1 in chagasic cardiomyopathy: molecular genetic evidence. Clin. Sci. (Lond.) 103 (Suppl. 48), 263S–266S.

Jelicks, L.A., Shirani, J., Wittner, M., Chandra, M., Weiss, L.M., Factor, S.M., et al., 1999. Application of cardiac gated magnetic resonance imaging in murine Chagas' disease. Am. J. Trop. Med. Hyg. 61, 207–214.

Jelicks, L.A., Chandra, M., Shirani, J., Shtutin, V., Tang, B., Christ, G.J., et al., 2002a. Cardioprotective effects of phosphoramidon on myocardial structure and function in murine Chagas' disease. Int. J. Parasitol. 32, 1497–1506.

Jelicks, L.A., Chandra, M., Shtutin, V., Petkova, S.B., Tang, B., Christ, G.J., et al., 2002b. Phosphoramidon treatment improves the consequences of chagasic heart disease in mice. Clin. Sci. (Lond.) 103 (Suppl. 48), 267S–271S.

Judenhofer, M.S., Wehrl, H.F., Newport, D.F., Catana, C., Siegel, S.B., Becker, M., et al., 2008. Simultaneous PET-MRI: a new approach for functional and morphological imaging. Nat. Med. 14, 459–465.

Junqueira Junior, L.F., Beraldo, P.S., Chapadeiro, E., Jesus, P.C., 1992. Cardiac autonomic dysfunction and neuroganglionitis in a rat model of chronic Chagas' disease. Cardiovasc. Res. 26, 324–329.

Kierszenbaum, F., 1980. Protection of congenitally athymic mice against *Trypanosoma cruzi* infection by passive antibody transfer. J. Parasitol. 66, 673–675.

Koeberle, F., 1968. Chagas' disease and Chagas' syndromes: the pathology of American trypanosomiasis. Adv. Parasitol. 6, 63–116.

Labrador-Hernandez, M., Suarez-Graterol, O., Romero-Contreras, U., Rumenoff, L., Rodriguez-Bonfante, C., Bonfante-Cabarcas, R., 2008. The cholinergic system in cyclophosphamide-induced Chagas dilated myocardiopathy in *Trypanosoma cruzi*-infected rats: an electrocardiographic study. Invest. Clin. 49, 207–224.

Maletto, B.A., Gruppi, A., Moron, G., Pistoresi-Palencia, M.C., 1996. Age-associated changes in lymphoid and antigen-presenting cell functions in mice immunized with *Trypanosoma cruzi* antigens. Mech. Ageing Dev. 88, 39–47.

McHardy, N., 1978. Effect of sex of mice in relation to their response to immunization with vaccines prepared from *Trypanosoma cruzi*. Trans. R. Soc. Trop. Med. Hyg. 72, 201–202.

Milei, J., Bolomo, N.J., Vazquez, A., Nagle, C.A., 1982. Normal and pathological electrocardiographic patterns in the *Cebus* monkey. J. Med. Primatol. 11, 10–19.

Mori, T., Yoon, H.S., Iizuka, F.H., Myung, J.M., Sato, H.R., Silva, M.F., et al., 1995. Intestinal transit and opaque enema study in chagasic mice. Rev. Hosp. Clin. Fac. Med. Sao Paulo 50, 63–66.

Morris, S.A., Barr, S., Weiss, L., Tanowitz, H., Wittner, M., Bilezikian, J.P., 1991. Myocardial beta-adrenergic adenylate cyclase complex in a canine model of chagasic cardiomyopathy. Circ. Res. 69, 185–195.

Nagajyothi, F., Zhao, D., Machado, F.S., Weiss, L.M., Schwartz, G.J., Desruisseaux, M.S., et al., 2010. Crucial role of the central leptin receptor in murine *Trypanosoma cruzi* (Brazil strain) infection. J. Infect. Dis. 202, 1104–1113.

Ny, L., Li, H., Mukherjee, S., Persson, K., Holmqvist, B., Zhao, D., et al., 2008. A magnetic resonance imaging study of intestinal dilation in *Trypanosoma cruzi*-infected mice deficient in nitric oxide synthase. Am. J. Trop. Med. Hyg. 79, 760–767.

Perez, A.R., Fontanella, G.H., Nocito, A.L., Revelli, S., Bottasso, O.A., 2009. Short treatment with the tumour necrosis factor-alpha blocker infliximab diminishes chronic chagasic myocarditis in rats without evidence of *Trypanosoma cruzi* reactivation. Clin. Exp. Immunol. 157, 291–299.

Petkova, S.B., Huang, H., Factor, S.M., Pestell, R.G., Bouzahzah, B., Jelicks, L.A., et al., 2001. The role of endothelin in the pathogenesis of Chagas' disease. Int. J. Parasitol. 31, 499–511.

Postan, M., Bailey, J.J., Dvorak, J.A., McDaniel, J.P., Pottala, E.W., 1987. Studies of *Trypanosoma cruzi* clones in inbred mice. III. Histopathological and electrocardiographical responses to chronic infection. Am. J. Trop. Med. Hyg. 37, 541–549.

Prado, C.M., Fine, E.J., Koba, W., Zhao, D., Rossi, M.A., Tanowitz, H.B., et al., 2009. Micropositron emission tomography in the evaluation of *Trypanosoma cruzi*-induced heart disease: comparison with other modalities. Am. J. Trop. Med. Hyg. 81, 900–905.

Ramirez, L.E., Brener, Z., 1987. Evaluation of the rabbit as a model for Chagas' disease. I. Parasitological studies. Mem. Inst. Oswaldo Cruz 82, 531–536.

Scremin, L.H., Corbett, C.E., Laurenti, M.D., Nunes, E.V., Gama-Rodrigues, J.J., Okumura, M., 1999. Megabladder in experimental Chagas disease: pathological features of the bladder wall. Rev. Hosp. Clin. Fac. Med. Sao Paulo 54, 43–46.

Souza, A.P., Jelicks, L.A., Tanowitz, H.B., Olivieri, B.P., Medeiros, M.M., Oliveira, G.M., et al., 2010. The benefits of using selenium in the treatment of Chagas disease: prevention of right ventricle chamber dilatation and reversion of *Trypanosoma cruzi*-induced acute and chronic cardiomyopathy in mice. Mem. Inst. Oswaldo Cruz 105, 746–751.

Tanowitz, H.B., Wittner, M., Morris, S.A., Zhao, W., Weiss, L.M., Hatcher, V.B., et al., 1999. The putative mechanistic basis for the modulatory role of endothelin-1 in the altered vascular tone induced by *Trypanosoma cruzi*. Endothelium 6, 217–230.

Tanowitz, H.B., Huang, H., Jelicks, L.A., Chandra, M., Loredo, M.L., Weiss, L.M., et al., 2005. Role of endothelin 1 in the pathogenesis of chronic chagasic heart disease. Infect. Immun. 73, 2496–2503.

Taylor-Robinson, A., 2010. Validity of modelling cerebral malaria in mice: argument and counter argument. J. Neuroparasitol. 1, Article ID N100601.

Teixeira, A.R., Figueiredo, F., Rezende Filho, J., Macedo, V., 1983. Chagas' disease: a clinical, parasitological, immunological, and pathological study in rabbits. Am. J. Trop. Med. Hyg. 32, 258–272.

Trischmann, T., Tanowitz, H., Wittner, M., Bloom, B., 1978. *Trypanosoma cruzi*: role of the immune response in the natural resistance of inbred strains of mice. Exp. Parasitol. 45, 160–168.

Zabalgoitia, M., Ventura, J., Lozano, J.L., Anderson, L., Carey, K.D., Hubbard, G.B., et al., 2004. Myocardial contrast echocardiography in assessing microcirculation in baboons with Chagas disease. Microcirculation 11, 271–278.

CHAPTER 10

The Genome and Its Implications

Santuza M. Teixeira,* Najib M. El-Sayed,† and Patrícia R. Araújo*

Contents

Abstract

Trypanosoma cruzi has a heterogeneous population composed of a pool of strains that circulate in the domestic and sylvatic cycles. Genome sequencing of the clone CL Brener revealed a highly repetitive genome of about 110 Mb containing an estimated 22,570 genes. Because of its hybrid nature, sequences representing the two haplotypes have been generated. In addition, a repeat content close to 50% made the assembly of the estimated 41 pairs of chromosomes quite challenging. Similar to other trypanosomatids, the organization of *T. cruzi* chromosomes was found to be very peculiar, with protein-coding genes organized in long polycistronic transcription units encoding 20 or more proteins in one strand separated by strand switch regions. Another remarkable

* Departamento de Bioquímica e Imunologia, Universidade Federal de Minas Gerais, Belo Horizone, MG, Brazil
† Department of Cell Biology and Molecular Genetics, Center for Bioinformatics and Computational Biology, University of Maryland, College Park, Maryland, USA

Advances in Parasitology, Volume 75
ISSN 0065-308X, DOI: 10.1016/B978-0-12-385863-4.00010-1

feature of the *T. cruzi* genome is the massive expansion of surface protein gene families. Because of the high genetic diversity of the *T. cruzi* population, sequencing of additional strains and comparative genomic and transcriptome analyses are in progress. Five years after its publication, the genome data have proven to be an essential tool for the study of *T. cruzi* and increasing efforts to translate this knowledge into the development of new modes of intervention to control Chagas disease are underway.

10.1. GENOME ORGANIZATION, GENE CONTENT AND GENE EXPRESSION MECHANISMS

In 2005, the first draft sequence of the *Trypanosoma cruzi* genome, along with the genome sequences of *Trypanosoma brucei* and *Leishmania major*, also known as the Tri-tryp genomes, were published by an international consortium of laboratories that included three genome sequencing centres (data available at www.EuPathdB.org; http://tritrypdb.org/tritrypdb/), The Institute for Genomic Research (Rockville, USA), The Seattle Biomedical Research Institute (Seattle, USA) and Karolinska Institute (Stockholm, Sweden) and 80 researchers from 14 countries that contributed to the data analysis. CL Brener, a hybrid strain which is a representative of one of the six *T. cruzi* lineages, named DTU VI (Zingales et al., 2009) was chosen as the reference strain. It was only after the genome sequencing had began that it became clear that CL Brener is a hybrid resulting from fusion of genotypes from strains belonging to *T. cruzi* II and III groups (de Freitas et al., 2006), and with some evidence of chromosomal triploidy. Without the knowledge of such important information, the choice of the clone CL Brener for the *T. cruzi* genome project was based on five characteristics: (i) it was isolated from the domiciliary vector *Triatoma infestans*; (ii) its pattern of infectivity in mice is very well known; (iii) it has preferential tropism for heart and muscle cells; (iv) it shows a clear acute phase in accidentally infected humans; and (v) it is susceptible to drugs used clinically in Chagas disease (Zingales et al., 1997). Also, several genomic studies have been performed previously with this strain including karyotype analyses (Branche et al., 2006), physical maps and the generation of ESTs (expressed sequence tags) from all major stages of the parasite life cycle (Brandao et al., 1997; Cano et al., 1995; Cerqueira et al., 2005; Henriksson et al., 1995; Porcel et al., 2000; Verdun et al., 1998).

The *T. cruzi* CL Brener diploid genome, estimated at 110.7 Mb, was sequenced using the WGS (whole genome shotgun) strategy. Because it is a hybrid genome showing high level of allelic polymorphism, much higher sequence coverage than the usual 8–10× coverage was required in order to distinguish the ambiguities derived from allelic variations from sequencing errors. With 14× coverage, a final assembly with 5489 scaffolds built by 8740 contigs was described in the draft sequence (El-Sayed et al., 2005a). In contrast to the genomes of *T. brucei* and *L. major*, the CL Brener sequence is represented by a redundant data set since homologous regions displaying high level of polymorphism were assembled separately, hence generating two sets of contigs, each corresponding to one haplotype. To identify the two haplotypes, reads from the genome of the cloned Esmeraldo strain, which is a member of one of the CL Brener parental group (DTU II; de Freitas et al., 2006), were generated. Thus, the two haplotypes in the annotation data of the CL Brener genome were referred as "Esmeraldo-like" or "non-Esmeraldo-like".

In an effort to arrive at a single chromosome model for the CL Brener genome, Weatherly et al. (2009) generated consensus versions of each homologous chromosome pair from contigs assigned as Esmeraldo- and non-Esmeraldo-like haplotypes. Initially, these authors based on the synteny maps for the *T. brucei* chromosomes to assemble 11 pairs of homologous "*T. brucei*-like" chromosomes. Then, *T. cruzi* chromosome-size pieces were constructed after mapping both ends of Bacterial Artificial Chromosome (BAC) clones that link contigs or scaffolds in the proper orientation. Ultimately, 41 chromosomes were assembled, a number that is similar to the predicted number of *T. cruzi* chromosomes based on studies of pulsed-field gel electrophoresis (PFGE) analyses (Branche et al., 2006). The scaffolding generated by Weatherly et al. (2009) contains 90% of the genes annotated in the draft genome. As discussed in the next section, the genome organization in *T. cruzi* is largely syntenic with the other Tri-tryp genomes (*T. brucei* and *L. major*) (Fig. 10.1), with most species-specific genes such as surface protein gene families, occurring at nonsyntenic chromosome-internal and sub-telomeric regions (El-Sayed et al., 2005b).

The haploid *T. cruzi* genome has an estimated number of 12,000 genes. Similar to other kinetoplastid genomes, the organization of the *T. cruzi* genome is reminiscent of bacterial operons, with protein-coding genes densely packed within directional clusters in one strand separated by strand switch regions (i.e. changes of the coding strand). Transcription initiates bidirectionally between two divergent gene clusters (Martinez-Calvillo et al., 2003, 2004), producing polycistronic pre-mRNAs which are subsequently processed. Remarkably, with the exception of the spliced leader (SL) promoter, no promoter is recognized by RNA polymerase II and only a few transcription factors have been identified (Cribb and Serra, 2009; Cribb et al., 2010). Even more surprisingly, although orthologs of all conserved components of the RNA polymerase II complex were identified in the Tri-tryp genome (Ivens et al., 2005), transcription of some trypanosomatid genes such as *VSG* and *procyclin* genes of *T. brucei* is mediated by RNA polymerase I, as are transfected genes containing a Pol I promoter or transfected genes integrated into a locus controlled by Pol I (Gunzl et al., 2003). Once the polycistronic pre-mRNA is produced, two coupled reactions allow the generation of mature monocistronic

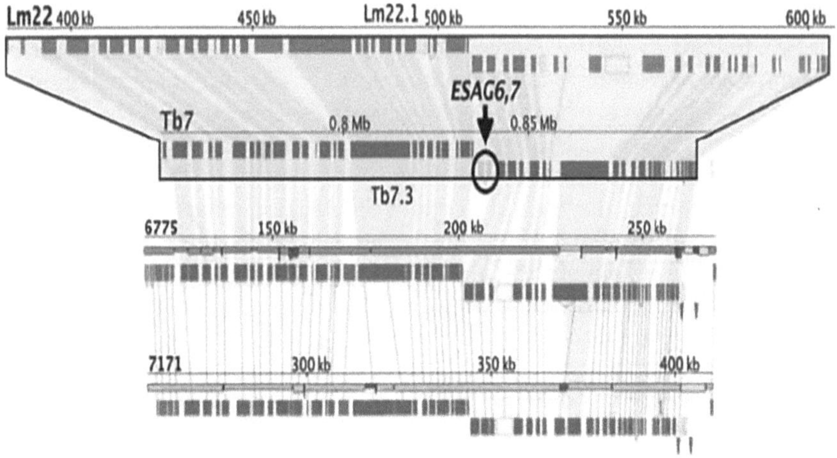

FIGURE 10.1 *Genome organization of trypanosomatids.* Alignment of segments of chromosome 7 of *T. brucei* (Tb7), chromosome 22 of *L. major* (Lm22) and a scaffold of a *T. cruzi* chromosome is shown (El-Sayed et al., 2005a,b). In these segments, two clusters of *T. brucei*, *L. major* and *T. cruzi* genes, coloured in red, purple and blue, respectively, are encoded in opposite strands, with a strand switch region corresponding to the position of the *T. brucei*-specific *ESAG* genes. High levels of gene synteny between the three genomes can be depicted from this alignment, as well as the presence of species-specific genes (represented by the *T. brucei ESAG* genes 6 and 7). The two different haplotypes in the *T. cruzi* CL Brener genome, denominated Esmeraldo- and non-Esmeraldo-like, are also shown in the representation of the *T. cruzi* chromosome scaffold.

transcripts: *trans*-splicing and polyadenylation (reviewed by Teixeira and daRocha, 2003). Therefore, every trypanosomatid mature mRNA presents a capped sequence of identical 39 nucleotides in the 5′-end named SL and the process whereby the SL is attached to the transcript is denominated *trans*-splicing (Liang et al., 2003). Whilst no sequence consensus for polyadenylation or SL addition was found, several studies have demonstrated that polypyrimidine-rich tracts located within intergenic regions guide both reactions, SL addition and polyadenylation, resulting in mature mRNAs (Liang et al., 2003; Fig. 10.2). Sequence requirements involved in the trypanosomatid mRNA processing have been more thoroughly investigated by comparing ESTs and/or cDNAs with genomic sequences (Benz et al., 2005; Campos et al., 2008; Smith et al., 2008). More recently, using high-throughput RNA sequencing, or RNAseq, other groups identified 5′ splice-acceptor sites and polyadenylation sites for a large number of *T. brucei* genes, revealing an extensive heterogeneity of 5′- and 3′-ends of the respective mRNAs (Siegel et al., 2010). Based on genomic sequences comparisons with ESTs and full-length cDNAs, Campos and colleagues determined the average distances between the SL addition and

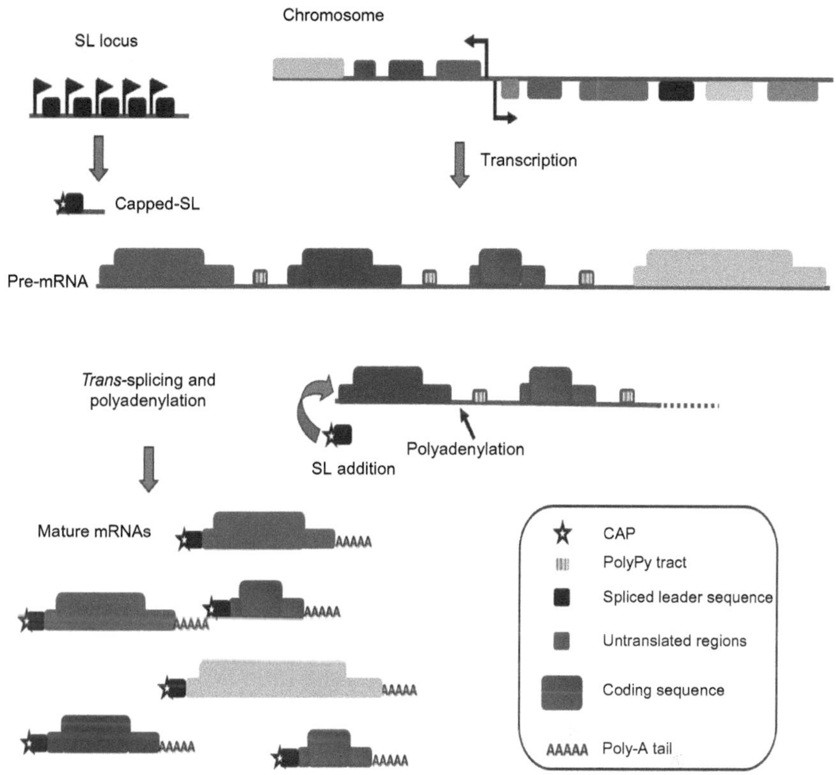

FIGURE 10.2 *mRNA transcription and processing in trypanosomatids.* Genes arranged in tandem are transcribed as polycistronic pre-mRNAs, which are processed by *trans*-splicing and polyadenylation reactions. Polypyrimidine tracts found in intergenic regions guide the insertion of capped-SL sequence at 5′-end and poly-A tail at 3′-end of transcripts generating monocistronic, mature mRNAs that accumulate at different levels in the cytoplasm. (See Color Section.)

polyadenylation site from the polypyrimidine tract, as well as the average sizes of 5′- and 3′-untranslated regions (UTRs) of *T. cruzi* genes (Campos et al., 2008). In addition to providing additional insights into gene expression mechanisms in these organisms, these predictions became useful tools to optimize transfection vectors that allow the expression of foreign genes in trypanosomatids, as discussed in the following sections.

As indicated before, one of the main characteristics revealed with the complete sequence of the *T. cruzi* genome is the dramatic expansion of families encoding surface proteins (El-Sayed et al., 2005a). Also accounting for the large proportion of repetitive sequences (50% of the genome) are long terminal repeat (LTR) and non-LTR retroelements and other subtelomeric repeats. The largest protein gene family encodes a group of surface proteins known as *trans*-sialidase (TS), with 1430 members. TSs are surface molecules identified as virulence factors of *T. cruzi* that are responsible for transferring sialic acid from sialoglycoconjugates from the host to the terminal β-galactose on the *T. cruzi* mucins. *MASP* (mucin-associated surface protein), with a total of 1377 members, represents the second largest *T. cruzi* gene family. Although MASP sequences correspond to approximately 6% of the parasite diploid genome, they were only identified during the annotation of the *T. cruzi* genome. MASPs are Glicophosphatidylinositol-anchored (GPI-anchored) surface proteins, preferentially expressed in trypomastigotes and characterized by highly conserved N- and C-terminal domains and a strikingly variable and repetitive central region (Bartholomeu et al., 2009). Together with *mucin* and *GP63* gene families, this group of four gene families accounts for approximately 17% of the total of protein-coding genes. They are organized as dispersed clusters of tandem and interspersed repeats. Other large families consist of the previously described *RHS* and *DGF-1* genes which, similar to the *TS* genes, are found mostly at sub-telomeric locations. The *T. cruzi* genome also includes large families encoding glycosyltransferases, protein kinase and phosphatases, kinesins, amino acid transporters and helicases, in addition to several gene families encoding hypothetical proteins (El-Sayed et al., 2005a).

Due to collapse of nearly identical repeats, not all copies of repetitive genes were included in the original genome assembly. In 2007, Arner et al. (2007) described an analysis of the total genomic repetitive content of protein-coding sequences and concluded that 18% of all protein-coding sequences exist in 14 or more copies. These authors proposed that an additional of 20,000 gene variants, including allelic variants, should be added to the *T. cruzi* genome database. These estimations, based on the alignment of shotgun reads of the genomic sequences and sequence coverage, showed, for example, that genes coding monoglyceride lipase, which were represented once in the genome assembly, are actually present in approximately 50 copies, whereas the flagellar calcium binding protein (FCBP), annotated as present in eight copies in the genome, has a more correct estimated number of 66 copies. Strikingly, not only surface antigens are repetitive, but also genes involved in a variety of cellular functions. Besides evasion of host immune system, an increased expression level, in the absence of strong promoters, may be a driving force resulting in the existence of highly repetitive gene families in the *T. cruzi* genome.

As a consequence of polycistronic transcription and the rarity of RNA polymerase II promoters on individual genes, expression of most trypanosomatid genes is regulated at the post-transcriptional level (reviewed in Haile and Papadopoulou, 2007). Global gene expression profiling (microarray) studies have shown that during its life cycle, mRNA levels from over 50% of the *T. cruzi* genes are up- or down-regulated (Minning et al., 2009). Similar to what is found in yeast and human cells, the rates of mRNA degradation and translation in trypanosomes are greatly influenced by sequence motifs present in UTRs which are recognized by components of the translation apparatus or the mRNA degradation machinery. Studies on a few *T. cruzi* genes that are regulated are beginning to unveil the elements involved in post-transcriptional control of gene expression, and this aspect of the *T. cruzi* biology is discussed elsewhere in this issue of *Advances in Parasitology*.

In trypanosomatids, the mitochondrial genome consists of a distinct mass of concatenated DNA known as the kinetoplast DNA (kDNA), present in a location adjacent to the basal body of the flagellum, inside the single tubular mitochondrion (Westenberger et al., 2006). Trypanosome kDNA comprises approximately 20–25% of the total cellular DNA and consists of a highly structured disk-shaped network composed of thousands of concatenated minicircles of 0.5–10 kb and dozens of concatenated maxicircles of 20–40 kb. Whereas minicircle sequences are present exclusively in kinetoplastids, maxicircles are the homologues of mtDNA molecules found in other eukaryotes (Lukes et al., 1997). Since the *T. cruzi* genome project took the approach of WGS sequencing of clones from libraries prepared with fragments derived from total cell DNA preparations, BLAST search of the primary reads readily identified sequences of the CL Brener and Esmeraldo strains with identity to previously known sequences of kDNA from *T. cruzi* and *T. brucei*. In an article that followed the *T. cruzi* genome publication, Westenberger et al. (2006) described the assembly of contigs that generated the complete sequence of CL Brener and Esmeraldo maxicircle DNAs (Westenberger et al., 2006). Similar to other trypanosomatid mitochondrial genes, sequence analyses showed that *T. cruzi* maxicircle contains frameshift errors in most of their genes, which are corrected at the RNA level by a complex U-insertion/deletion process known as RNA editing (Hajduk et al., 1993). Key elements of this process, gRNAs, are encoded mainly by minicircles, but few gRNA sequences are also present in maxicircles. They hybridize to the 3′-end of a target message and direct U insertion and deletion by the so-called editosome machinery. *T. cruzi* maxicircles are 25 kb in size and contain 18 tightly clustered mitochondrial protein-coding genes and two rRNA genes that are syntenic with previously sequenced maxicircles of *T. brucei* and *Leishmania tarentolae*. Fifteen of 18 protein-coding genes are edited. Outside the coding region, strain-specific repetitive regions and a variable region that is unique for each strain were identified, in which a 300 bp conserved elements may serve as an origin of replication (Westenberger et al., 2006).

10.2. COMPARATIVE GENOME ANALYSES

A comparison of the genomes of *T. cruzi* (CL Brener) with the two other reference trypanosomatid genomes, *T. brucei* (Berriman et al., 2005) and *L. major* (Ivens et al., 2005), has allowed the community to gain insights into the genetic and evolutionary bases of the shared and distinct lifestyles of these parasites. Probably, the most striking observation is that the three genomes display high levels of synteny (Fig. 10.1) and share a conserved set of approximately 6200 genes, 94% of which are arranged in syntenic directional gene clusters (El-Sayed et al., 2005b). An alignment of the deduced protein sequences of the majority of the clusters of orthologous genes across the three organisms reveals an average 57% identity between *T. cruzi* and *T. brucei*, and 44% identity between *T. cruzi* and *L. major*, and reflects the expected phylogenetic relationships (Haag et al., 1998; Lukes et al., 1997; Stevens et al., 1999; Wright et al., 1999). Species-specific genes, such as *T. brucei ESAG* genes 6 and 7 depicted in Fig. 10.1, are found in non-syntenic regions. Most species-specific genes are found to occur at non-syntenic chromosome—internal and sub-telomeric regions and consist of members of large surface antigen families. Structural RNAs, retroelements and gene family expansion are often associated with the breaks in conservation of gene synteny (El-Sayed et al., 2005b).

Those multigene family expansions are generally species-specific and most pronounced in the *T. cruzi* genome. The large majority encode surface proteins, such as TSs, MASPs, *T. cruzi* mucins (TcMUC), GP63, among others, and likely play a role in parasite–hosts interactions (El-Sayed et al., 2005b). The *T. cruzi* surface protein-encoding genes are often clustered into large arrays that can be as large as 600 kb in length and appear to be preferentially associated with large chromosomes (Baida et al., 2006; Bartholomeu et al., 2009; Di Noia et al., 1995; Vargas et al., 2004). Considering their location at regions of synteny breaks, it is likely that these arrays were subject to extensive rearrangements during the parasite's evolution. It is also likely that much of the striking polymorphism among the *T. cruzi* isolates that is reflected in several epidemiological and pathological aspects of Chagas disease are due, in part, to variability within these regions. Whole genome comparisons of distinct *T. cruzi* lineages would allow investigating this further.

The advent of next-generation sequencing technologies has ushered a new era in comparative sequencing, allowing the beginning of the exploration of a wide range of evolutionary and pathological questions within the *T. cruzi* lineage. An effort initiated and funded by the National Institutes of Health/National Institutes of Allergy and Infectious Diseases (NIAID) and the National Human Genome Research Institute (NHGRI) is aimed at sequencing additional isolates from the three main groups of trypanosomatid pathogens, including six first priority isolates/strains of *T. cruzi*. Those strains prioritized for sequencing include *T. cruzi* Silvio X10 (*T. cruzi* I), Esmeraldo (*T. cruzi* II), 3869 (*T. cruzi* III), Can III (*T. cruzi* IV), NRcl3 (*T. cruzi* V) and Tula cl2 (*T. cruzi* VI). They were strategically selected according to two main principles: coverage of the major subgroups within *T. cruzi* (Zingales et al., 2009) and coverage of closely related strains/isolates with clearly different pathogenesis.

This comparative sequencing initiative will begin addressing some of the outstanding questions in the pathogenesis of *T. cruzi*. It will reveal genome content and features associated with the ability of different strains or isolates to cause widely varied clinical manifestations and uncover any metabolic, regulatory or genetic networks associated with disease. Chagas disease presents with a wide variety of clinical outcomes, and the genetic bases of the diversity of clinical outcomes in these parasites are largely unknown. One example, it has been shown that the major lineages of *T. cruzi* exhibit significant differences in pathogenic potential. *T. cruzi* I, for example, is generally less pathogenic for humans, has a lower acute infectious profile, has a lower rate of progression and causes pathology in different organs. Comparison of at least one *T. cruzi* I isolate (e.g. Silvio X10) with the other isolates will provide an opportunity to discover the genetic basis of these phenomena. Other questions related to the genetic bases of the phenotypic variation (cell cycle, host range, vector selection, method of invasion, effects on the invaded cells, levels of parasitemia, etc.) will also be addressed. Whereas it is quite well established that the differences among *T. cruzi* isolates are genetically programmed, it is not yet established which genes or gene networks confer these different phenotypes. Thus, obtaining a good draft sequence, with the subsequent gene annotation and metabolic and other network reconstructions of these isolates (*T. cruzi* I Silvio X10, *T. cruzi* II Esmeraldo, *T. cruzi* III 3869, *T. cruzi* IV Can III, *T. cruzi* V NRcl3 and *T. cruzi* VI Tula cl2), will provide a basis for a comparison that will identify the genetic roots of these differences and constitute the first step towards a better understanding of their biology and pathogenesis.

10.3. ANTIGEN DISCOVERY AND IDENTIFICATION OF OTHER PARASITE MOLECULES INVOLVED IN HOST–PARASITE INTERACTIONS

In the first reports describing the construction and analyses of *T. cruzi* DNA libraries, most groups were interested in identifying sequences encoding *T. cruzi* antigens using screening protocols that select clones reacting with sera from patients or infected animals. Using the immunoscreening approach, a number of *T. cruzi* genes encoding antigens relevant for serodiagnosis have been isolated in several laboratories (DaRocha et al., 2002; Hoft et al., 1989; Ibanez et al., 1988). Among the positive clones identified, a large proportion encodes proteins with repetitive amino acid domains, and for several of them, it was demonstrated that the repetitive domains contain the epitopes that are targets of the B-cell response (Fontanella et al., 2008; Pais et al., 2008). Several of these antigens have been used to develop improved methods for immunodiagnostic based on recombinant proteins (da Silveira et al., 2001). These efforts are still needed, since current methods for diagnosis of Chagas disease such as enzyme-linked immunoassays, indirect immunofluorescence assays and indirect hemagglutination assays usually employ *T. cruzi* epimastigote forms or total protein extracts as the antigen. Frequently, these results can be inconclusive or doubtful depending on the commercial diagnostic assay used, and this uncertainty has serious consequences for blood screening. It is well known that false-positive reactions often result from cross-reactivity with other parasites, mainly *Leishmania* antigens. Among the antigens frequently identified in immunoscreenings and which have been used in studies towards the development of new tests for diagnosis, are members of the TS super family, which contain variable numbers of C-terminal 12 amino acids repeats (the so-called SAPA repeats), ribosomal proteins, heat-shock proteins, the FCBP, the flagellar protein FRA and the cytoplasmic protein CRA (da Silveira et al., 2001). The immunodominance of antigens carrying tandem repeat domains has been confirmed by a recent systematic survey of the *T. cruzi* genome that revealed that it is particularly rich in genes encoding proteins containing large repeats. In their report, Goto et al. (2008) identified, in addition to previously characterized *T. cruzi* antigens, a number of uncharacterized tandem repeat proteins which were also found to possess significant antigenicity.

Besides helping designing improved methods for serodiagnosis, several immunodominant antigens have been tested as candidates for the development of a vaccine against Chagas disease (Garg and Tarleton, 2002; Haolla et al., 2009). The presence of a large repertoire of proteins with tandem amino acid repeats among the immunodominant antigens prompts researchers to investigate whether they might contribute to a protective immunological response, host susceptibility, disease outcomes or pathogenicity. Global genomic analyses for the presence of repetitive domains in the genome of other *T. cruzi* strains will be highly informative if their variability and number of repeats can be correlated with the biological characteristics of the strains regarding the infection. In a first attempt towards this goal, Pais et al. (2008) examined two antigens that are recognized by antibodies from Chagas disease patients and found that antigens from strains belonging to *T. cruzi* II have repetitive domains that are larger and more variable than in *T. cruzi* I strains. This difference may be relevant for the outcome of the infection, since two recent studies showed that mice vaccinated with recombinant antigens such as TS (Fontanella et al., 2008) and the cystein protease cruzipain (Cazorla et al., 2010), from which the immunodominant repeats were deleted, were highly protected against *T. cruzi* infection. Similar to TS, the major *T. cruzi* cysteine proteinase, cruzipain, has a catalytic N-terminal domain and a C-terminal extension with unknown function but which is highly immunogenic (Cazorla et al., 2010).

In spite of some controversy regarding whether autoimmunity is part of the mechanism of pathogenesis leading to Chagas disease, it is now well established that *T. cruzi* parasite persistence in the heart is a major contributor to disease development, and that reducing parasite load would alleviate disease progression (Marin-Neto et al., 2007). Because of that, studies towards vaccine development experienced a new boost in recent years and are now being conducted by several laboratories with attention being given to the potential of therapeutic vaccines with the goal of reducing parasite load (this is discussed in-depth in another review in this issue of *Advances in Parasitology*). In the experimental model of Chagas disease, these studies have clearly established that a Th1 immune response characterized by IFN-γ production is required for parasite control. The role of CTL CD8+ T cells, as key players for protecting animals in vaccination experiments, has also become clear. It seems also apparent that a multi-component vaccine is needed for an effective immune protection. However, while studies performed in the past few years have greatly contributed to the understanding of the elements that are important for protective immunity in Chagas disease, only a very small and selected set of parasite molecules has been evaluated as antigen candidates. Among the antigens tested using different vaccination protocols are the cysteine protease cruzipain, amastigote surface protein, ASP-1 and ASP-2, the *T. cruzi* 24 kDa antigen, Tc24, the *T. cruzi* 52 kDa antigen, Tc5 and members of the TSs, TSA-1 and TSSA (for a recent review, see Cazorla et al., 2009). Therefore, there is a clear need for testing other antigens and antigen combinations as well as new formulations that include more efficient adjuvants. It is likely, given antigenic diversity between strains, that a successful vaccine, even if based on one protein, will need to include several strain-specific variants of the protein to provide protection for the spectrum of isolates found in endemic regions. Genomic and proteomic data combined with expression analyses of parasite antigens and bioinformatic approaches that can predict the presence of B and T cell epitopes can now be used in multiple ways for vaccine development.

A recent bioinformatic analysis of glycosylphosphatidylinositol-anchored molecules predicted from genomic data revealed that approximately 12% of *T. cruzi* genes possibly encode GPI-anchored proteins, and these are concentrated in few large multigene families, such as MASP, mucin, TS/gp85, mucin-like and gp63 (Nakayasu et al., 2009). Besides being important components involved in host–parasite interactions, GPI-anchored proteins may be released continually by low numbers of parasites that are present during the chronic phase of Chagas disease and thus may represent a potent immune-stimulatory group of molecules. The immunostimulatory activity of protozoa-derived GPI anchors and their related structure called glycoinositolphospholipids (GIPLs) has been well documented (Ropert and Gazzinelli, 2000). The identification of genes involved in the biosynthesis of GPI anchors in *T. cruzi* (M. S. C. unpublished) and the genetic manipulation of parasites aiming at generating knockout mutants related to the GPI pathway will certainly contribute to the understanding of the role of this molecules in the immune response to this parasite.

The availability of genomic sequence also allowed searching for new targets of the cellular immune response using bioinformatics and high-throughput methods such as testing of gene pools for immunostimulatory molecules (Dumonteil, 2009; Tarleton, 2005). Using a trypomastigote cDNA expression library, several new antigen candidates were identified by immunizing mice with pools of cDNAs and challenging with trypomastigotes (Tekiel et al., 2009). Among the 28 sequences that were found to improve *in vivo* protection, 19 of them encoded hypothetical proteins or unannotated *T. cruzi* open reading frames. Immunoscreenings of pools of cDNA for their recognition by T cells have also been successfully used. Martin et al. (2006) found that dominant parasite peptides recognized by CD8+ T cells in *T. cruzi*-infected mice and humans are encoded by members of the TS family. These studies demonstrated that a large number of new vaccine candidates still wait to be better characterized.

The weakened immunogenicity of highly purified recombinant antigens compared to attenuated live organisms has highlighted the need to search for novel adjuvant formulations. With our growing knowledge of the interplay between the innate and the adaptive immune systems, the roles of other molecules as immune potentiators are being investigated. Among the new promising adjuvants that are being tested, the Toll-like receptor 9 (TLR-9) ligand CpG DNA has been documented to stimulate cytokine production from immune cells *in vitro* and to give a better performance to vaccine formulations *in vivo* (Pashine et al., 2005). In a recent report, Bartholomeu et al. (2008) described a search for immunostimulatory DNA sequences containing CpG motifs in the *T. cruzi* genome (Bartholomeu et al., 2008). Interestingly, it was found that the retrotransposon VIPER element and the *TcMUC* genes were enriched for these sequences. It was showed that synthetic oligonucleotides containing sequences corresponding to CpG motifs derived from the *T. cruzi* genome stimulate IL-12 production by dendritic cells *in vitro*. Further, *T. cruzi* derived CpG dramatically enhances the ability of both CD8 and CD4+ cells to produce IFN-γ in immunized mice. Together with the development of viral vectors as recombinant live vaccines, chemically defined TLR agonists as immunological adjuvants became part of the arsenal necessary to induce the T-cell-mediated immunity that is needed to control infection by intracellular parasites such as *T. cruzi*. As discussed in the next section (and in another chapter in this issue of *Advances in Parasitology*), genetic manipulation of the parasite became also a powerful new tool to identify other molecules involved in parasite interaction with the host immune system.

10.4. MANIPULATING THE *TRYPANOSOMA CRUZI* GENOME AND THE PERSPECTIVES OF DEVELOPING NEW TOOLS FOR THE STUDY OF CHAGAS DISEASE

Since the first report describing the cloning of a *T. cruzi* gene in 1986 (Peterson et al., 1986), until the completion of the *T. cruzi* genome, molecular studies in this parasite advanced gene by gene, and in most cases, they were driven by the interest of several groups to identify molecules that are targets of the immune response in Chagas disease. Before the development of transfection protocols that allowed direct manipulation of the *T. cruzi* genome, these studies were limited to sequence analyses and partial descriptions of gene function or the activity of bacterial derived recombinant proteins. Soon after the first reports describing transfection experiments in *T. brucei* and in *Leishmania* in the early 1990s, a transfection protocol for *T. cruzi* was published by Lu and Buck (1991). It should be noted that these experiments were conducted in the absence of information regarding the sequences required for gene expression in these organisms (Laban and Wirth, 1989). It was not until the late 1990s that the elements involved with gene expression in *T. cruzi* and other trypanosomatids were identified, and improved transfection vectors that promote high levels of expression of foreign genes were developed. Using a vector containing a segment of the SL gene placed upstream of the bacterial *CAT* (*chloranfenicolacetyltransferase*) gene, Lu and Buck (1991) were able to detect CAT activity in transfected *T. cruzi* epimastigotes. Soon thereafter, Kelly et al. (1992) described the pTEX vector which has flanking sequences derived from the two tandemly repeated *glyceraldehyde-3-phosphate dehydrogenase (GAPDH)* genes, providing signals for *trans*-splicing and polyadenylation of the transfected gene. This first generation of vectors allowed the selection of stable transfectants through the expression of a drug-resistance marker. As reported in similar experiments with *Leishmania*, episomal plasmids replicate in *T. cruzi* in the form of large concatemers and remain stable in the presence of drug selection. Although these earlier vectors contained all the sequences necessary for the expression of the exogenous mRNA, the lack of promoter elements resulted in relatively low levels of expression of the reporter genes. The introduction of sequences derived from the ribosomal RNA promoter (Martinez-Calvillo et al., 1997; Teixeira et al., 1995; Tyler-Cross et al., 1995) resulted in a new generation of vectors, yielding expression levels in epimastigotes of at least two orders of magnitude greater when compared to vectors without promoter elements. Moreover, these vectors were found to be integrated, by homologous recombination, into the rRNA locus in the *T. cruzi* genome. Interestingly, whereas stable transfectants of *T. cruzi* and *L. major* can be achieved using episomal vectors, with

T. brucei this is not the case. In fact, pTEX can be used to transfect several species of *Leishmania* spp., but not *T. brucei* or *Crithidia fasciculata* (Taylor et al., 1994). As it became clear later, bidirectional transcription initiates randomly within the plasmid vector, and the long transcript generated is processed according to the rules of *trans*-splicing and polyadenylation. It has been speculated that, in *T. cruzi* and some *Leishmania* species, gene expression from episomal vectors is possible because of the absence of components of the RNAi machinery which would degrade double strand RNAs that are generated from the bidirectional plasmid transcription (Lye et al., 2010).

Early experiments aimed at identifying promoter regions in the *T. cruzi* genome using plasmids containing DNA fragments derived from intergenic regions of various genes inserted upstream from the luciferase reporter gene showed that the levels of luciferase activity resulting from transfections with these constructs were similar to the levels found in parasites transfected with a plasmid in which most of the trypanosome sequences were deleted and only a 73-bp fragment containing a *trans*-splicing additional signal was left upstream from the luciferase gene (Teixeira et al., 1995). Therefore, to obtain basal expression of episomal constructs in *T. cruzi*, the only *cis*-acting element that is required is a splice leader (SL) acceptor site, which was defined as a dinucleotide AG preceded by at least 10 pyridimines inserted 5′ of the coding region of the gene of interest. A similar sequence can also provide the signal for polyadenylation if inserted downstream from the gene (see Teixeira and DaRocha, 2003). Several improvements both in the vector design, with the inclusion of rRNA promoter, and in transfection protocols greatly enhanced the efficiency of genetic manipulation in *T. cruzi* (DaRocha et al., 2004b).

The first contribution resulting from genetic manipulation of the trypanosome genome was the identification of the elements involved with basic mechanisms of gene expression. As indicated before, no promoter sequences are present in trypanosome and because of polycistronic transcription, two coupled processing reactions, *trans*-splicing and polyadenylation, are required to generate mature monocistronic mRNA. Much before the identification of sequences necessary for polyadenylation or SL addition, through bioinformatic analyses of genome and transcriptome data, the major characteristics of the SL addition and polyadenylation signals were discovered by transfecting *T. brucei* and *L. major* with different reporter genes (LeBowitz et al., 1993; Matthews et al., 1994). Soon thereafter, experiments aiming at identifying regulatory elements controlling gene expression in *T. cruzi* were published by a few groups studying post-transcriptional mechanisms controlling the expression of stage-specific genes. To identify the elements involved in post-transcriptional control of gene expression in *T. cruzi*, we and others have used transient transfection and stable transfection protocols to test the effect of sequences corresponding to 5′- and 3′-UTR from different genes on the expression of a reporter gene (D'Orso and Frasch 2001; Teixeira et al., 1995).

Gene knockout experiments are powerful tools to determine gene function. Protocols that allowed reverse genetic manipulation of the *T. cruzi* genome have been used in only a limited number of studies that revealed the function of parasite genes and their role in the complex interactions with its hosts. In contrast to the large number of reports in *T. brucei* and in different *Leishmania* species, only a dozen genes have been experimentally characterized by reverse genetics in *T. cruzi*. The discovery that the RNAi machinery is not functional in *T. cruzi*, in contrast to the African trypanosomes (DaRocha et al., 2004a) highlights the importance of the development of strategies to knockout *T. cruzi* genes in order to access gene function. The gene encoding the flagellar adhesion molecule, *GP72*, the homologue of the *T. brucei FLA-1*, was the first *T. cruzi* gene to be analysed through gene deletion (Cooper et al., 1993). A role of GP72 in flagellum adhesion became evident in null mutants that showed parasites with their flagellum detached from the cell body. This phenotype is quite similar to the phenotype observed in *T. brucei* expressing dsRNA containing FLA1 sequences (LaCount et al., 2000). For all *T. cruzi* knockout genes described so far, disruption was achieved through homologous recombination, using a DNA cassette that has one of the three drug selectable markers, G418, hygromycin or puromycin, flanked by the coding sequence or the UTRs of the target gene. This is, however, a slow, time-consuming protocol in which drug-resistant parasites are obtained after the first round of transfection which disrupts the first allele followed by a second round of transfection with a vector containing a second selectable marker flanked by sequences of the second allele. Each round of transfection and drug selection usually takes 30–40 days. Given that allelic copies of most genes in the CL Brener genome vary in sequence by as much as 1.5%, carefully designed vectors containing sequence specific for the each allele need to be constructed. Moreover, gene knockout experiments have been hindered in *T. cruzi* by the fact that a large number of genes are encoded by multigene families. Thus, with all these limitations, it is not surprising that, after the release of the complete genome sequence, still a limited number of reports describing phenotypes of *T. cruzi* knockout parasites have been reported. In some few cases, where it is assumed that the gene is essential, haploid deficiency resulted in phenotypes that can also revealed interesting results regarding gene function (Campos et al., 2010; MacRae et al., 2006).

New protocols describing alternative methodologies to facilitate genetic manipulation in *T. cruzi* are indeed very welcome. Recently, Xu et al. (2009) described two approaches that could be used to improve these methodologies: a one-step-PCR strategy that was found to be the fastest method for production of knockout constructs, but that requires gene-specific sequences flanking the drug-resistant marker with more than 80 nucleotides. However, the use of the Gateway Technology (Invitrogen) to prepare the gene deletion constructs seems to be amenable to use as part of a higher throughput gene knockout project (Xu et al., 2009). The Gateway system has also been used by Batista et al. (2010) who described a platform that allows the exchange of various elements, such as promoters, fusion tags, intergenic regions and drug selectable markers to construct various types of vectors to be use in *T. cruzi* transfections. Another major improvement that allowed better control of genetic manipulation in these parasites was the development of inducible expression of gene products with the tetracycline repressor. This system, initially developed for *T. brucei*, requires the generation of transgenic parasites expressing the tetracycline repressor of *E. coli*. Tetracycline-dependent expression of a reporter gene cloned downstream from the *tet* operator (Wirtz et al., 1999) has been successfully described in *T. cruzi* (DaRocha et al., 2004b; Taylor and Kelly, 2006). The control of gene expression over a range of four orders of magnitude in response to variations in tetracycline concentration became an excellent tool for dissecting the functions of essential genes and for the expression of toxic gene products. Thus, we have now a much more broad collection of vectors that can be used to perform genetic manipulation in *T. cruzi*, including vectors containing sequences that allow the integration of the transfected gene into different loci of the parasite genome (DaRocha et al., 2004b; Vazquez and Levin, 1999).

As an alternative to gene knockout, several groups have described the analysis of phenotypic changes in parasites over-expressing a particular gene. Phenotypic analysis of parasites over-expressing the cysteine proteinase showed that they had an enhanced ability to undergo metacyclogenesis (Tomas et al., 1997). Metacyclic forms expressing trypomastigote-specific TS on the surface escaped earlier from the vacuole and differentiated earlier into amastigotes than non-transfected metacyclics (Rubin-de-Celis et al., 2006). Epimastigotes over-expressing genes encoding the NADPH-cytochrome P450 reductases showed a significant role for TcCPR-B and TcCPR-C in the sterol biosynthetic pathway in *T. cruzi* (De Vas et al., 2011). Similarly, a role of the RNA binding protein in controlling mRNA stability was also revealed in parasites over-expression of TcUBP-1 (D'Orso and Frasch, 2001). Using similar strategies, the involvement of the *RAD51* gene and genes encoding different DNA polymerases in the *T. cruzi* DNA metabolism has been studied by our group: we showed evidence for a role of *RAD51* in the unusually high *T. cruzi* resistance to ionizing radiation (Regis-da-Silva et al., 2006) and the activities of DNA polymerase in oxidative damage as well as of DNA polymerase beta and polymerase kappa in mitochondrial DNA maintenance (de Moura et al., 2009; Lopes Dde et al., 2008; Rajao et al., 2009).

Expression of foreign genes in *T. cruzi* can also be used to study the possibility of using an avirulent strain of the parasite to develop new vaccine protocols. The CL-14 clone is an attenuated strain, at least fourfold less infective than the parental CL strain (Atayde et al., 2004). Previous studies also showed that CL-14 trypomastigotes, instead of producing disease, are able to efficiently induce protective immunity against subsequent challenge with a highly virulent strain, preventing mortality, development of parasitemia and symptoms of the disease in mice (Lima et al., 1991, 1995). Recently, Gazzinelli and colleagues (R. T. G., personal communication) have shown that expressing a foreign antigen in CL-14 resulted in a strong immune response against this antigen. Although the basis of the attenuated, less-infective phenotype of CL-14 still needs to be thoroughly investigated, genetic manipulation of this strain has already became an attractive tool for studies towards a better understanding of the role of different parasite components in the complex process involved in protective immunity. A current hypothesis is that activation of TLRs and other innate immune receptors, during the initial contact between host cells and the intact parasite, is an essential event that leads to long-lasting and robust cellular immunity, as well as the production of antibodies, which are required for an efficient protective immunity.

The elucidation of critical pathways such as DNA replication and repair, polycistronic RNA transcription and editing, as well as the roles of numerous parasite gene families encoding surface protein, protein kinases and phosphatases that are now afforded by analysis of the *T. cruzi* genome promise to reveal novel targets for studies towards development of new trypanocidal drugs and methods to prevent infection. A better understanding of gene function and cellular processes that are distinct from the typical eukaryotic machinery may also open new possibilities for studies towards targeted drug development, which can be combined with high-throughput approaches in the searching for new vaccine antigens candidates. Although it is still too early to evaluate the impact that genome sequencing has had on drug and vaccine development, it is now clear that the genomic information is helping us to increase our understanding on several aspects of *T. cruzi* biology, host–parasite interactions and immunity to infection.

REFERENCES

Arner, E., Kindlund, E., Nilsson, D., Farzana, F., Ferella, M., Tammi, M.T., et al., 2007. Database of *Trypanosoma cruzi* repeated genes: 20,000 additional gene variants. BMC Genomics 8, 391.

Atayde, V.D., Neira, I., Cortez, M., Ferreira, D., Freymuller, E., Yoshida, N., 2004. Molecular basis of non-virulence of *Trypanosoma cruzi* clone CL-14. Int. J. Parasitol. 34, 851–860.

Baida, R.C., Santos, M.R., Carmo, M.S., Yoshida, N., Ferreira, D., Ferreira, A.T., et al., 2006. Molecular characterization of serine-, alanine- and proline-rich proteins of *Trypanosoma cruzi* and their possible role in host cell infection. Infect. Immun. 74, 1537–1546.

Bartholomeu, D.C., Ropert, C., Melo, M.B., Parroche, P., Junqueira, C.F., Teixeira, S.M., et al., 2008. Recruitment and endo-lysosomal activation of TLR9 in dendritic cells infected with *Trypanosoma cruzi*. J. Immunol. 181, 1333–1344.

Bartholomeu, D.C., Cerqueira, G.C., Leao, A.C., daRocha, W.D., Pais, F.S., Macedo, C., et al., 2009. Genomic organization and expression profile of the mucin-associated surface protein (masp) family of the human pathogen *Trypanosoma cruzi*. Nucleic Acids Res. 37, 3407–3417.

Batista, M., Marchini, F.K., Celedon, P.A., Fragoso, S.P., Probst, C.M., Preti, H., et al., 2010. A high-throughput cloning system for reverse genetics in *Trypanosoma cruzi*. BMC Microbiol. 10, 259.

Benz, C., Nilsson, D., Andersson, B., Clayton, C., Guilbride, D.L., 2005. Messenger RNA processing sites in *Trypanosoma cruzi*. Mol. Biochem. Parasitol. 143, 125–134.

Berriman, M., Ghedin, E., Hertz-Fowler, C., Blandin, G., Renauld, H., Bartholomeu, D.C., et al., 2005. The genome of the African trypanosome *Trypanosoma cruzi*. Science 309, 416–422.

Branche, C., Ochaya, S., Aslund, L., Andersson, B., 2006. Comparative karyotyping as a tool for genome structure analysis of *Trypanosoma cruzi*. Mol. Biochem. Parasitol. 147, 30–38.

Brandao, A., Urmenyi, T., Rondinelli, E., Gonzalez, A., de Miranda, A.B., Degrave, W., 1997. Identification of transcribed sequences (ESTs) in the *Trypanosoma cruzi* genome project. Mem. Inst. Oswaldo Cruz 92, 863–866.

Campos, P.C., Bartholomeu, D.C., DaRocha, W.D., Cerqueira, G.C., Teixeira, S.M., 2008. Sequences involved in mRNA processing in *Trypanosoma cruzi*. Int. J. Parasitol. 38, 1383–1389.

Campos, P.C., Silva, V.G., Furtado, C., Machado-Silva, A., Darocha, W.D., Peloso, E.F., et al., 2010. *Trypanosoma cruzi* MSH2: functional analyses on different parasite strains provide evidences for a role on the oxidative stress response. Mol. Biochem. Parasitol. 176, 8–16.

Cano, M.I., Gruber, A., Vazquez, M., Cortes, A., Levin, M.J., Gonzalez, A., et al., 1995. Molecular karyotype of clone CL Brener chosen for the *Trypanosoma cruzi* genome project. Mol. Biochem. Parasitol. 71, 273–278.

Cazorla, S.I., Frank, F.M., Malchiodi, E.L., 2009. Vaccination approaches against *Trypanosoma cruzi* infection. Expert Rev. Vaccines 8, 921–935.

Cazorla, S.I., Frank, F.M., Becker, P.D., Arnaiz, M., Mirkin, G.A., Corral, R.S., et al., 2010. Redirection of the immune response to the functional catalytic domain of the cystein proteinase cruzipain improves protective immunity against *Trypanosoma cruzi* infection. J. Infect. Dis. 202, 136–144.

Cerqueira, G.C., DaRocha, W.D., Campos, P.C., Zouain, C.S., Teixeira, S.M., 2005. Analysis of expressed sequence tags from *Trypanosoma cruzi* amastigotes. Mem. Inst. Oswaldo Cruz 100, 385–389.

Cooper, R., de Jesus, A.R., Cross, G.A., 1993. Deletion of an immunodominant *Trypanosoma cruzi* surface glycoprotein disrupts flagellum-cell adhesion. J. Cell Biol. 122, 149–156.

Cribb, P., Serra, E., 2009. One- and two-hybrid analysis of the interactions between components of the *Trypanosoma cruzi* spliced leader RNA gene promoter binding complex. Int. J. Parasitol. 39, 525–532.

Cribb, P., Esteban, L., Trochine, A., Girardini, J., Serra, E., 2010. *Trypanosoma cruzi* TBP shows preference for C/G-rich DNA sequences *in vitro*. Exp. Parasitol. 124, 346–349.

da Silveira, J.F., Umezawa, E.S., Luquetti, A.O., 2001. Chagas disease: recombinant *Trypanosoma cruzi* antigens for serological diagnosis. Trends Parasitol. 17, 286–291.

DaRocha, W.D., Bartholomeu, D.C., Macedo, C.D., Horta, M.F., Cunha-Neto, E., Donelson, J.E., et al., 2002. Characterization of cDNA clones encoding ribonucleoprotein antigens expressed in *Trypanosoma cruzi* amastigotes. Parasitol. Res. 88, 292–300.

DaRocha, W.D., Otsu, K., Teixeira, S.M., Donelson, J.E., 2004a. Tests of cytoplasmic RNA interference (RNAi) and construction of a tetracycline-inducible T7 promoter system in *Trypanosoma cruzi*. Mol. Biochem. Parasitol. 133, 175–186.

DaRocha, W.D., Silva, R.A., Bartholomeu, D.C., Pires, S.F., Freitas, J.M., Macedo, A.M., et al., 2004b. Expression of exogenous genes in *Trypanosoma cruzi:* improving vectors and electroporation protocols. Parasitol. Res. 92, 113–120.

de Freitas, J.M., Augusto-Pinto, L., Pimenta, J.R., Bastos-Rodrigues, L., Goncalves, V.F., Teixeira, S.M., et al., 2006. Ancestral genomes, sex, and the population structure of *Trypanosoma cruzi*. PLoS Pathog. 2, e24.

de Moura, M.B., Schamber-Reis, B.L., Passos Silva, D.G., Rajao, M.A., Macedo, A.M., Franco, G.R., et al., 2009. Cloning and characterization of DNA polymerase eta from *Trypanosoma cruzi*: roles for translesion bypass of oxidative damage. Environ. Mol. Mutagen. 50, 375–386.

De Vas, M.G., Portal, P., Alonso, G.D., Schlesinger, M., Flawia, M.M., Torres, H.N., et al., 2011. The NADPH-cytochrome P450 reductase family in *Trypanosoma cruzi* is involved in the sterol biosynthesis pathway. Int. J. Parasitol. 41, 99–108.

Di Noia, J.M., Sanchez, D.O., Frasch, A.C., 1995. The protozoan *Trypanosoma cruzi* has a family of genes resembling the mucin genes of mammalian cells. J. Biol. Chem. 270, 24146–24149.

D'Orso, I., Frasch, A.C., 2001. TcUBP-1, a developmentally regulated U-rich RNA-binding protein involved in selective mRNA destabilization in trypanosomes. J. Biol. Chem. 276, 34801–34809.

Dumonteil, E., 2009. Vaccine development against *Trypanosoma cruzi* and *Leishmania* species in the post-genomic era. Infect. Genet. Evol. 9, 1075–1082.

El-Sayed, N.M., Myler, P.J., Bartholomeu, D.C., Nilsson, D., Aggarwal, G., Tran, A.N., et al., 2005a. The genome sequence of *Trypanosoma cruzi*, etiologic agent of Chagas disease. Science 309, 409–415.

El-Sayed, N.M., Myler, P.J., Blandin, G., Berriman, M., Crabtree, J., Aggarwal, G., et al., 2005b. Comparative genomics of trypanosomatid parasitic protozoa. Science 309, 404–409.

Fontanella, G.H., De Vusser, K., Laroy, W., Daurelio, L., Nocito, A.L., Revelli, S., et al., 2008. Immunization with an engineered mutant *trans*-sialidase highly protects mice from experimental *Trypanosoma cruzi* infection: a vaccine candidate. Vaccine 26, 2322–2334.

Garg, N., Tarleton, R.L., 2002. Genetic immunization elicits antigen-specific protective immune responses and decreases disease severity in *Trypanosoma cruzi* infection. Infect. Immun. 70, 5547–5555.

Goto, Y., Carter, D., Reed, S.G., 2008. Immunological dominance of *Trypanosoma cruzi* tandem repeat proteins. Infect. Immun. 76, 3967–3974.

Gunzl, A., Bruderer, T., Laufer, G., Schimanski, B., Tu, L.C., Chung, H.M., et al., 2003. RNA polymerase I transcribes procyclin genes and variant surface glycoprotein gene expression sites in *Trypanosoma cruzi*. Eukaryot. Cell 2, 542–551.

Haag, J., O'HUigin, C., Overath, P., 1998. The molecular phylogeny of trypanosomes: evidence for an early divergence of the Salivaria. Mol. Biochem. Parasitol. 91, 37–49.

Haile, S., Papadopoulou, B., 2007. Developmental regulation of gene expression in trypanosomatid parasitic protozoa. Curr. Opin. Microbiol. 10, 569–577.

Hajduk, S.L., Harris, M.E., Pollard, V.W., 1993. RNA editing in kinetoplastid mitochondria. FASEB J. 7, 54–63.

Haolla, F.A., Claser, C., de Alencar, B.C., Tzelepis, F., de Vasconcelos, J.R., de Oliveira, G., et al., 2009. Strain-specific protective immunity following vaccination against experimental *Trypanosoma cruzi* infection. Vaccine 27, 5644–5653.

Henriksson, J., Porcel, B., Rydaker, M., Ruiz, A., Sabaj, V., Galanti, N., et al., 1995. Chromosome specific markers reveal conserved linkage groups in spite of extensive chromosomal size variation in *Trypanosoma cruzi*. Mol. Biochem. Parasitol. 73, 63–74.

Hoft, D.F., Kim, K.S., Otsu, K., Moser, D.R., Yost, W.J., Blumin, J.H., et al., 1989. *Trypanosoma cruzi* expresses diverse repetitive protein antigens. Infect. Immun. 57, 1959–1967.

Ibanez, C.F., Affranchino, J.L., Macina, R.A., Reyes, M.B., Leguizamon, S., Camargo, M.E., et al., 1988. Multiple *Trypanosoma cruzi* antigens containing tandemly repeated amino acid sequence motifs. Mol. Biochem. Parasitol. 30, 27–33.

Ivens, A.C., Peacock, C.S., Worthey, E.A., Murphy, L., Aggarwal, G., Berriman, M., et al., 2005. The genome of the kinetoplastid parasite, *Leishmania major*. Science 309, 436–442.

Kelly, J.M., Ward, H.M., Miles, M.A., Kendall, G., 1992. A shuttle vector which facilitates the expression of transfected genes in *Trypanosoma cruzi* and *Leishmania*. Nucleic Acids Res. 20, 3963–3969.

Laban, A., Wirth, D.F., 1989. Transfection of *Leishmania enriettii* and expression of chloramphenicol acetyltransferase gene. Proc. Natl. Acad. Sci. USA 86, 9119–9123.

LaCount, D.J., Bruse, S., Hill, K.L., Donelson, J.E., 2000. Double-stranded RNA interference in *Trypanosoma cruzi* using head-to-head promoters. Mol. Biochem. Parasitol. 111, 67–76.

LeBowitz, J.H., Smith, H.Q., Rusche, L., Beverley, S.M., 1993. Coupling of poly(A) site selection and *trans*-splicing in *Leishmania*. Genes Dev. 7, 996–1007.

Liang, X.H., Haritan, A., Uliel, S., Michaeli, S., 2003. *Trans–cis* splicing in trypanosomatids: mechanism, factors, and regulation. Eukaryot. Cell 2, 830–840.

Lima, M.T., Jansen, A.M., Rondinelli, E., Gattass, C.R., 1991. *Trypanosoma cruzi*: properties of a clone isolated from CL strain. Parasitol. Res. 77, 77–81.

Lima, M.T., Lenzi, H.L., Gattass, C.R., 1995. Negative tissue parasitism in mice injected with a noninfective clone of *Trypanosoma cruzi*. Parasitol. Res. 81, 6–12.

Lopes Dde, O., Schamber-Reis, B.L., Regis-da-Silva, C.G., Rajao, M.A., Darocha, W.D., Macedo, A.M., et al., 2008. Biochemical studies with DNA polymerase beta and DNA polymerase beta-PAK of *Trypanosoma cruzi* suggest the involvement of these proteins in mitochondrial DNA maintenance. DNA Repair (Amst.) 7, 1882–1892.

Lu, H.Y., Buck, G.A., 1991. Expression of an exogenous gene in *Trypanosoma cruzi* epimastigotes. Mol. Biochem. Parasitol. 44, 109–114.

Lukes, J., Jirku, M., Dolezel, D., Kral'ova, I., Hollar, L., Maslov, D.A., 1997. Analysis of ribosomal RNA genes suggests that trypanosomes are monophyletic. J. Mol. Evol. 44, 521–527.

Lye, L.F., Owens, K., Shi, H., Murta, S.M., Vieira, A.C., Turco, S.J., et al., 2010. Retention and loss of RNA interference pathways in trypanosomatid protozoans. PLoS Pathog. 6, e1001161.

MacRae, J.I., Obado, S.O., Turnock, D.C., Roper, J.R., Kierans, M., Kelly, J.M., et al., 2006. The suppression of galactose metabolism in *Trypanosoma cruzi* epimastigotes causes changes in cell surface molecular architecture and cell morphology. Mol. Biochem. Parasitol. 147, 126–136.

Marin-Neto, J.A., Cunha-Neto, E., Maciel, B.C., Simoes, M.V., 2007. Pathogenesis of chronic Chagas heart disease. Circulation 115, 1109–1123.

Martin, D.L., Weatherly, D.B., Laucella, S.A., Cabinian, M.A., Crim, M.T., Sullivan, S., et al., 2006. CD8+ T-Cell responses to *Trypanosoma cruzi* are highly focused on strain-variant *trans*-sialidase epitopes. PLoS Pathog. 2, e77.

Martinez-Calvillo, S., Lopez, I., Hernandez, R., 1997. pRIBOTEX expression vector: a pTEX derivative for a rapid selection of *Trypanosoma cruzi* transfectants. Gene 199, 71–76.

Martinez-Calvillo, S., Yan, S., Nguyen, D., Fox, M., Stuart, K., Myler, P.J., 2003. Transcription of *Leishmania major* Friedlin chromosome 1 initiates in both directions within a single region. Mol. Cell 11, 1291–1299.

Martinez-Calvillo, S., Nguyen, D., Stuart, K., Myler, P.J., 2004. Transcription initiation and termination on *Leishmania major* chromosome 3. Eukaryot. Cell 3, 506–517.

Matthews, K.R., Tschudi, C., Ullu, E., 1994. A common pyrimidine-rich motif governs *trans*-splicing and polyadenylation of tubulin polycistronic pre-mRNA in trypanosomes. Genes Dev. 8, 491–501.

Minning, T.A., Weatherly, D.B., Atwood, J., 3rd, Orlando, R., Tarleton, R.L., 2009. The steady-state transcriptome of the four major life-cycle stages of *Trypanosoma cruzi*. BMC Genomics 10, 370.

Nakayasu, E.S., Yashunsky, D.V., Nohara, L.L., Torrecilhas, A.C., Nikolaev, A.V., Almeida, I.C., 2009. GPIomics: global analysis of glycosylphosphatidylinositol-anchored molecules of *Trypanosoma cruzi*. Mol. Syst. Biol. 5, 261.

Pais, F.S., DaRocha, W.D., Almeida, R.M., Leclercq, S.Y., Penido, M.L., Fragoso, S.P., et al., 2008. Molecular characterization of ribonucleoproteic antigens containing repeated amino acid sequences from *Trypanosoma cruzi*. Microbes Infect. 10, 716–725.

Pashine, A., Valiante, N.M., Ulmer, J.B., 2005. Targeting the innate immune response with improved vaccine adjuvants. Nat. Med. 11, S63–68.

Peterson, D.S., Wrightsman, R.A., Manning, J.E., 1986. Cloning of a major surface-antigen gene of *Trypanosoma cruzi* and identification of a nonapeptide repeat. Nature 322, 566–568.

Porcel, B.M., Aslund, L., Pettersson, U., Andersson, B., 2000. *Trypanosoma cruzi*: a putative vacuolar ATP synthase subunit and a CAAX prenyl protease-encoding gene, as examples of gene identification in genome projects. Exp. Parasitol. 95, 176–186.

Rajao, M.A., Passos-Silva, D.G., DaRocha, W.D., Franco, G.R., Macedo, A.M., Pena, S.D., et al., 2009. DNA polymerase kappa from *Trypanosoma cruzi* localizes to the mitochondria, bypasses 8-oxoguanine lesions and performs DNA synthesis in a recombination intermediate. Mol. Microbiol. 71, 185–197.

Regis-da-Silva, C.G., Freitas, J.M., Passos-Silva, D.G., Furtado, C., Augusto-Pinto, L., Pereira, M.T., et al., 2006. Characterization of the *Trypanosoma cruzi* Rad51 gene and its role in recombination events associated with the parasite resistance to ionizing radiation. Mol. Biochem. Parasitol. 149, 191–200.

Ropert, C., Gazzinelli, R.T., 2000. Signaling of immune system cells by glycosylphosphatidylinositol (GPI) anchor and related structures derived from parasitic protozoa. Curr. Opin. Microbiol. 3, 395–403.

Rubin-de-Celis, S.S., Uemura, H., Yoshida, N., Schenkman, S., 2006. Expression of trypomastigote *trans*-sialidase in metacyclic forms of *Trypanosoma cruzi* increases parasite escape from its parasitophorous vacuole. Cell. Microbiol. 8, 1888–1898.

Siegel, T.N., Hekstra, D.R., Wang, X., Dewell, S., Cross, G.A., 2010. Genome-wide analysis of mRNA abundance in two life-cycle stages of *Trypanosoma cruzi* and identification of splicing and polyadenylation sites. Nucleic Acids Res. 38, 4946–4957.

Smith, M., Blanchette, M., Papadopoulou, B., 2008. Improving the prediction of mRNA extremities in the parasitic protozoan *Leishmania*. BMC Bioinformatics 9, 158.

Stevens, J.R., Noyes, H.A., Dover, G.A., Gibson, W.C., 1999. The ancient and divergent origins of the human pathogenic trypanosomes, *Trypanosoma brucei* and *T. cruzi*. Parasitology 118 (Pt 1), 107–116.

Tarleton, R.L., 2005. New approaches in vaccine development for parasitic infections. Cell. Microbiol. 7, 1379–1386.

Taylor, M.C., Kelly, J.M., 2006. pTcINDEX: a stable tetracycline-regulated expression vector for *Trypanosoma cruzi*. BMC Biotechnol. 6, 32.

Taylor, M.C., Kelly, J.M., Chapman, C.J., Fairlamb, A.H., Miles, M.A., 1994. The structure, organization, and expression of the *Leishmania donovani* gene encoding trypanothione reductase. Mol. Biochem. Parasitol. 64, 293–301.

Teixeira, S.M., daRocha, W.D., 2003. Control of gene expression and genetic manipulation in the Trypanosomatidae. Genet. Mol. Res. 2, 148–158.

Teixeira, S.M., Kirchhoff, L.V., Donelson, J.E., 1995. Post-transcriptional elements regulating expression of mRNAs from the amastin/tuzin gene cluster of *Trypanosoma cruzi*. J. Biol. Chem. 270, 22586–22594.

Tekiel, V., Alba-Soto, C.D., Gonzalez Cappa, S.M., Postan, M., Sanchez, D.O., 2009. Identification of novel vaccine candidates for Chagas' disease by immunization with sequential fractions of a trypomastigote cDNA expression library. Vaccine 27, 1323–1332.

Tomas, A.M., Miles, M.A., Kelly, J.M., 1997. Overexpression of cruzipain, the major cysteine proteinase of *Trypanosoma cruzi*, is associated with enhanced metacyclogenesis. Eur. J. Biochem. 244, 596–603.

Tyler-Cross, R.E., Short, S.L., Floeter-Winter, L.M., Buck, G.A., 1995. Transient expression mediated by the *Trypanosoma cruzi* rRNA promoter. Mol. Biochem. Parasitol. 72, 23–31.

Vargas, N., Pedroso, A., Zingales, B., 2004. Chromosomal polymorphism, gene synteny and genome size in *T. cruzi* I and *T. cruzi* II groups. Mol. Biochem. Parasitol. 138, 131–141.

Vazquez, M.P., Levin, M.J., 1999. Functional analysis of the intergenic regions of TcP2beta gene loci allowed the construction of an improved *Trypanosoma cruzi* expression vector. Gene 239, 217–225.

Verdun, R.E., Di Paolo, N., Urmenyi, T.P., Rondinelli, E., Frasch, A.C., Sanchez, D.O., 1998. Gene discovery through expressed sequence Tag sequencing in *Trypanosoma cruzi*. Infect. Immun. 66, 5393–5398.

Weatherly, D.B., Boehlke, C., Tarleton, R.L., 2009. Chromosome level assembly of the hybrid *Trypanosoma cruzi* genome. BMC Genomics 10, 255.

Westenberger, S.J., Cerqueira, G.C., El-Sayed, N.M., Zingales, B., Campbell, D.A., Sturm, N.R., 2006. *Trypanosoma cruzi* mitochondrial maxicircles display species- and strain-specific variation and a conserved element in the non-coding region. BMC Genomics 7, 60.

Wirtz, E., Leal, S., Ochatt, C., Cross, G.A., 1999. A tightly regulated inducible expression system for conditional gene knock-outs and dominant-negative genetics in *Trypanosoma brucei*. Mol. Biochem. Parasitol. 99, 89–101.

Wright, A.D., Li, S., Feng, S., Martin, D.S., Lynn, D.H., 1999. Phylogenetic position of the kinetoplastids, Cryptobia bullocki, Cryptobia catostomi, and Cryptobia salmositica and monophyly of the genus *Trypanosoma* inferred from small subunit ribosomal RNA sequences. Mol. Biochem. Parasitol. 99, 69–76.

Xu, D., Brandan, C.P., Basombrio, M.A., Tarleton, R.L., 2009. Evaluation of high efficiency gene knockout strategies for *Trypanosoma cruzi*. BMC Microbiol. 9, 90.

Zingales, B., Pereira, M.E., Oliveira, R.P., Almeida, K.A., Umezawa, E.S., Souto, R.P., et al., 1997. *Trypanosoma cruzi* genome project: biological characteristics and molecular typing of clone CL Brener. Acta Trop. 68, 159–173.

Zingales, B., Andrade, S.G., Briones, M.R., Campbell, D.A., Chiari, E., Fernandes, O., et al., 2009. A new consensus for *Trypanosoma cruzi* intraspecific nomenclature: second revision meeting recommends TcI to TcVI. Mem. Inst. Oswaldo Cruz 104, 1051–1054.

CHAPTER 11

Genetic Techniques in *Trypanosoma cruzi*

Martin C. Taylor,* **Huan Huang,**[†] and **John M. Kelly***

Contents

Abstract

It is almost 20 years since genetic manipulation of *Trypanosoma cruzi* was first reported. In this time, there have been steady improvements in the available vector systems, and the applications

* Department of Pathogen Molecular Biology, London School of Hygiene and Tropical Medicine, London, United Kingdom
† Department of Pathology, Albert Einstein College of Medicine, Bronx, New York, USA

Advances in Parasitology, Volume 75
ISSN 0065-308X, DOI: 10.1016/B978-0-12-385863-4.00011-3

of the technology have been extended into new areas. Episomal vectors have been modified to enhance the level of expression of transfected genes and to facilitate the sub-cellular location of their products. Integrative vectors have been adapted to allow the development of inducible expression systems and the construction of vectors which enable genome modification through telomere-associated chromosome fragmentation. The uses of reverse genetic approaches to dissect peroxide metabolism and the mechanisms of drug activity and resistance in *T. cruzi* are illustrated in this chapter as examples of how the technology has been used to investigate biological function. Although there remains scope to improve the flexibility of these systems, they have made valuable contributions towards exploiting the genome sequence data and providing a greater understanding of parasite biology and the mechanisms of infection.

11.1. INTRODUCTION

Since the 1970s, biomedical research has been transformed by several important technical advances. These include the development of recombinant DNA procedures, exceptional progress in genome sequencing methodologies, huge increases in computing capacity and, more recently, high-throughput post-genome technologies. In parallel, the continuing development and refinement of techniques which facilitate genetic manipulation has allowed the generation of comprehensive data sets on the biological function of genes, both individually and collectively. Systematic attempts to genetically manipulate trypanosomatids were initiated in mid-1980s, when it had become apparent that the increasing flow of data produced using the new recombinant DNA technologies would remain largely descriptive in the absence of transformation procedures. In this chapter, we outline how reverse genetic approaches applicable to *Trypanosoma cruzi* were developed, discuss the properties of the tools now available, and describe how, despite some limitations, these have proved to be crucial to advances in our understanding of biological function.

11.2. GENETIC TOOLS APPLICABLE TO *TRYPANOSOMA CRUZI*

11.2.1. Background

Initial attempts to genetically manipulate trypanosomatids were complicated by an incomplete understanding of how these organisms regulate gene expression. At the time, it had only just become apparent that protein-coding genes were subject to polycistronic transcription and that *trans*-splicing of the expressed transcripts results in the addition of a 39-nucleotide 5′-spliced leader sequence to each mRNA. Therefore, the first transfection experiments were largely empirical, carried out in the absence of information on where transcription was initiated and which sequences might be required for RNA processing. Preliminary progress in this area was achieved by transient transfection of *Leptomonas seymouri* (Bellofatto and Cross, 1989) and *Leishmania enrietti* (Laban and Wirth, 1989) using electroporation. In these experiments, no attempt was made to select stable transformants, rather uptake and expression of an exogenous chloramphenicol transferase (*cat*) gene was monitored on the basis of enzyme activity. These experiments helped define the genetic context needed for expression of transfected genes. In *L. seymouri*, the 5′-upstream region of the mini-exon genes and 3′-downstream of an α-tubulin gene were used as flanking sequences. With *L. enrietti*, the 5′- and 3′-flanking regions were both derived from α-tubulin. Since these early transfection experiments, electroporation has remained the method of choice for introducing exogenous DNA into trypanosomatids.

The first reports of stable trypanosomatid transformation involved the use of episomal vectors which conferred G418 resistance on *Leishmania*, following expression of neomycin phosphotransferase (*neo*^{r}) genes. Flanking sequences from the dihydrofolate reductase-thymidylate synthase (Kapler et al., 1990) and α-tubulin genes (Laban et al., 1990) were used in the plasmid vectors. Within transformed parasites, these constructs were propagated in multiple extrachromosomal copies, often forming large circular episomes made up of head-to-tail repeats. Subsequent studies have shown that in *Leishmania*, specific origins of replication are not required for vector propagation and that expression of transfected genes is not promoter driven. Rather, transcription initiation appears to be stochastic, with a spliced leader site and an associated upstream polypyrimidine stretch being the requirements for expression (Curotto de Lafaille et al., 1992). Episomal transfection vectors have even been constructed that completely lack *Leishmania*-derived sequences (Papadopoulou et al., 1994). This situation contrasts with *Trypanosoma brucei*, where transient expression from episomes is promoter driven (Clayton et al., 1990; Rudenko et al., 1990; Zomerdijk et al., 1990).

When integration of transfected DNA into the *Leishmania* genome was first reported (Cruz and Beverley, 1990), it was shown to be mediated by homologous recombination. This is the predominant mechanism involved in transformation when linearised DNA, containing a drug-selectable marker flanked by the appropriate targeting sequences, is used for electroporation. Similarly, with *T. brucei*, targeted integration of vector DNA into the genomes of both procylic- and bloodstream-form parasites could be readily achieved (Carruthers et al., 1993; ten Asbroek et al., 1990). In contrast to *Leishmania* and *T. cruzi* (below), stable transformation of *T. brucei* with episomal vectors has proved to be problematic, with the requirements for autonomous replication appearing to be considerably more stringent (Patnaik et al., 1993; ten Asbroek et al., 1993).

11.2.2. The initial development of *Trypanosoma cruzi* transfection procedures

Transfection of *T. cruzi* was first achieved by electroporation of epimastigotes, using a transient expression construct in which the *cat* gene had been placed downstream of an intact mini-exon gene repeat (Lu and Buck, 1991). These experiments demonstrated that electroporation was applicable to *T. cruzi*, and that the requirements for expression of transfected genes seemed to be more similar to *Leishmania* than to *T. brucei*.

The first reported stable transformation of *T. cruzi* involved the use of the pTEX expression vector (Kelly et al., 1992; Fig. 11.1). This *neo*^{r}-based episomal construct was designed using flanking sequences derived from the tandemly repeated glycosomal glyceraldehyde-3-phosphate dehydrogenase (*gGAPDH*) genes (Kendall et al., 1990). pTEX was replicated within the parasite predominantly as large circular elements made up of

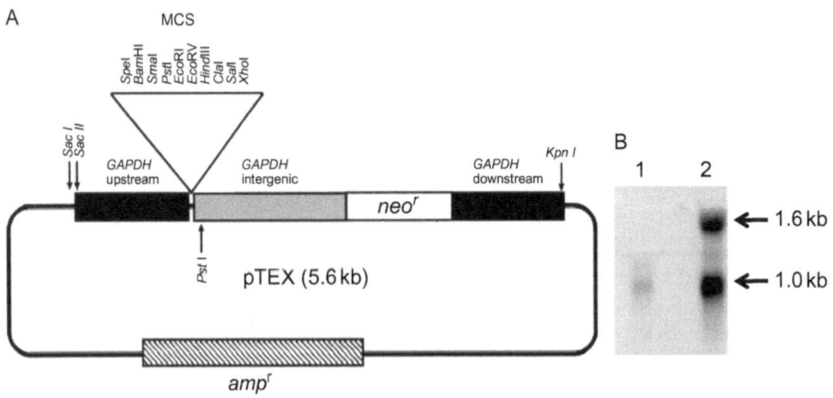

FIGURE 11.1 *The Trypanosoma cruzi expression vector pTEX (5.6 kb).* (A) Map of the construct. The multiple cloning site (MCS) and the *neo*^{r} gene are flanked by the 5′-upstream and 3′-downstream regions of the *T. cruzi* glycosomal *GAPDH* genes (Kendall et al., 1990). The plasmid backbone and *amp*^{r} gene are indicated. Genes inserted into the MCS can be expressed at high levels in transfected parasites. (B) pTEX-mediated over-expression of mitochondrial peroxidase *TcMPX* RNA in *T. cruzi* epimastigotes. Northern blot: lane 1, wild type; lane 2, over-expressing cell line. The 1.0/1.6 kb transcripts in lane 2 result from alternative polyadenylation sites provided by both the insert and the vector. Over-expression of *TcMPX* confers resistance to exogenous hydrogen peroxide (Wilkinson et al., 2000).

multiple head-to-tail repeats. The copy number and the level of expression of foreign genes inserted into the multiple cloning site (Fig. 11.1) could be enhanced significantly by culturing transformed cells in medium containing increased levels of G418. This is probably due to the selective advantage conferred on those daughter cells which contain a higher vector copy number, a phenomenon which occurs as a result of random segregation. The pTEX shuttle vector could also be used to transform *Leishmania*, but not *T. brucei*. In both *Leishmania* and *T. cruzi*, transfected genes were *trans*-spliced at the site used during the post-transcriptional processing of *gGAPDH*. *T. cruzi* was also found to support stable integration of transfected DNA via homologous recombination. The first reported experiments described the targeted disruption of the *PUB12.5* polyubiquitin locus (Hariharan et al., 1993) and the *TCR27* gene (Otsu et al., 1993), which encodes an antigen containing 14 amino acid repeats. In the latter case, although null mutants were viable, they grew more slowly within infected mammalian cells (Otsu et al., 1995).

The development of both integrative and episomal transformation systems for *T. cruzi* represented an important technical breakthrough which opened the way to the application of reverse genetics experiments. The surface glycoprotein Gp72 was one of the first proteins whose biological function was identified using these transfection-based techniques (Cooper et al., 1993). Null mutants were characterised by an abnormal flagellar phenotype in which attachment to the parasite cell membrane was disrupted. This was associated with a greatly reduced ability to survive within the triatomine insect vector. The role of Gp72 was confirmed by reintroduction of the gene on an episomal expression vector. This resulted in complementation of the mutant phenotype, including the restoration of normal flagellar morphology (Nozaki and Cross, 1994).

Genes that encode resistance to hygromycin, phleomycin, puromycin and tunicamycin have now been added to the list of selectable markers available for work on *T. cruzi*. However, one major limitation of *T. cruzi* transfection technology has been apparent since the beginning. The time taken to generate cloned transformants is approximately 6–8 weeks, four times longer than required for *Leishmania*, and eight times longer than is necessary for bloodstream form *T. brucei* (Kelly et al., 1995).

11.2.3. Additions and improvements to the *Trypanosoma cruzi* genetic "tool-box"

Over the years, efforts have been made to extend the repertoire of *T. cruzi* transfection vectors and to increase the range of their applications. In one of the first attempts, Martínez-Calvillo et al. (1997) modified the pTEX expression vector (Fig. 11.1) by insertion of an 800-bp ribosomal DNA fragment upstream of the multiple cloning site. The resulting construct (pRIBOTEX) shortened by 2 weeks the time required for selection of drug-resistant parasites, and there was a modest increase in the level of marker gene expression. Interestingly, this vector was not maintained as an episome, rather it integrated into the ribosomal DNA locus. The level of expression achievable with pRIBOTEX was further enhanced by insertion of a DNA fragment from the upstream region of the *TcP2beta H1* gene into a location adjacent to the putative ribosomal promoter element, to produce the construct pTREX (Vazquez and Levin, 1999). This sequence contains a splice acceptor site which appears to be highly efficient. The pTEX vector has also been modified to provide a rapid method for identifying the sub-cellular location of proteins (Tibbetts et al., 1995). An oligonucleotide, corresponding to the 10 amino acid epitope 9E10 (EQK-LISEEDL) of human c-myc, was inserted into the multiple cloning site (Fig. 11.1) so that genes of interest could be ligated in-frame. Following transfection, the expressed protein, tagged with the epitope at the carboxyl terminus, can be localised within the parasite using immunofluorescence microscopy. In a parallel approach, episomal expression vectors have been modified by inclusion of green (GFP) or red (RFP) fluorescent protein sequences, which can be used to identify the sub-cellular location of fused proteins, following parasite transfection (Wilkinson et al., 2002a).

In addition to these expression vectors, a *T. cruzi* cosmid shuttle vector (pcos-TL) has been produced (Kelly et al., 1994). Cosmids are modified plasmids that have been engineered to allow the selective cloning of recombinant molecules containing DNA inserts of between 30 and 45 kb. Following transfection of *T. cruzi*, recombinant pcos-TL molecules are maintained at high copy as circular extrachromosomal elements. Genes contained within the large insert fragments are co-expressed at high levels (Tomas et al., 1997).

The constitutive expression vectors described above have limitations which restrict their use for studying gene function. Inappropriate expression of some proteins can result in a lethal or deleterious phenotype, and the use of approaches based on expression of dominant-negative mutant proteins can be problematic. These issues, together with the inability to perform conditional knockout experiments, indicated a need to develop systems for expressing *T. cruzi* transgenes in a controlled and repressible manner. In *T. brucei*, inducible expression systems were constructed based on the ability of the bacterial tetracycline repressor protein (tetR) to block T7 RNA polymerase-mediated transcription from an integrated T7 promoter in the absence of tetracycline (Wirtz and Clayton, 1995; Wirtz et al., 1999). Import of the genetic machinery for tetracycline-regulatable expression into the parasite was necessary because trypanosomes lack inducible transcription units that might be easily adaptable for this purpose.

The feasibility of developing this type of inducible expression system for *T. cruzi* was demonstrated by transient transfection experiments (Wen et al., 2001). Following this, stable tetracycline-inducible expression was described, using an approach where the T7 polymerase and *tetR* genes were inserted into the tubulin locus under the control of a ribosomal RNA reporter (DaRocha et al., 2004a). However, detailed characterisation of this cell line, to assess the parameters of inducible expression and the effect of placing a strong pol I promoter within a polycistronic transcription unit, was not undertaken. To circumvent potential problems associated with integration at an endogenously transcribed locus, an alternative strategy has been reported. The T7 polymerase and *tetR* genes were expressed from an episome, and the cassette containing the regulatable T7 promoter was inserted into a non-transcribed ribosomal RNA spacer region, upstream of the pol I-mediated transcription start site (Taylor and Kelly, 2006). Expression of reporter genes under these conditions proved to be tetracycline-inducible and tightly regulated (Fig. 11.2). The applicability of the system was further verified in a study of the role of mitochondrial iron superoxide dismutase in protecting *T. cruzi* from programmed cell death (Piacenza et al., 2007).

One possible limitation of inducible expression systems, particularly in the context of conditional knockout experiments, is that the kinetics of repression depend on the level of turnover of the protein of interest. A method for promoting rapid destabilisation of specific proteins has recently been described (Banaszynski et al., 2006). It involves expression of the target protein as a fusion with the destabilisation domain (ddFKBP) of the "rapamycin-binding protein". In the absence of the synthetic ligand Shield-1, proteins bearing this domain are rapidly degraded by the cytoplasmic proteosome. For example, in *Toxoplasma gondii*, addition of the ddFKBP sequence to the amino terminus of yellow fluorescent protein (YFP) or the carboxyl terminus of GFP results in degradation of these fusions within 6 h of the removal of 1 μM Shield-1 (Herm-Götz et al., 2007). Both the pTEX and pTREX vectors have been modified to facilitate expression of transfected proteins in *T. cruzi* tagged at either the amino or carboxyl termini with the ddFKBP domain. Preliminary results indicate that ligand-controlled destabilisation is feasible (H.Huang et al., unpublished data). Selective stabilisation/destabilisation of transfected YFP fusion constructs was readily achievable, with the addition of Shield-1 (4 μM) resulting in epimastigotes that are reversibly fluorescent. Huang et al. are currently optimising this inducible system.

Transfection vectors have also been used to study aspects of chromosome structure and function in *T. cruzi*. The construct pTEX-CF (Fig. 11.3) was designed to facilitate telomere-associated chromosome fragmentation (Obado et al., 2005), thereby enabling the deletion of defined regions of chromosomal DNA and the generation of partially monosomic cell

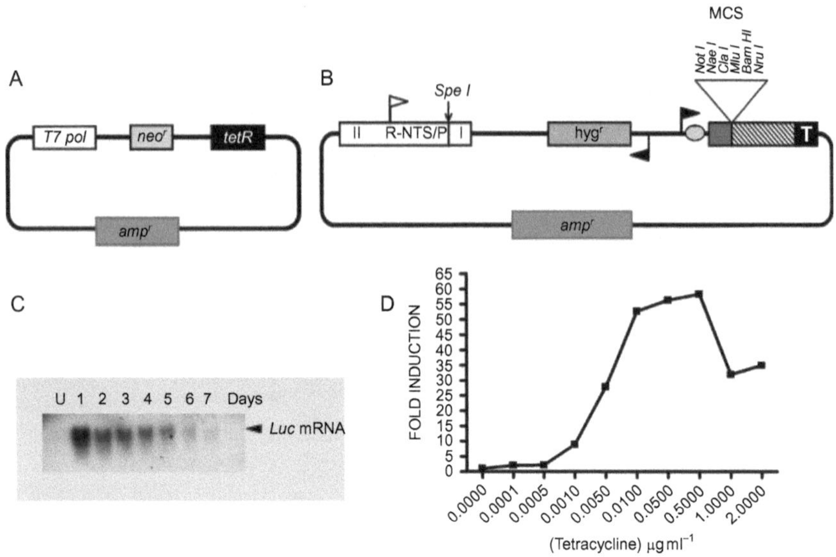

FIGURE 11.2 *Inducible expression of transfected genes in Trypanosoma cruzi.* (A) Simplified map of the pLEW vector (Wirtz et al., 1999) which contains the genes encoding T7 polymerase, G418 resistance (*neo*^{r}) and the tetracycline repressor (*tetR*). (B) The inducible expression vector pTcINDEX (Taylor and Kelly, 2006). The grey box adjacent to the MCS identifies the ribosomal protein P2β splice acceptor site (Vazquez and Levin, 1999). The hatched box indicates the *T. cruzi* actin intergenic region. The black box (T) is the T7 transcriptional terminator. The black flag represents the T7 promoter and the oval identifies the location of the *tet* operator. R-NTS/P is the ribosomal non-transcribed spacer and promoter region used for targeting. Roman numerals I and II indicate the two halves of the targeting sequence, cloned in opposite orientation to that in the genome. The white flag indicates the location of the pol I transcription start site (Martínez-Calvillo and Hernández, 1994). Following insertion of a gene of interest into the MCS, the construct can be linearised with *Spe*I to facilitate targeting into the ribosomal non-transcribed spacer region of parasites transformed with pLEW. (C) Induction of luciferase mRNA by tetracycline. RNA was prepared from pTcINDEX-*luc* transformed epimastiogotes each day (1–7) following a single dose of tetracycline (5 μg ml^{-1}). Lane U is the uninduced lane. (D) Effect of tetracycline concentration on level of luciferase activity. Epimastigotes were treated with different concentrations for 24 h and luciferase activity was measured and normalised to the amount of protein (Taylor and Kelly, 2006).

lines. The approach involves targeted integration by single-crossover, with the new telomere of the fragmented chromosome supplied by the vector (Fig. 11.3). In an attempt to delineate putative centromeric regions, we used this approach to generate parasite cell lines containing a series of truncated versions of chromosomes 1 and 3. (Obado et al., 2005, 2007). In each case, single GC-rich transcriptional "strand-switch regions" (11 kb, chromosome 1) and (16 kb, chromosome 3), composed predominantly of

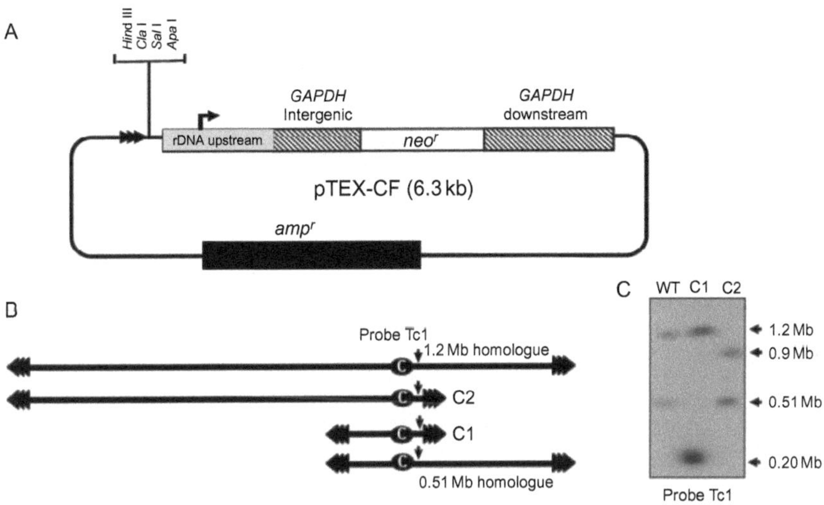

FIGURE 11.3 (A) The chromosome fragmentation vector pTEX-CF (6.3 kb). The vector was constructed as described in Obado et al. (2005). The location and direction of telomeric repeats are indicated by horizontal arrowheads. Following insertion of the targeting fragment into the MCS, the construct can be used for transfection of *T. cruzi* after linearisation with the appropriate restriction enzyme. (B) Exploring the organisation of chromosome 1. In the *T. cruzi* CL Brener strain, chromosome 1 exists as homologues of 0.51 and 1.2 Mb. Using a pTEX-CF construct to delete the right arm of the chromosome, we were able to demonstrate that the major size difference between the chromosome 1 homologues is the result of the insertion/deletion of 0.7 Mb of DNA into/from the left arm of the chromosome (Obado et al., 2005). (C) Southern blot of *T. cruzi* chromosomal DNA separated by pulse field gel electrophoresis. Lane 1, wild-type parasites identifying the 0.51 and 1.2 Mb homologues; lane 2, cell line in which the right arm of the 0.51 Mb homologue has been deleted 5 kb upstream of probe Tc1; and lane 3, cell line where the 1.2 Mb homologue has been deleted at the corresponding site.

degenerate retrotransposons, were found to be essential for mitotic stability. Consistent with this, etoposide-mediated cleavage sites, which are biochemical markers of centromere location, were also mapped to these domains in both chromosomes (Obado et al., 2007).

In addition to the development of new vector systems, several attempts have been made to enhance the efficiency and flexibility of *T. cruzi* transformation procedures. Using an agarose plating technique, Mondragon et al. (1999) were able to optimise conditions which allowed the isolation of parasite colonies in 21–28 days, with a transformation efficiency as high as 10^{-5} cells μg^{-1} of DNA. Expression of GFP has also been used to monitor transfection efficiency and to optimise parameters such as the electroporation buffer, the amount of DNA and the growth phase of the parasites used in the experiment (Ramirez et al., 2000). With similar approaches, DaRocha et al. (2004b) have developed electroporation procedures which result in up to 8% of the parasites expressing red fluorescence, following a transient transfection assay.

Another step, which can be time consuming when undertaking genetic manipulation of *T. cruzi*, is the generation of constructs, particularly when high-throughput deletion experiments are planned. Recently, it has been reported that a Multisite Gateway strategy can be adapted to enhance the efficiency of this process, particularly when used in combination with the AMAXA Nucleofector electroporation device (Xu et al., 2009). The Gateway cloning system, which is based on recombination rather than ligation, has also been used to facilitate the construction of a series of vectors which can be used for sub-cellular localisation of *T. cruzi* proteins and for tandem affinity purification of protein complexes (Batista et al., 2010).

11.2.4. Why is RNA interference technology not applicable to *Trypanosoma cruzi*?

Molecular biology has been revolutionised in the past decade by the discovery of RNA interference (RNAi) and the ever-increasing number of small regulatory RNA molecules. RNAi is widespread in eukaryotes and has functions that include gene regulation and the protection of cells from viruses and transposons (Ullu et al., 2004). The RNAi process is initiated within cells by the production, or introduction, of double-stranded RNA (dsRNA), which leads to the degradation of the homologous mRNA transcript. Briefly, long dsRNA is processed by the ribonuclease III DICER into 21–25 bp short interfering RNAs (siRNAs). The siRNAs are then loaded onto the RNA-induced silencing complex (RISC), at the heart of which is the protein Argonaute. The Argonaute binds the siRNA and the passenger strand is removed, leaving a single-stranded siRNA free to base pair with the cognate mRNA. When the cognate mRNA is bound by RISC, the endonuclease (SLICER) activity of Argonaute cleaves it in two, and the mRNA fragments are then degraded by cellular nucleases. This leads to down-regulation of the corresponding protein.

RNAi-based procedures have been widely exploited as a tool for exploring gene function. *T. brucei* is particularly amenable to this approach (Alsford and Horn, 2008), which has produced numerous insights into gene function. However, RNAi has not been detected in *T. cruzi*, despite numerous attempts (DaRocha et al., 2004a), and the associated genetic modification approaches have therefore not been applicable. The reason for this became clear when the trypanosomatid genome sequences were published; *T. cruzi* lacks genes for both of the DICER-like proteins DCL1 and DCL2 (Patrick et al., 2009; Shi et al., 2006) and the

Argonaute protein found in *T. brucei* (Durand-Dubief and Bastin, 2003; Shi et al., 2004) and is incapable of mounting an RNAi response to dsRNA. Examination of syntenic regions in the trypanosome genomes indicates that the relevant genes are completely missing from *T. cruzi* (e.g. Fig. 11.4), without even the pseudogene remnants found in *Leishmania major*. Interestingly, although Old World *Leishmania* species lack RNAi machinery, it is clear that *Leishmania braziliensis* and other *Viannia* species have intact and functional genes for the DICER-like proteins and Argonaute (Lye et al., 2010; Peacock et al., 2007). This suggests that *T. cruzi* and the Old World *Leishmania* species lost their RNAi machinery independently, subsequent to their divergence from *T. brucei* and the *Viannia* complex, respectively.

The absence of RNAi machinery in *T. cruzi* may explain why this parasite can be transformed with promoter-less circular episomes, whereas in *T. brucei*, chromosomal integration of foreign DNA is usually required. In *T. cruzi* and *Leishmania*, both episomal DNA strands are transcribed, a phenomenon which may reflect the more relaxed requirements for initiation of pol II-mediated transcription in trypanosomatids. In *T. brucei*, where RNAi is present, transcription of both strands will induce an RNAi response, which would act to "knockdown" episomally derived mRNAs. The question then arises as to why *T. cruzi* and *Leishmania* lost their RNAi machinery during evolution. Superficially, the pathway is beneficial in controlling transposon and viral proliferation. One explanation, in the case of *Leishmania* at least, is that portions of the genome can readily undergo amplification as extrachromosomal elements (Leprohon et al., 2009; Ubeda et al., 2008). This appears to occur

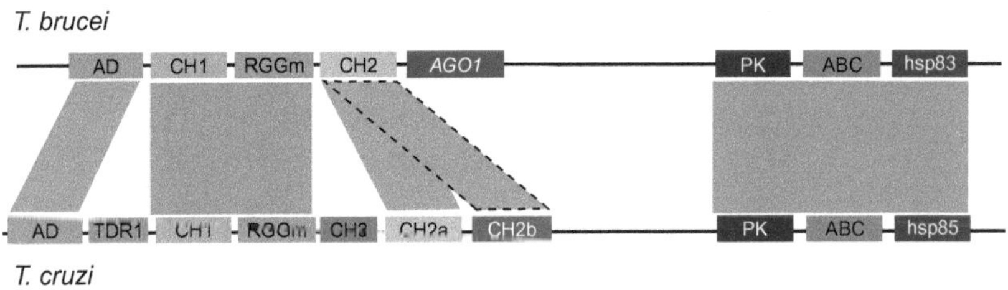

FIGURE 11.4 *Synteny between the T. brucei Argonaute locus (chromosome 10) and the corresponding region of the T. cruzi genome (chromosome 37).* Protein coding genes are indicated by coloured boxes. AD, adenosine deaminase; CH, conserved hypothetical; RGGm, RNA-binding protein; PK, protein serine/threonine kinase; ABC, ATP-binding cassette transporter; hsp83/85, heat shock protein 83 homologue. The *T. brucei* Argonaute gene (*AGO1*) (Tb927.10.10840) essential for RNAi is shown in red. The corresponding sequence is missing from the *T. cruzi* genome. In *T. cruzi*, the conserved hypothetical CH2 (Tc00.1047053509105.100) appears to have undergone a duplication/diversification event. Sequences downloaded from GeneDB.org.

randomly, so that within a population, individual cells can contain different amplicons. This mechanism can operate to allow individual cells, within an otherwise clonal population, to survive changes in the environment. One consequence is the ease with which drug-resistant parasites can be selected. In an organism with an RNAi pathway, transcription from these amplicons would have to be promoter-controlled to ensure that only one strand was transcribed. Trypanosomatid genes generally do not have individual promoters; therefore, loss of the RNAi response is almost a prerequisite for this type of extrachromosomal gene amplification system. In contrast, *T. brucei* depends on stringent transcriptional control of its variant surface glycoprotein expression to avoid immune elimination and cannot afford to support random extrachromosomal amplification/transcription. Therefore, maintenance of a functional RNAi system has not been selected against.

Whatever the reason, the evolutionary loss of RNAi by *T. cruzi* has allowed the scientific community to develop simple episome-based expression systems. Conversely, it has deprived us of a very useful reverse genetics tool. However, there are instances where *T. cruzi* genes can be used in combination with RNAi to address biological function. Sequence heterogeneity between orthologues means that *T. cruzi* genes expressed in a *T. brucei* background are often resistant to RNAi-mediated depletion of the corresponding host gene and can be used in complementation experiments to rescue the "knockdown" phenotype. Examples of this include functional analysis *T. brucei* flagellar rod protein 2, where motility of the flagellum could be rescued by expression of the *T. cruzi* equivalent (Rusconi et al., 2005), and studies on the role of topoisomerase-II in chromosome segregation (Obado et al., 2010).

11.3. THE USE OF GENETIC TECHNIQUES TO INVESTIGATE *TRYPANOSOMA CRUZI* OXIDATIVE DEFENCE AND DRUG-RESISTANCE MECHANISMS

11.3.1. Background

Aerobic organisms are exposed to a range of reactive oxygen species (ROS) produced by endogenous metabolic processes and extensive mechanisms have evolved to combat their deleterious effects. *T. cruzi* can also be subject to ROS generated by the host immune system and drug metabolism. The mechanisms used to combat oxidative stress in *T. cruzi*, and other trypanosomatids, differ significantly from those in humans. This, together with a widely held view that *T. cruzi* was deficient in aspects of peroxide metabolism, suggested that these defence systems might be a source of potential targets for chemotherapeutic intervention.

As a result, enzymes with a role in protecting the parasite from oxidative stress were amongst the first to be subjected to functional analysis using genetic techniques.

11.3.2. Dissection of peroxide metabolism

Trypanosomes have both enzymatic and non-enzymatic mechanisms for defence against peroxides (Irigoín et al., 2008; Piacenza et al., 2009). The parasite-specific thiol trypanothione (N^1,N^8-bisglutathionylspermidine) is the most important component of the non-enzymatic system. It has a role as a free radical scavenger and assumes the functions normally played by glutathione in most other eukaryotes. Trypanothione reductase (TR) is central to peroxide metabolism and acts by maintaining trypanothione in its reduced form. Peroxide detoxification in *T. cruzi* involves a number of overlapping and compartmentalised trypanothione-dependent redox pathways in which the peroxidases have complimentary substrate specificities (Fig. 11.5). To investigate the functional importance of trypanothione, the *Leishmania donovani* TR gene was expressed at high levels in *T. cruzi* (Kelly et al., 1993). Transformed cells were characterised by a greatly increased level of TR activity (14- to 18-fold) and by an enhanced ability to regenerate the reduced form of the thiol, $T[SH]_2$. However, the transformed parasites did not exhibit increased resistance to agents that induce oxidative stress and did not metabolise H_2O_2 more rapidly than non-transformed cells. These experiments, therefore, suggested that under this set of conditions, trypanothione availability is not a rate-limiting factor in the detoxification of H_2O_2. Consistent with this, in *T. brucei* it has been found that the levels of TR activity must be reduced by >90% to have a deleterious effect (Krieger et al., 2000).

Similar approaches have been taken to investigate the functional significance of the trypanothione-dependent cytosolic (TcCPX) and mitochondrial (TcMPX) 2-Cys peroxiredoxins (Fig. 11.5). Over-expression of both enzymes in *T. cruzi* was found to protect the parasite from exogenous H_2O_2 and *t*-butyl hydroperoxide, indicating that the level of these enzymes is a rate-limiting factor within their respective sub-cellular compartments (Wilkinson et al., 2000). These experiments also suggest that exogenous peroxides gain access to the cytosol and the mitochondrion and that enhanced peroxide metabolising capacity at these sites can protect against cellular damage. Parasites over-expressing 2-Cys peroxiredoxins also exhibit greater virulence (Piñeyro et al., 2008). This results from increased survival within infected cells (both phagocytic and non-phagocytic), rather than from changes to invasive capacity. The mechanisms involved result from the enhanced ability to detoxify cytosolic and diffusible reactive oxygen and nitrogen species. Survival within activated macrophages seems to be highly dependent on the efficiency

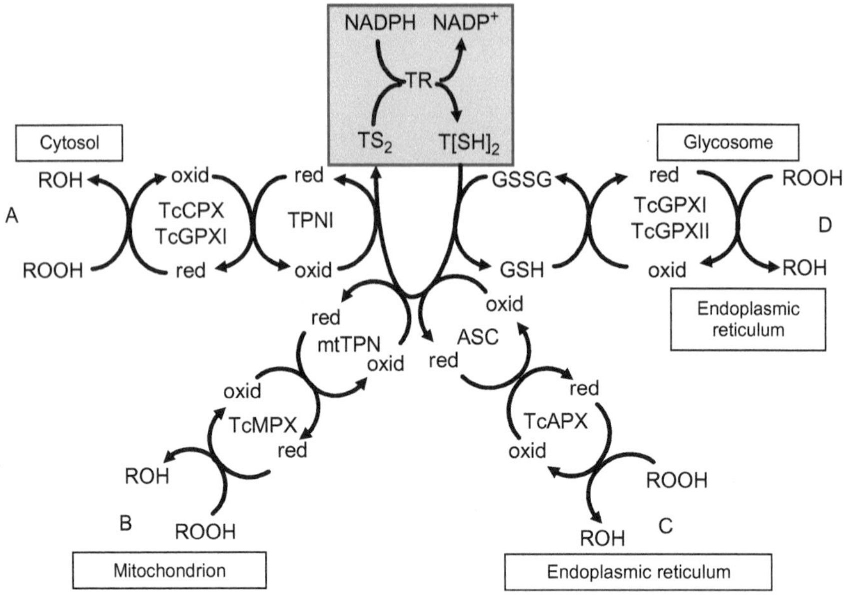

FIGURE 11.5 *Enzyme-mediated peroxide metabolism in T. cruzi.* The compartmentalised nature of the pathways is indicated. Trypanothione disulphide (TS_2) is maintained in its reduced form, dihydrotrypanothione ($T[SH]_2$), by trypanothione reductase (TR) (shaded region). $T[SH]_2$ transfers reducing equivalents to the tryparedoxin, glutathione or ascorbate pathways. (A, B) The tryparedoxin pathways: cytosolic peroxiredoxin (TcCPX) can metabolise H_2O_2 and alkyl hydroperoxides using the tryparedoxin TcTPNI as an electron donor. The mitochondrial tryparedoxin (TcMPX) may function using a mitochondrial tryparedoxin (mtTPN). TcTPNI is also an electron donor to TcGPXI, and under physiological conditions may be the major source. (C) Ascorbate-dependent pathway: ascorbate (ASC) is reduced by $T[SH]_2$ via non-enzymatic interactions. H_2O_2 is detoxified by TcAPX, a plant-like heme-containing peroxidase in the ER. (D) Glutathione-dependent pathways: oxidised glutathione (GSSG) interacts with $T[SH]_2$ by enzymatic and non-enzymatic mechanisms to generate reduced glutathione (GSH). GSH then drives the metabolism of fatty acid, phospholipid (TcGPXI and TcGPXII) and short-chain hydroperoxides (TcGPXI) to the corresponding alcohol (ROH). Both enzymes are members of the non-selenium phospholipid hydroperoxide glutathione peroxidase family.

with which the peroxidases reduce peroxynitrite to nitrite (Piacenza et al., 2008). The use of genetic approaches has therefore been an important factor in identification of these antioxidant pathways as determinants of virulence.

Genetic techniques have also been used to shed light on the biological roles of the *T. cruzi* peroxidases TcGPXI and TcGPXII (Fig. 11.5). These enzymes are members of the phospholipid hydroperoxide non-selenium glutathione-dependent subgroup of peroxidases and can be distinguished from each other on the basis of both sub-cellular location and substrate specificity (Wilkinson et al., 2002a,b). TcGPXI is localised to the cytosol and glycosomes, whereas TcGPXII is an ER protein. Both can metabolise fatty acid and phospholipid hydroperoxides, but only TcGPXI can metabolise short-chain hydroperoxides. Over-expression of these enzymes in *T. cruzi* confers resistance to exogenous H_2O_2, even though this oxidant cannot be metabolised by either. This suggests that their role may be to minimise the effects of secondary oxidation within their respective compartments, by preventing damage caused by lipid peroxidation.

In addition to TcGPXII, a second peroxidase has been localised within the *T. cruzi* ER, a plant-like ascorbate-dependent hemoperoxidase (TcAPX; Wilkinson et al., 2002c). This enzyme has a substrate specificity restricted to H_2O_2, an activity that seems to complement TcGPXII in providing the ER with protection against a range of oxidant challenges. Over-expression of TcAPX confers resistance to exogenous H_2O_2; however, unlike the 2-Cys peroxiredoxins, this does not result in increased resistance to peroxynitrite (Piacenza et al., 2008). To determine if TcAPX activity was essential for parasite viability, we attempted to generate *TcAPX* null mutants. This proved not to be possible, unless deletion of the second allele was carried out using cells where an additional copy of *TcAPX* was expressed from an episome (M. C. Taylor, unpublished data). This type of outcome is usually taken as evidence that the corresponding gene is essential. In this instance though, when parasites harbouring the episomal copy were cultured continuously in the absence of the selective drug, null mutants which had lost the episome could be isolated. Our interpretation is that loss of TcAPX activity is probably deleterious to *T. cruzi* and negates the isolation of null mutants under the selection conditions used following transfection. However, loss of the episome in an actively growing population of null mutants is possible because these conditions may permit metabolic adaptation. This finding highlights that the inability to generate *T. cruzi* null mutants should no longer be considered as evidence for an essential gene.

11.3.3. Identifying the mechanisms of drug resistance

Nifurtimox and benznidazole are the front line drugs used to treat Chagas disease. They are characterised by toxic side effects and their efficacy against the chronic stage of the infection is limited (Wilkinson and Kelly, 2009). Both these nitroheterocyclic compounds function as prodrugs, and to have cytotoxic effects, they must undergo nitroreductase-mediated activation. Their precise mode of action has been the subject of research for more than 30 years and until recently has remained unclear.

Two main hypotheses were proposed. The first was based on observations that activation of both drugs can lead to the generation of ROS, a process that involves a one electron reduction catalysed by a type II nitroreductase activity. However, experiments involving transfection-mediated over-expression of TR and the five *T. cruzi* peroxidases (Fig. 11.5) have failed to find an association between up-regulation of these pathways and protection against the trypanocidal activity of nitroheterocyclic drugs (Wilkinson and Kelly, 2009).

A second mechanism was proposed, based on the activation of nitrofurans by FMN-dependent oxygen-insensitive type I nitroreductases in bacteria. This involves two-electron reduction to form a hydroxylamine derivative, which upon reaction with nitrenium cations, can promote DNA breakage. Evidence that such a mechanism might operate in trypanosomes came from the observation that nifurtimox-resistant *T. cruzi* selected in the laboratory were found to have lost a chromosome containing a gene encoding a type I nitroreductase (TcNTR; Wilkinson et al., 2008). To confirm this, insertional disruption of a copy of *TcNTR* was found to result in a resistance profile similar to the laboratory-generated strain: three- to fivefold resistance to nifurtimox and other heterocyclic drugs, including benznidazole. As predicted, deletion of the second *TcNTR* allele gave rise to parasites with an even greater level of resistance. Fortunately, from a public health perspective, the null mutants displayed a non-infectious phenotype. These genetic experiments clearly identify *TcNTR* as an important determinant of drug activity and show that cross-resistance (at least up to fivefold) to the front line drugs can arise by a straightforward mechanism.

11.4. CONCLUDING REMARKS

Transfection-based techniques have long been established as a routine research tool in the *T. cruzi* field. In combination with the data from the trypanosomatid genome projects, they have provided new insights into fundamental aspects of parasite biology and infection. Continued development has enhanced the utility of the technology and extended the range of questions that can be addressed. However, the flexibility of reverse genetic approaches applicable to *T. cruzi* still lags behind those that are available for work on *T. brucei*. This is mainly due to the absence of RNAi machinery and the time-consuming effort necessary to generate transformants. Neither of these issues is likely to be resolved easily. Nevertheless, as outlined in this chapter, refinement and modification of the current systems offer the prospect of more robust technology that will find wider applications.

ACKNOWLEDGEMENTS

J. M. K. and M. C. T. gratefully acknowledge the support of the Wellcome Trust (Grant Number 084175). H. H. is funded by National Institutes of Health Grant AI 058893.

REFERENCES

Alsford, S., Horn, D., 2008. Single-locus targeting constructs for reliable RNAi and transgene expression in *Trypanosoma brucei*. Mol. Biochem. Parasitol. 161, 76–79.

Banaszynski, L.A., Chen, L.C., Maynard-Smith, L.A., Ooi, A.G., Wandless, T.J., 2006. A rapid, reversible, and tunable method to regulate protein function in living cells using synthetic small molecules. Cell 126, 995–1004.

Batista, M., Marchini, F.K., Celedon, P.A.F., Fragoso, S.P., Probst, C.M., Preti, H., et al., 2010. A high-throughput cloning system for reverse genetics in *Trypanosoma cruzi*. BMC Microbiol. 10, 259.

Bellofatto, V., Cross, G.A., 1989. Expression of a bacterial gene in a trypanosomatid protozoan. Science 244, 1167–1169.

Carruthers, V.B., van der Ploeg, L.H., Cross, G.A., 1993. DNA-mediated transformation of bloodstream-form *Trypanosoma brucei*. Nucleic Acids Res. 21, 2537–2538.

Clayton, C.E., Fueri, J.P., Itzhaki, J.E., Bellofatto, V., Sherman, D.R., Wisdom, G.S., et al., 1990. Transcription of the procyclic acidic repetitive protein genes of *Trypanosoma brucei*. Mol. Cell. Biol. 10, 3036–3047.

Cooper, R., de Jesus, A.R., Cross, G.A., 1993. Deletion of an immunodominant *Trypanosoma cruzi* surface glycoprotein disrupts flagellum-cell adhesion. J. Cell Biol. 122, 149–156.

Cruz, A., Beverley, S.M., 1990. Gene replacement in parasitic protozoa. Nature 348, 171–173.

Curotto de Lafaille, M.A., Laban, A., Wirth, D.F., 1992. Gene expression in *Leishmania*: analysis of essential 5′ DNA sequences. Proc. Natl. Acad. Sci. USA 89, 2703–2707.

DaRocha, W.D., Otsu, K., Teixeira, S.M., Donelson, J.E., 2004a. Tests of cytoplasmic RNA interference (RNAi) and construction of a tetracycline-inducible T7 promoter system in *Trypanosoma cruzi*. Mol. Biochem. Parasitol. 133, 175–186.

DaRocha, W.D., Silva, R.A., Bartholomeu, D.C., Pires, S.F., Freitas, J.M., Macedo, A.M., et al., 2004b. Expression of exogenous genes in *Trypanosoma cruzi*: improving vectors and electroporation protocols. Parasitol. Res. 92, 113–120.

Durand-Dubief, M., Bastin, P., 2003. TbAGO1, an argonaute protein required for RNA interference, is involved in mitosis and chromosome segregation in *Trypanosoma brucei*. BMC Biol. 1, 2.

Hariharan, S., Ajioka, J., Swindle, J., 1993. Stable transformation of *Trypanosoma cruzi*: inactivation of the PUB12.5 polyubiquitin gene by targeted gene disruption. Mol. Biochem. Parasitol. 57, 15–30.

Herm-Götz, A., Agop-Nersesian, C., Münter, S., Grimley, J.S., Wandless, T.J., Frischknecht, F., et al., 2007. Rapid control of protein level in the apicoplexan *Toxoplasma gondii*. Nat. Methods 4, 1003–1005.

Irigoín, F., Cibils, L., Comini, M.A., Wilkinson, S.R., Flohé, L., Radi, R., 2008. Insights into the redox biology of *Trypanosoma cruzi*: trypanothione metabolism and oxidant detoxification. Free Radic. Biol. Med. 45, 733–742.

Kapler, G.M., Coburn, C.M., Beverley, S.M., 1990. Stable transfection of the human parasite *Leishmania major* delineates a 30-kilobase region sufficient for extrachromosomal replication and expression. Mol. Cell. Biol. 10, 1084–1094.

Kelly, J.M., Ward, H.M., Miles, M.A., Kendall, G., 1992. A shuttle vector which facilitates the expression of transfected genes in *Trypanosoma cruzi* and *Leishmania*. Nucleic Acids Res. 20, 3963–3969.

Kelly, J.M., Taylor, M.C., Smith, K., Hunter, K.J., Fairlamb, A.H., 1993. Phenotype of recombinant *Leishmania donovani* and *Trypanosoma cruzi* which overexpress trypanothione reductase: sensitivity towards agents that are thought to induce oxidative stress. Eur. J. Biochem. 218, 29–37.

Kelly, J.M., Das, P., Tomas, A.M., 1994. An approach to functional complementation by introduction of large DNA fragments into *Trypanosoma cruzi* and *Leishmania donovani* using a cosmid shuttle vector. Mol. Biochem. Parasitol. 65, 51–62.

Kelly, J.M., Taylor, M.C., Rudenko, G., Blundell, P.A., 1995. Transfection of the African and American trypanosomes. In: Nickoloff, J.A. (Ed.), Electroporation Protocols for Microorganisms. Methods in Molecular Biology, Vol. 47. Humana Press, New Jersey, pp. 349–359.

Kendall, G., Wilderspin, A.F., Ashall, F., Miles, M.A., Kelly, J.M., 1990. *Trypanosoma cruzi* glycosomal glyceraldehyde-3-phosphate dehydrogenase does not conform to the "hotspot" topogenic signal model. EMBO J. 9, 2751–2758.

Krieger, S., Schwarz, W., Ariyanayagam, M.R., Fairlamb, A.H., Krauth-Siegel, R.L., Clayton, C., 2000. Trypanosomes lacking trypanothione reductase are avirulent and show increased sensitivity to oxidative stress. Mol. Microbiol. 35, 542–552.

Laban, A., Wirth, D.F., 1989. Transfection of *Leishmania enriettii* and expression of chloramphenicol acetyltransferase gene. Proc. Natl. Acad. Sci. USA 86, 9119–9123.

Laban, A., Tobin, J.F., Curotto de Lafaille, M.A., Wirth, D.F., 1990. Stable expression of the bacterial *neo*^{r} gene in *Leishmania enriettii*. Nature 343, 572–574.

Leprohon, P., Legare, D., Raymond, F., Madore, E., Hardiman, G., Corbeil, J., et al., 2009. Gene expression modulation is associated with gene amplification, supernumerary chromosomes and chromosome loss in antimony-resistant *Leishmania infantum*. Nucleic Acids Res. 37, 1387–1399.

Lu, H.Y., Buck, G.A., 1991. Expression of an exogenous gene in *Trypanosoma cruzi* epimastigotes. Mol. Biochem. Parasitol. 44, 109–114.

Lye, L.-F., Owens, K., Shi, H., Murta, S.M.F., Vieira, A.C., Turco, S.J., et al., 2010. Retention and loss of RNA interference pathways in trypanosomatid protozoans. PLoS Pathog. 6, e1001161.

Martínez-Calvillo, S., Hernández, R., 1994. *Trypanosoma cruzi* ribosomal DNA: mapping of a putative distal promoter. Gene 142, 243–247.

Martínez-Calvillo, S., López, I., Hernández, R., 1997. pRIBOTEX expression vector: a pTEX derivative for a rapid selection of *Trypanosoma cruzi* transfectants. Gene 199, 71–76.

Mondragon, A., Wilkinson, S.R., Taylor, M.C., Kelly, J.M., 1999. Optimisation of conditions for growth of wild-type and genetically transformed *Trypanosoma cruzi* on agarose plates. Parasitology 118, 461–467.

Nozaki, T., Cross, G.A., 1994. Functional complementation of glycoprotein 72 in a *Trypanosoma cruzi* glycoprotein 72 null mutant. Mol. Biochem. Parasitol. 67, 91–102.

Obado, S.O., Taylor, M.C., Wilkinson, S.R., Bromley, E.V., Kelly, J.M., 2005. Functional mapping of a trypanosome centromere by chromosome fragmentation identifies a 16 kb GC-rich transcriptional "strand-switch" domain as a major feature. Genome Res. 15, 36–43.

Obado, S.O., Bot, C., Nilsson, D., Andersson, B., Kelly, J.M., 2007. Repetitive DNA is associated with centromeric domains in *Trypanosoma brucei* but not *Trypanosoma cruzi*. Genome Biol. 8, R37.

Obado, S.O., Bot, C., Echeverry, M.C., Bayona, J.C., Alvarez, V.E., Taylor, M.C., Kelly, J.M., 2010. Centromere-associated topoisomerase activity in bloodstream form *Trypanosoma brucei*. Nucleic Acids Res. 39, 1023–1033.

Otsu, K., Donelson, J.E., Kirchhoff, L.V., 1993. Interruption of a *Trypanosoma cruzi* gene encoding a protein containing 14-amino acid repeats by targeted insertion of the neomycin phosphotransferase gene. Mol. Biochem. Parasitol. 57, 317–330.

Otsu, K., Donelson, J.E., Kirchhoff, L.V., 1995. *Trypanosoma cruzi*: interruption of both alleles of a gene encoding a protein containing 14-amino-acid repeats by targeted insertion of *NEO*^{r} and *HYG*^{r}. Exp. Parasitol. 81, 529–535.

Papadopoulou, B., Roy, G., Ouellette, M., 1994. Autonomous replication of bacterial DNA plasmid oligomers in *Leishmania*. Mol. Biochem. Parasitol. 65, 39–49.

Patnaik, P.K., Kulkarni, S.K., Cross, G.A., 1993. Autonomously replicating single-copy episomes in *Trypanosoma brucei* show unusual stability. EMBO J. 12, 2529–2538.

Patrick, K.L., Shi, N.G., Kolev, K., Ersfeld, C., Tschudi, C., Ullu, E., 2009. Distinct and overlapping roles for two Dicer-like proteins in the RNA interference pathways of the ancient eukaryote *Trypanosoma brucei*. Proc. Natl. Acad. Sci. USA 106, 17933–17938.

Peacock, C.S., Seeger, K., Harris, D., Murphy, L., Ruiz, J.C., Quail, M.A., et al., 2007. Comparative genomic analysis of three *Leishmania* species that cause diverse human disease. Nat. Genet. 39, 839–847.

Piacenza, L., Irigoín, F., Alvarez, M.N., Peluffo, G., Taylor, M.C., Kelly, J.M., et al., 2007. Mitochondrial superoxide radicals mediate programmed cell death in *Trypanosoma cruzi*: cytoprotective action of mitochondrial Fe-superoxide dismutase overexpression. Biochem. J. 403, 323–334.

Piacenza, L., Peluffo, G., Alvarez, M.N., Kelly, J.M., Wilkinson, S.R., Radi, R., 2008. Peroxiredoxins play a major role in protecting *Trypanosoma cruzi* against macrophage- and endogenously derived peroxynitrite. Biochem. J. 410, 359–368.

Piacenza, L., Alvarez, M.N., Peluffo, G., Radi, R., 2009. Fighting the oxidative assault: the *Trypanosoma cruzi* journey to infection. Curr. Opin. Microbiol. 12 (4), 415–421.

Ramirez, M.I., Yamauchi, L.M., de Freitas, L.H., Uemura, H., Jr., Schenkman, S., 2000. The use of the green fluorescent protein to monitor and improve transfection in *Trypanosoma cruzi*. Mol. Biochem. Parasitol. 111, 235–240.

Piñeyro, M.D., Parodi-Talice, A., Arcari, T., Robello, C., 2008. Peroxiredoxins from *Trypanosoma cruzi*: virulence factors and drug targets for treatment of Chagas disease? Gene 408, 45–50.

Rudenko, G., Le Blancq, S., Smith, J., Lee, M.G., Rattray, A., Van der Ploeg, L.H., 1990. Procyclic acidic repetitive protein (PARP) genes located in an unusually small alpha-amanitin-resistant transcription unit: PARP promoter activity assayed by transient DNA transfection of *Trypanosoma brucei*. Mol. Cell. Biol. 10, 3492–3504.

Rusconi, F., Durand-Dubief, M., Bastin, P., 2005. Functional complementation of RNA interference mutants in trypanosomes. BMC Biotechnol. 5, 6.

Shi, H., Djikeng, A., Tschudi, C., Ullu, E., 2004. Argonaute protein in the early divergent eukaryote *Trypanosoma brucei*: control of small interfering RNA accumulation and retroposon transcript abundance. Mol. Cell. Biol. 24, 420–427.

Shi, H., Tschudi, C., Ullu, E., 2006. An unusual Dicer-like1 protein fuels the RNA interference pathway in *Trypanosoma brucei*. RNA 12, 2063–2072.

Taylor, M.C., Kelly, J.M., 2006. A stable tetracycline-regulated gene expression system for *Trypanosoma cruzi*. BMC Biotechnol. 6, 32.

ten Asbroek, A.L., Ouellette, M., Borst, P., 1990. Targeted insertion of the neomycin phosphotransferase gene into the tubulin gene cluster of *Trypanosoma brucei*. Nature 348, 174–175.

ten Asbroek, A.L., Mol, C.A., Kieft, R., Borst, P., 1993. Stable transformation of *Trypanosoma brucei*. Mol. Biochem. Parasitol. 59, 133–142.

Tibbetts, R.S., Klein, K.G., Engman, D.M., 1995. A rapid method for protein localization in trypanosomes. Exp. Parasitol. 80, 572–574.

Tomas, A.M., Miles, M.A., Kelly, J.M., 1997. Overexpression of cruzipain, the major cysteine proteinase of *Trypanosoma cruzi* is associated with enhanced metacyclogenesis. Eur. J. Biochem. 244, 596–603.

Ubeda, J.M., Legare, D., Raymond, F., Ouameur, A.A., Boisvert, S., Rigault, P., et al., 2008. Modulation of gene expression in drug resistant *Leishmania* is associated with gene amplification, gene deletion and chromosome aneuploidy. Genome Biol. 9, R115.

Ullu, E., Tschudi, C., Chakraborty, T., 2004. RNA interference in protozoan parasites. Cell. Microbiol. 6, 509–519.

Vazquez, M.P., Levin, M.J., 1999. Functional analysis of the intergenic regions of TcP2beta gene loci allowed the construction of an improved *Trypanosoma cruzi* expression vector. Gene 239, 217–225.

Wen, L.M., Xu, P., Benegal, G., Carvaho, M.R., Butler, D.R., Buck, G.A., 2001. *Trypanosoma cruzi*: exogenously regulated gene expression. Exp. Parasitol. 97, 196–204.

Wilkinson, S.R., Kelly, J.M., 2009. Trypanocidal drugs: mechanisms, resistance and new targets. Expert Rev. Mol. Med. 11 (e31), 1–24.

Wilkinson, S.R., Temperton, N.J., Mondragon, A., Kelly, J.M., 2000. Distinct mitochondrial and cytosolic enzymes mediate trypanothione-dependent peroxide metabolism in *Trypanosoma cruzi*. J. Biol. Chem. 275, 8220–8225.

Wilkinson, S.R., Meyer, D.J., Taylor, M.C., Bromley, E.V., Miles, M.A., Kelly, J.M., 2002a. The *Trypanosoma cruzi* enzyme TcGPXI is a glycosomal peroxidase and can be linked to trypanothione reduction by glutathione or tryparedoxin. J. Biol. Chem. 277, 17062–17071.

Wilkinson, S.R., Taylor, M.C., Touitha, S., Mauricio, I.L., Meyer, D.J., Kelly, J.M., 2002b. TcGPXII, a glutathione-dependent *Trypanosoma cruzi* peroxidase with substrate specificity restricted to fatty acid and phospholipid hydroperoxides, is localised to the endoplasmic reticulum. Biochem. J. 364, 787–794.

Wilkinson, S.R., Obado, S.O., Mauricio, I.L., Kelly, J.M., 2002c. *Trypanosoma cruzi* expresses a plant-like ascorbate-dependent haemoperoxidase localized to the endoplasmic reticulum. Proc. Natl. Acad. Sci. USA 99, 13453–13458.

Wilkinson, S.R., Taylor, M.C., Horn, D., Kelly, J.M., Cheeseman, I., 2008. A mechanism for cross-resistance to nifurtimox and benznidazole in trypanosomes. Proc. Natl. Acad. Sci. USA 105, 5022–5027.

Wirtz, E., Clayton, C., 1995. Inducible gene expression in trypanosomes mediated by a prokaryotic repressor. Science 268, 1179–1183.

Wirtz, E., Leal, S., Ochatt, C., Cross, G.A., 1999. A tightly regulated inducible expression system for conditional gene knock-outs and dominant-negative genetics in *Trypanosoma brucei*. Mol. Biochem. Parasitol. 99, 89–101.

Xu, D., Brandán, C.P., Basombrío, M.A., Tarleton, R.L., 2009. Evaluation of high efficiency gene knockout strategies for *Trypanosoma cruzi*. BMC Microbiol. 9, 90.

Zomerdijk, J.C., Ouellette, M., ten Asbroek, A.L., Kieft, R., Bommer, A.M., Clayton, C.E., et al., 1990. The promoter for a variant surface glycoprotein gene expression site in *Trypanosoma brucei*. EMBO J. 9, 791–801.

CHAPTER 12

Nuclear Structure of *Trypanosoma cruzi*

Sergio Schenkman,*,† **Bruno dos Santos Pascoalino,*** and **Sheila C. Nardelli***

Contents

* Departamento de Microbiologia, Imunologia e Parasitologia, Universidade Federal de São Paulo, São Paulo, Brazil
† Center for Tropical and Emerging Diseases, University of Georgia, Athens, Georgia, USA

Advances in Parasitology, Volume 75
ISSN 0065-308X, DOI: 10.1016/B978-0-12-385863-4.00012-5

Abstract

The presence of nucleus in living organisms characterizes the Eukaryote domain. The nucleus compartmentalizes the genetic material surrounded by a double membrane called nuclear envelope. The nucleus has been observed since the advent of the light microscope, and sub-compartments such as nucleoli, diverse nuclear bodies and condensed chromosomes have been later recognized, being part of highly organized and dynamic structure. The significance and function of such organization has increased with the understanding of transcription, replication, DNA repair, recombination processes. It is now recognized as consequence of adding complexity and regulation in more complex eukaryotic cells. Here we provide a description of the actual stage of knowledge of the nuclear structure of *Trypanosoma cruzi.* As an early divergent eukaryote, it presents unique and/or reduced events of DNA replication, transcription and repair as well as RNA processing and transport to the cytosol. Nevertheless, it shows peculiar structure changes accordingly to the cell cycle and stage of differentiation. *T. cruzi* proliferates only as epimastigote and amastigote stages, and when these forms differentiate in trypomastigote forms, their cell cycle is arrested. This arrested stage is capable of invading mammalian cells and of surviving harsh conditions, such as the gut of the insect vector and mammalian macrophages. Transcription and replication decrease during transformation in trypomastigotes implicating large alterations in the nuclear structure. Recent evidences also suggest that *T. cruzi* nucleus respond to oxidative and nutritional stresses. Due to the phylogenetic proximity with other well-known trypanosomes, such as *Trypanosoma brucei* and *Leishmania major*, they are expected to have similar nuclear organization, although differences are noticed due to distinct life cycles, cellular organizations and the specific adaptations for surviving in different host environments. Therefore, the general features of *T. cruzi* nuclear structure regarding unique characteristics of this protozoan parasite will be described.

12.1. GENERAL ASPECTS OF NUCLEAR ORGANIZATION IN EUKARYOTIC CELLS

12.1.1. Nuclear components

The cell nucleus contains DNA, which constitutes the genomic material and is combined with highly conserved proteins, the histones. This structure is called chromatin and establishes the basic unit of the nuclear organization. Several levels of chromatin condensation occur depending on the function of each DNA portion. For example, portions being transcribed into RNA are usually less condensed, forming what is defined as euchromatin, while transcriptionally silenced regions involved in chromatin structure and gene silencing are highly packed. This later is called heterochromatin and is maintained by the association of specific proteins (Grewal and Jia, 2007). When cells divide, the chromatin duplicates and eventually condenses forming chromosomes that are segregated into each resulting daughter cell. Each chromosome is formed by a linear portion of genomic material containing repetitive sequences at their extremities, called telomeres. Telomeres maintain chromosome stability by either promoting efficient DNA replication at the extremities or avoiding exchanges between different chromosomes (Gomes et al., 2010). For cell division, condensed chromosomes attach to cytoskeleton components, required to segregate each copy of the duplicated material to the progeny. The anchoring sites contain specific chromatin components associated with defined and/or repetitive DNA sequences known as centromeres (Mehta et al., 2010).

In interphase, that is, when cells are not dividing, chromosomes are much less condensed and several structures can be seen inside the nucleus. One of the first recognized structures was the nucleolus, where the ribosomal RNAs are transcribed, processed and assembled in ribonuclear protein (RNP) complexes (Boisvert et al., 2007; Sirri et al., 2008). The nucleolus also contains distinguishable domains. The fibrillar centre, contains RNA polymerase I (RNA Pol I) transcribing the ribosomal DNA, which is surrounded by the dense fibrillar component, a place though to congregate the ribosomal RNA processing. Both are enclosed by the granular component, a region where pre-ribosomes assemble. The nucleolus including these domains is easily visualized by transmission electron microscopy as an electron dense region, similar to the heterochromatin containing structures.

In addition to ribosomal RNA, other RNA species are also part of nuclear structures. For example, pre-mRNAs and small nuclear RNA (snRNA) assemble in protein structures forming RNPs. These RNPs are involved in RNA processing, which includes addition of capping modifications at the beginning of each transcribed mRNA and removal of noncoding intervening sequences, a process known as splicing. RNA processing is coupled with the events of transcription, and these processes appear to be located in perichromatin fibrils, as seen by electron microscopy (Hocine et al., 2010). These perichromatin fibrils surround structures rich in RNA processing factors that are also distinguished by electron microscopy as interchromatin granules. These granules correspond to "speckles" stained by immunofluorescence when antibodies to RNA processing and splicing factors are employed. In mammalian cells, between 20 and 50 speckles are seen per nucleus and it is proposed that they are involved in recycling processing factors and in the control of gene expression (Spector and Lamond, 2010).

The eukaryotic nucleus is enclosed by a double membrane structure contiguous with the endoplasmic reticulum, named nuclear envelope (NE). The NE contains pores formed by large protein complexes, known as nuclear pore complexes (NPCs), which allow and mediate the transport of proteins and ribonucleoproteins complexes in and out from the nucleus (Hetzer, 2010). The NPC also controls signalling for cell cycle control and gene expression. In metazoans, lamins, which are type V intermediate filaments, form a nuclear skeleton that is localized between the inner NE membranes and peripheral heterochromatin. Lamins are found associated with heterochromatin, probably anchoring the chromosomes to the envelope. They also appear to interact with several transcription, replication and repair enzymatic complexes in the nucleoplasm. Lamin filaments are contiguous with the cytosolic cytoskeleton holding chromosome distribution and sustaining several nuclear processes (Dechat et al., 2010). This skeleton has been associated with the concept that the nucleus contains an insoluble matrix, defined mainly as the remains after extraction with deoxyribonuclease, ribonuclease and high salt concentrations. Observations that replicating and transcribed DNA, as well as the machineries involved in these processes are associated with the nuclear matrix, suggested that it would form a scaffold for these nuclear activities (Albrethsen et al., 2009). However, it has not been possible to demonstrate that a structured network exists in live cells. The current view is that it corresponds to dynamic association that remains aggregated upon cell lysis with detergents or fixation when observed by optic and electron microscopy.

12.1.2. Chromatin structure and organization

Two copies of each histone (H2A, H2B, H3 and H4) form one nucleosome wrapping about 160 bp of DNA, which is the basic unit of the 10-μm fibers of chromatin. The binding of histone H1 to each nucleosome provides further compaction and is responsible for the formation of higher-ordered structures such as the 30 μm fibres observed *in vitro*. More compacted structures are assembled by the presence of specific proteins and RNPs interacting with modified histones and DNA, forming the heterochromatin at defined regions of the genome. These regions contain facultative silenced genes, or constitutive structured portions of the genome such as telomeres and centromeres (for a general review about chromatin, see Campos and Reinberg, 2009). Further condensation, forming chromosome structures during mitosis and meiosis, is dependent on the participation of other cross-linking proteins named condensins and cohesins (Woodcock and Ghosh, 2010). How these components interact and promote the formation of chromosomes is still a matter of speculation in the field.

Histone H1 is the most divergent histone and is the one that possesses more variants. It presents three domains: the central conserved globular domain sided by N- and C-terminals unfolded portions. Phosphorylation of these domains affects the interaction of histone H1 with the nucleosome and mediates chromatin compaction (Woodcock et al., 2006). Histone H4 is the most conserved histone with few variants, probably because it participates in more interactions with other histones in the nucleosome structure. In contrast, several variants of histone H3 are found, each one with specific roles in the chromatin structure. For example, a variant of histone H3, called CENP-A, is present in centromeric chromatin instead of histone H3. Histone H2A and H2B are more divergent among species. Several histone H2A variants are well characterized and are recruited to sites with specific transcriptional control, chromatin remodelling and repair of DNA damages.

The N-terminal portions of histones and the C-terminal portion of histone H2A are exposed outside the nucleosome structure and are subjected to diverse post-translational modifications such as methylation, acetylation, phosphorylation, ubiquitination, sumoylation, citrullination and proline isomerization (Peterson and Laniel, 2004). These modifications act in an interdependent way, generating innumerable combinations that can diversely affect the chromatin structure and several nuclear processes such as removal/deposition of histones, transcription, replication and DNA repair (Strahl and Allis, 2000), who proposed the existence of a histone modification code. Moreover, each modification can facilitate or inhibit that other residues are modified. They are dynamic, changing upon intra- and extracellular signals (Berger, 2007), being recognized by regulatory factors that bind to the chromatin. For example, chromo domain-containing proteins bind to methylated residues, bromo domain to acetylated residues and 14-3-3 proteins to phosphorylated sites (Taverna et al., 2007). Some of these factors are part of multimeric enzymes that further modify the histones. They also promote the assembly of specific enzymatic machineries at defined chromatin regions. Beyond histones, diverse proteins associate with the chromatin depending also on post-translational modifications. Among them, there are proteins involved in chromatin assembly and remodelling such as high-mobility group (HMG) proteins involved in DNA replication, DNA repair, DNA transcription, RNA processing and export (Bianchi and Agresti, 2005; Stros, 2010).

12.1.3. The nuclear organization as a dynamic structure

The eukaryotic nucleus although lacking internal membranes is seen as a highly organized structure with defined domains, as observable by various microscope techniques for more than a 100 years. Such sub-compartmentalization suggests that each one of the nuclear domains and nuclear bodies is involved in specific functions. These nuclear bodies occupy defined positions relative to each other, which are maintained after each cell division cycle, in a pattern specific for each cell type. Chromosomes occupy defined positions in the nucleus, known as chromosome territories depending on the cell type and function. This structured pattern seems to obey functional roles and responds to alterations in the environment, metabolic and growth state of the cells, indicating that the nuclear organization is related to the functional state of the cells (Branco and Pombo, 2006).

Recent studies, based on the dynamic analysis, revealed a large degree of motility of nuclear components arguing against a fixed nuclear structure. Rather, the organization reflects a functional state and is the consequence of the assembly of DNA replication, transcription and repair, and also of RNA processing enzymes and export machineries. For example, replication and transcription factories can be detected by fluorescence techniques, and these machineries assemble non-contiguous regions of the genome (Chagin et al., 2010; Chakalova and Fraser, 2010). This organization also depends on the chromatin structure and histone post-translation modifications, which create local environments that allow the presence of activating or repressing factors. The NE and nuclear pore components serve as anchors, attaching defined regions such as telomeres, centromeres and non-constitutive heterochromatin. Overall, these multiple factors act to establish a complex organization that reflects the actual set of nuclear activities in eukaryotic cells.

12.2. THE NUCLEUS OF *TRYPANOSOMA CRUZI*

12.2.1. The nucleus and Chagas' disease

T. cruzi is an early divergent organism that presents differences in nuclear processes regarding other eukaryotes. It has primitive mechanisms concerning DNA replication, transcription and repair. Consequently, the nuclear structure and chromatin organization should display peculiar characteristics. The sequencing of *T. cruzi* genome (El Sayed et al., 2005) has provided new insights in understanding the biology of this parasite. It also became an important source of information to prevent and treat

Chagas' disease. Due to the complexity of the parasite, with a large number of repetitive sequences and a high degree of variability among different isolates, the assembled genome has not been fully solved. Nevertheless, the new set of information will allow the identification of new drug targets, the reasons and consequences of strain variability and how the parasite can adapt and survive to cause the disease. In this sense, studies on the role of the nuclear structure and chromatin modifications are one aspect that can help in attaining these tasks.

T. cruzi reproduces by binary fission in the gut of the insect vector as an epimastigote form and in the cytosol of mammalian cells as an amastigote form. In these two situations, the parasite displays a spherical nucleus with an evident and central nucleolus (de Souza, 2002; de Souza and Meyer, 1974; Souza, 2009). When the nucleus was compared between epimastigotes and amastigotes generated from released trypomastigotes, there are clear differences in size (Fig. 12.1). The reasons for this difference are not understood and might be related to differences in ploidy between these two stages. Reductive division as well as nuclear fusion has not been described in *T. cruzi* although evidences of genome exchange (Gaunt et al., 2003) and hybridization events during evolution were found (Ienne et al., 2010; Pena et al., 2009). Alternatively, the different nuclear

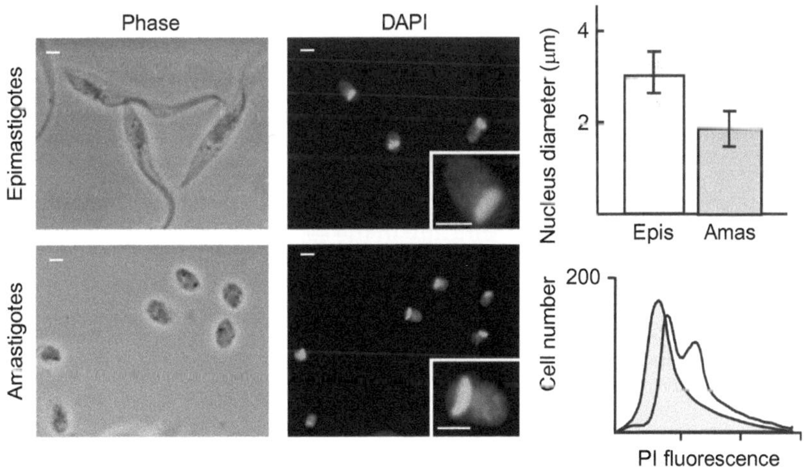

FIGURE 12.1 *Nucleus size variation and DNA content in epimastigotes and amastigotes.* The left panels show microscope images of epimastigotes and amastigotes differentiated from cell-derived trypomastigotes after medium acidification observed under phase microscopy and after staining with DAPI. Bars = 2 μm. The top right panel shows the mean ± standard deviation (n = 50) of the diameter size of epimastigote with a single flagellum (Epis) and amastigote (Amas) nuclei. The bottom panel shows cytometry analysis of the same parasites stained with propidium iodide.

sizes could reflect distinct cell activities. Under starvation conditions, the epimastigotes and amastigotes undergo transformation into trypomastigote forms. This happened at the end of the vector gut or inside mammalian cells cytoplasm filled with parasites. The cell size is dramatically reduced with a drastic change in the nuclear shape and organization. Trypomastigotes have decreased transcription activity (Elias et al., 2001), no replication (Elias et al., 2002), but express some of the DNA repair components (Machado et al., 2006). These and other peculiarities justify the importance in studying the nucleus of *T. cruzi*, in addition to works being performed in other trypanosomes, such as *Trypanosoma brucei* and *Leishmania* that certainly have similar but also quite different properties. In the following sections, known aspects of nuclear structure and function are described specifically for *T. cruzi*.

12.2.2. The cell cycle of the parasite

A unique aspect of *T. cruzi* is how dividing life cycle stages controls de progress of cell division cycle. In epimastigote form, the cell cycle steps have been determined with the demonstration that nuclear mitosis occurs after the separation of the duplicated kinetoplast (Elias et al., 2007). It is possible to distinguish epimastigotes before and after entry into G2 stage by the presence of a second flagellum. After mitosis, the cell undergoes cytokinesis with an asymmetrical growth of the parasite cell body. The cell cycle steps of replicating amastigote stage are still uncharacterized.

The control of the cell cycle in *T. cruzi* relies on the presence of cyclin-dependent kinases (Gomez et al., 1998, 2001; Santori et al., 2002), but the mechanisms involved in each step have not been identified. More progress have been made understanding the cell cycle control in *T. brucei* (Hammarton et al., 2003), but it is expected that due to differences in the cellular organization and specifically in the segregation of the kinetoplast, the cell cycle control would be species specific. For example, only the cell cycle of *T. cruzi* can be arrested by adding hydroxyurea, which inhibits nucleotide reductase, required for the formation of deoxyribonucleotides from ribonucleotides (Galanti et al., 1994).

12.2.3. Chromosome structure

Vickerman and Preston (1970) had shown that it is not possible to visualize chromosomes during trypanosome mitosis, which occurs without NE disruption as found in lower eukaryotes and fungi (Solari, 1995). Therefore, the *T. cruzi* chromosome structure has only been detected by molecular techniques. By pulse field gel electrophoresis, it was estimated that there are 64 individual chromosomes per cell (Cano et al., 1995). This number is stable during the parasite cell and life cycle (Galindo et al.,

2007) but varies across the different isolates (Henriksson et al., 2002). More recently, genomic sequencing analysis, synteny maps and sequence from BAC libraries allowed to assemble 41 chromosomes in the CL-Brener isolate (Weatherly et al., 2009). The presence of genes in at least two different chromosome size bands suggested that *T. cruzi* are diploid organisms (Gibson and Miles, 1986), which is recently supported by the analysis of the sequenced genome (El Sayed et al., 2005).

Telomeres are found at each chromosome extremities and contain GGATTT repeats of variable size among the different *T. cruzi* isolates, ranging from about 500 to 10,000 bp (Freitas-Junior et al., 1999). Subtelomere sequences are enriched with copies of large and variable family of genes as pseudo-genes and retrotransposons (Kim et al., 2005). Telomeres and subtelomeres regions contains β-d-glucopyranosyloxymethyluracil (base J), whose function seems related to control of gene expression and gene diversity (Ekanayake et al., 2007). When probed by fluorescent *in situ* hybridization, *T. cruzi* telomeres are located at the nucleus periphery (Elias, M.C. and Schenkman, S., unpublished results), suggesting that telomere associate with the NE. Telomerase enzyme activity forming large RNP complex (>600 kDa) has been identified in extracts of epimastigotes showing atypical enzymatic properties (Munoz and Collins, 2004). Some proteins involved in telomere maintenance, although identified in the genome, were not characterized yet (Table 12.1). It is interesting to observe some extent of variability among Esmeraldo and Non-Esmeraldo type of isolates, possibly explaining the differences in telomere size among the different *T. cruzi* isolates.

Centromere sequences are poorly evident in *T. cruzi*. By analysing the requirements for chromosomal stability, the localization of centromere was proposed to include GC-rich strand-switch domains composed predominantly of degenerate retrotransposons (Obado et al., 2007). Repetitive sequences of 195 bp with characteristics of α-satellite DNA, known to be part of centromeres in other eukaryotes, are found in *T. cruzi*. These sequences comprised up to 10% of the total DNA of the parasite depending on the isolate (Elias et al., 2003, 2005). They are present only in the larger chromosomes and whether they participate in the centromere formation or chromatin organization remains to be investigated. However, several proteins involved in the formation of mitotic spindle, particularly kinesins, were identified in the genome analysis demonstrating a high degree of conservation of these sequences among the eukaryotes (Table 12.1).

12.2.4. Chromatin organization in *Trypanosoma cruzi*

Nucleosomes are also the basic unit of the *T. cruzi* chromatin. It was shown by sucrose gradient, that a single nucleosome encompasses 200 bp of DNA (Astolfi et al., 1980). The chromatin of *T. cruzi* is organized

TABLE 12.1 Identified and annotated proteins participating in the telomere, centromere, nuclear pore, envelope, nuclear transport and the nucleolus of *T. cruzi* in comparison with *T. brucei*[a]

T. cruzi	Function	*T. brucei*	Function
Telomere proteins			
Tc00.1047053503643.10 (CLB-E)	KU70 protein, put.	Tb927.3.5030 (KU70)	KU70 protein
Tc00.1047053507093.72 (CLB-E)	Hypoth. protein, conserv.	Tb11.03.0760 (RAP1)	Repressor activator protein 1
Tc00.1047053508827.50 (CLB-NE)	DNA repair and recombination protein, mitochondrial precursor, put.	Tb11.01.3660 (TbPIF3)	DNA repair and recombination helicase protein PIF1, put.
Tc00.1047053503677.20 (CLB-E)	PIF1 helicase-like protein, put.	Tb11.01.6420 (TbPIF4)	DNA repair and recombination helicase protein PIF1, put.
Tc00.1047053506775.90 (CLB-E)	PIF1 helicase-like protein, put.	Tb11.02.4730 (TbPIF1)	DNA repair and recombination helicase protein PIF1, put.
Tc00.1047053506775.100 (CLB-E)	PIF1 helicase-like protein, put.	Tb11.02.4740 (TbPIF2)	DNA repair and recombination helicase protein PIF1, put.
Tc00.1047053511133.4 (CLB-E)	DNA repair and recombination helicase protein PIF1, put.	Tb927.10.910 (TbPIF6)	DNA repair and recombination helicase protein PIF1, put.
Tc00.1047053511491.50 (CLB-NE)	KU80 protein, put.	Tb927.6.1760 (KU80)	KU80 protein
Tc00.1047053511807.200 (CLB-NE)	Hypoth. protein, conserv.	Tb927.7.2170	Hypoth. protein, conserv.

Tc00.1047053505945.10 (CLB-E)	PIF1 helicase-like protein, put.	Tb927.8.3560 (TbPIF5)	DNA repair and recombination helicase
Tc00.1047053508567.80 (CLB-E)	DNA repair and recombination helicase protein PIF1, put.	Tb927.8.700 (TbPIF7)	DNA repair and recombination helicase protein PIF1, put.
Tc00.1047053508207.150 (CLB-E)	Silent information regulator 2, put. (SIR2RP1)	Tb927.7.1690 (SIR2RP1)	Silent information regulator 2
Tc00.1047053510719.200 (CLB-E)	Telomerase reverse transcriptase, put.	Tb11.01.1950	Telomerase reverse transcriptase, put.
Centromere protein			
Tc00.1047053510841.10 (CLB-E)	Mitotic centromere-associated kinesin (MCAK, pseudogene), put.	Tb927.4.3910 (Kif13-4)	MCAK-like kinesin, put.
Tc00.1047053504125.60 (CLB-E)	MCAK-like kinesin, put.	Tb11.02.2970 (Kif13-3)	MCAK-like kinesin, put.
Not found		Tbg972.4.4020	MCAK-like kinesin, put.
Not found		Tbg972.11.5980	MCAK-like kinesin, put.
Tc00.1047053506635.110 (CLB-E)	Kinesin-like protein, put.	Tb927.4.2730	Kinesin, put.
Tc00.1047053506635.120 (CLB-E)	Kinesin, put.		
Tc00.1047053508029.59 (CLB-NE)	Kinesin, put.		
Tc00.1047053510611.30 (CLB-E)	Kinesin, put.	Tb927.7.7260 (TbKIF9B)	Kinesin, put.
Tc00.1047053509149.80 (CLB-E)	Hypoth. protein, conserv.	Tb927.7.5040 (KIN-B)	Kinesin, put.

(*continued*)

TABLE 12.1 *(continued)*

T. cruzi	Function	*T. brucei*	Function
Tc00.1047053506895.40 (CLB-E)	MCAK-like kinesin, put.	Tb09.160.2260 (Kif-13-1)	Kinesin
Tc00.1047053506579.90 (CLB-E)	Hypoth. protein	Not found	
Nucleolus proteins			
Not found		Tb05.5K5.70	Nucleolar RNA helicase II, put.
Tc00.1047053503811.20 (CLB-E)	U3 small nucleolar ribonucleoprotein protein MPP10, put.	Tb927.3.3590	U3 small nucleolar ribonucleoprotein protein MPP10, put.
Tc00.1047053509951.10 (CLB-E)	Nucleolar protein, put.	Tb927.4.3840	Nucleolar protein, put.
Tc00.1047053507583.20 (CLB-NE)	Nucleolar protein, put.		
Tc00.1047053508205.20 (CLB-E)	Nucleolar RNA helicase II, put.	Tb927.5.4420	Nucleolar RNA helicase II, put.
Tc00.1047053507649.80 (CLB-NE)	Nucleolar RNA-binding protein, put.	Tb927.8.730	Nucleolar RNA-binding protein, put.
Tc00.1047053510859.17 (CLB-E)	Nucleolar RNA-binding protein, put.	Tb927.8.740 and Tb927.8.760 (Nopp44/46)	Nucleolar RNA-binding protein, truncated
Tc00.1047053510859.10 (CLB-E)	Nucleolar RNA-binding protein, put.		

Not found		Tb927.8.750	Nucleolar RNA-binding protein, put.
Tc00.1047053511573.58 (CLB-E)	Nucleolar protein, put.	Tb927.8.3750	Nucleolar protein, put.
Tc00.1047053506189.10 (CLB-E)	Nucleolar protein, put.		
Tc00.1047053511573.58 (CLB-E)	Nucleolar protein, put.		
Tc00.1047053504423.30 (CLB-E)	Hypoth. protein, conserv.	Tb09.160.1160 (NOP86) and Tb09.160.1180 (NOP66)	Nucleolar protein
Tc00.1047053508277.230 (CLB-E)	Nucleolar RNA-binding protein, put.	Tb09.160.3820	Nucleolar RNA-binding protein, put.
Tc00.1047053510289.6 (CLB-E)	Nucleolar RNA-binding protein, put.	Tb927.10.4740	Nucleolar RNA-binding protein, put.
Tc00.1047053510431.160 (CLB-E)	Nucleolar GTP-binding protein 1, put.	Tb11.02.0620 (NOG1)	Nucleolar GTP-binding protein 1
Tc00.1047053504643.20 (CLB-E)	Hypoth. protein, conserv.	Tb11.01.5500	U3 small nucleolar ribonucleoprotein protein IMP3, put.
Tc00.1047053503833.69 (CLB-E)	Ribosome biogenesis protein, put.	Tb927.10.14680	Ribosome biogenesis protein, put.
Tc00.1047053506925.510 (CLB-E)	RNA processing factor 1, put. (PIE8)	Tb11.03.0050	RNA processing factor 1, put.
Tc00.1047053511753.60 (CLB-E)	ESAG8-associated protein, put. (PUF7)	Tb927.6.2850 (PIE8)	ESAG8-associated protein, put.

(*continued*)

TABLE 12.1 *(continued)*

T. cruzi	Function	*T. brucei*	Function
Tc00.1047053511715.100 (CLB-E)	Pumilio/PUF RNA-binding protein 7, put.	Tb11.01.6600 (PUF7)	Pumilio/PUF RNA-binding protein 7, put.
Tc00.1047053510241.110 (CLB-E)	Hypoth. protein, conserv.	Tb09.211.0180	Hypoth. protein, conserv.
Tc00.1047053510761.60 (CLB-E)	Casein kinase II, put.	Tb09.211.4890	Casein kinase II, put.
Tc00.1047053509499.20 (CLB-E)	Beta propeller protein, put.	Tb927.8.1980	Hypoth. protein, conserv.
Tc00.1047053510105.50 (CLB-E)	Fibrillarin, put.	Tb927.10.7500 (NOP1)	Fibrillarin
Tc00.1047053508837.180 (Tc00.1047053508837.180)	DNA polymerase I alpha catalytic subunit, put.	Tb927.8.4880	DNA polymerase I, alpha catalytic subunit
Nuclear envelope proteins			
Tc00.1047053510597.40 (CLB-E)	Nucleoporin (NUP54/57), put.	(TbNup62) Tb927.4.5200	Nucleoporin (NUP54/57), put.
Tc00.1047053506247.70 (CLB-NE)	Nuclear pore complex protein (NUP155), put.	Tb927.10.8170	Nuclear pore complex protein (NUP155), put.
Tc00.1047053510181.50 (CLB-E)	Nucleoporin interacting component (NUP93), put.	Tb927.10.7060	Nucleoporin interacting component (NUP93), put.
Tc00.1047053508153.410 (CLB-NE)	Hypoth. protein, conserv.	(TbNup98) Tb927.3.3180	Nucleoporin
Tc00.1047053506591.69 (CLB-E)	Hypoth. protein, conserv.	(TbNup53b) Tb927.3.3540	Nucleoporin

Tc00.1047053507735.50 (CLB-E)	Hypoth. protein, conserv. (pseudogene)	(TbNup225) Tb927.4.2880	Nucleoporin
Tc00.1047053505009.10 (CLB-E)	Hypoth. protein, conserv.	(TbNup64) Tb927.4.4310	Nucleoporin
Tc00.1047053511809.60 (CLB-NE)	Hypoth. protein, conserv.	(TbNup132) Tb927.7.2300	Nucleoporin
Not found		(TbNup75) Tb927.8.8050	Nucleoporin
Tc00.1047053504769.80 (CLB-E)	Hypoth. protein, conserv.	(TbMlp-2) Tb09.160.0340	Nucleoporin
Tc00.1047053510759.180 (CLB-E)	Hypoth. protein, conserv.	(TbNup82) Tb09.211.4780	
Tc00.1047053507093.50 (CLB-E)	Hypoth. protein, conserv.	(TbMlp-1) Tb11.03.0810	Nucleoporin, myosin-like protein
Tc00.1047053506925.440 (CLB-E)	Nucleoporin (pseudogene), put, serine peptidase, Clan SP, family S59	(TbNup158) Tb11.03.0140	Nucleoporin
Tc00.1047053504153.330 (CLB-E)	Hypoth. protein, conserv.	(TbNup59) Tb11.02.0270	Nucleoporin
Tc00.1047053503887.10 (CLB-E)	Hypoth. protein, conserv.	(TbNup89) Tb11.02.0460	Nucleoporin
Tc00.1047053510431.340 (CLB-E)	Hypoth. protein, conserv.		
Tc00.1047053506227.220 (CLB-E)	Hypoth. protein, conserv.	(TbNup48) Tb11.02.2120	Nucleoporin
Tc00.1047053508831.150 (CLB-E)	Hypoth. protein, conserv.	(TbNup149) Tb11.01.2880	Nucleoporin

(continued)

TABLE 12.1 *(continued)*

T. cruzi	Function	*T. brucei*	Function
Tc00.1047053511671.60 (CLB-NE)	Surface antigen 2 (CA-2), put.	(TbNup140) Tb11.01.2885	Nucleoporin
Tc00.1047053504159.10 (CLB-E)	Hypoth. protein, conserv.	(TbNup53a) Tb11.01.7200	Nucleoporin
Tc00.1047053507037.60 (CLB-E)	Hypoth. protein, conserv.	(TbNup109) Tb11.01.7630	Nucleoporin
Tc00.1047053508815.140 (CLB-NE)	Protein transport protein Sec13, put.	Tb11.01.0420	Protein transport protein Sec13, put.
Tc00.1047053506525.20 (CLB-E)	Protein transport protein Sec13, put.	Tb927.10.14180	Protein transport protein Sec13, put.
Lamina proteins			
Not found		Tb927.2.4230	NUP-1 protein, put.
Tc00.1047053511617.9 (CLB-E)	NUP-1 protein (pseudogene), put.	Not found	
Tc00.1047053507969.60 (CLB-NE)	C-14 sterol reductase, put.	Tb11.01.7170	C-14 Sterol reductase/lamin B receptor
Nuclear transport proteins			
Tc00.1047053509455.80 (CLB-E)	GTP-binding nuclear protein rtb2, put.	Tb927.3.1120 (rtb2)	GTP-binding nuclear protein rtb2, put.
Tc00.1047053506945.30 (CLB-E)	CAS/CSE/importin domain protein, put.	Tb927.6.4740	Importin alpha re-exporter protein, put.
Tc00.1047053503579.50 (CLB-E)	Hypoth. protein, conserv.	Tb927.7.1460	Hypoth. protein, conserv.
Tc00.1047053508173.180 (CLB-NE)	Nuclear transport factor 2 protein (NFT2), put.	Tb927.7.5760 (NFT2)	Nuclear transport factor 2 protein, put.

Tc00.1047053511407.10 (CLB-E)	Nuclear transport factor 2, put.	Tb927.8.4280	Nuclear transport factor 2, put.
Tc00.1047053511367.220 (CLB-NE)	Hypoth. protein, conserv.	Tb927.10.2240	Hypoth. protein, conserv.
Tc00.1047053504105.150 (CLB-NE)	Importin beta-1 subunit, put.	Tb927.10.2900	Importin beta-1 subunit, put.
Tc00.1047053510181.50 (CLB-E)	Nucleoporin interacting component (NUP93), put.	Tb927.10.7060	Nucleoporin interacting component (NUP93), put.
Tc00.1047053506247.70 (CLB-NE)	Nuclear pore complex protein (NUP155), put.	Tb927.10.8170	Nuclear pore complex protein (NUP155), put.
Tc00.1047053506925.440 (CLB-E)	Nucleoporin (pseudogene), put.	Tb11.03.0140 (TbNup158)	Nucleoporin
Tc00.1047053507099.30 (CLB-E)	Ran-binding protein 1, put.	Tb11.02.0870	Ran-binding protein 1, put.
Tc00.1047053511725.150 (CLB-NE)	Exportin 1, put. (CRM1)	Tb11.01.5940 (XPO1)	Exportin 1
Tc00.1047053511529.9 (CLB-E)	Hypoth. protein, conserv.	Tb11.01.8030	Hypoth. protein, conserv.
Tc00.1047053504019.9 (CLB-E)	Hypoth. protein, conserv.		
Tc00.1047053421321.9 (CLB-E)	tRNA exportin, put.	Tb927.2.2240	tRNA exportin, put.
Tc00.1047053509965.110 (CLB-E)	Importin alpha, put.	Tb927.6.2640 (TbKap60)	Importin alpha subunit, put.
Tc00.1047053509161.90 (CLB-NE)	Hypoth. protein, conserv.	Tb11.01.5410	Hypoth. protein, conserv.

put, put; Hypoth. prot., conserv., Hypoth. prot., conserv.; CL Brener Esmeraldo, CLB-E, CL Brener Non-Esmeraldo. For simplicity, the only proteins of CL Brener Non-Esmeraldo are the ones not present in the Esmeraldo Haplotype and are shown in italicized and bold typeface.

[a] The data were obtained from Trytrip DB (http:/tritrypdb.org/tritrypdb/).

in filaments of nucleosomes arranged irregularly, not condensing in 30 nm fiber and being more sensible to nucleases as compared to superior eukaryotes (Hecker and Gander, 1985). Histones H2A, H2B, H3 and H4 form the nucleosome core structure (Hecker et al., 1994). The genes for each type of histone of *T. cruzi* were identified and found to be organized in tandem of 14–24 genes. They are expressed at the S phase of cell cycle undergoing polyadenylation, as found in lower eukaryotes (Recinos et al., 2001). The histones of *T. cruzi* present a globular domain flanked by divergent N- and C-terminal domains, sites of post-translational modifications (Elias et al., 2009). The histone H1 of *T. cruzi* presents only the region that corresponds to C-terminal domain, defined as the prototype of histone H1 in lower eukaryotes (Kasinsky et al., 2001). The absence of the globular domain and N-terminal domain can be one of the reasons of its weak association with the chromatin and absence of 30 nm fibres in this parasite as suggested previously (Toro and Galanti, 1988).

The first identified post-translational modification in *T. cruzi* histones was the phosphorylation of histone H1 in a single amino acid ($S_{12}{}^{P}$PKK), a motif recognized by cyclin-dependent protein kinases (da Cunha et al., 2005). The role of histone H1 phosphorylation is poorly defined, but in general, it promotes the dissociation from the DNA (Raghuram et al., 2009), which could allow the binding of chromatin condensing factors as found in the mitosis of higher eukaryotes. *T. cruzi* histone becomes phosphorylated in trypomastigotes (Marques Porto et al., 2002) and when parasites enter the DNA replication phase of the cell cycle (Gutiyama et al., 2008), compatible with the nuclear reorganization seen in those conditions.

The first evidence that the core nucleosomes could be modified in *T. cruzi* was got through the incorporation of radiolabelled acetic acid and methyl-methionine, both precursors of the acetylation and methylation, respectively, in histones. Histones H4 and H2A were preferentially labelled with [^{3}H] acetate, while histones H3, H2B and H4, to a less extent, with [^{3}H] methyl-methionine, indicating that histones H4 and H2A are mainly acetylated, while histones H3 and H2B are preferentially methylated (da Cunha et al., 2006). The presence and localization of the modifications in the histone H4 was confirmed by mass spectrometry showing that most of the histone H4 is acetylated at lysine 4. Other minor acetylations occur in lysines 10, 14 and 57. The first alanine at the N-terminus is methylated, lysine 18 is mono-methylated and arginine 53 is dimethylated. Although histones of *T. cruzi* are divergent of the higher eukaryotes, it resembles the ones of *T. brucei*, where an extensive analysis of histone modifications has been made (Mandava et al., 2007).

To understand the role of histone modifications in *T. cruzi*, chromatin immunoprecipitation (CHIP) assays have been performed showing a preferential acetylation of histone H4 at lysines 4, 10 and 14 and trimethylation of histone H3 at the region of reading frames inversion in chromosomes, probably sites related to transcription initiation (Respuela et al., 2008). No enrichment was observed in promoters of ribosomal RNA or spliced leader (SL) RNA genes. The use of specific antibodies to the modified histone H4 revealed that the less abundant modifications (K10 and K14) are present in less compacted chromatin regions and increase in conditions that affect the chromatin structure (Nardelli et al., 2009).

Specific enzymes that catalyse addition and removal of histone modifications were detected in the database of *T. cruzi*. These enzymes were studied in *T. brucei* (Horn, 2007) and were shown to be important in controlling transcriptional events and antigenic variation (Figueiredo et al., 2009). However, very little information is known about the *T. cruzi* histone-modifying enzymes. In the databank, six different histone acetylases (HATs) are found, one of them, HAT4 from the MYST family, is absent in *T. brucei*. Also at least six different histone deacetylases are present including the NAD-dependent enzyme Sir2protein, which participates in the telomere structure (Table 12.1).

Modified histones of *T. cruzi* are recognized by proteins that contain bromo domains (BD). One of these proteins was identified in *T. cruzi* (TcBD factor 2) and found to interact *in vitro* with acetylated forms of histones H2A and H4 (Villanova et al., 2009). By immunofluorescence analysis, it appears as punctuated structures distributed in the nucleoplasm that matches the localization of histone H4 acetylated at lysines 10 and 14. Assays of CHIP had confirmed the interaction of TcBD factor 2 with nucleosomes enriched in histones with H4K10ac. Several other bromo domain-containing proteins are annotated in the *T. cruzi* genome databank, but their functions are presently unknown. Some of their orthologues were characterized in *T. brucei* as proteins participating in the transcription initiation together with histone H4 and H3 variants (Siegel et al., 2009). In addition, few proteins with chromo domains, known to interact with methylated histones, although present in trypanosome genome, were characterized.

12.2.5. Nucleolus

T. cruzi nucleolus has been examined by electron microscopy 3D reconstruction showing the presence of dense fibrillar and granular components but not fibrillar centres (Lopez-Velazquez et al., 2005). The size of nucleolus is increased in exponentially growing epimastigotes as compared to stationary cells (Nepomuceno-Mejia et al., 2010). Non-phosphorylated histone H1 is concentrated in the nucleolus (Gutiyama et al., 2008). It becomes phosphorylated during cell cycle progression until mitosis, then dispersing through the entire nucleoplasm upon cytokinesis. As shown for histone H1, a nucleolus artificial fusion protein, consisting in the first segment of histone H2b in fusion with GFP, also disperses (Elias et al., 2001), suggesting that the nucleolus disperses in mitosis as found in other eukaryotes. Targeting signals for nucleolar proteins appear to depend on the presence of stretches of basic amino acids (Gluenz et al., 2007), a finding that could explain why a fusion containing the first amino acids of histone H2B promotes the deliver to the nucleolus as it does not assemble in nucleosomes. The nucleolus disappears when epimastigotes transform in metacyclics (Ramirez et al., 2000) and reappears as soon as metacyclics invade mammalian cells (Gluenz et al., 2007), compatible with the low level of transcription and translation in trypomastigote forms. It is, however, unknown how the cells control the levels of transcription during differentiation. Several nucleolus proteins are identified in the *T. cruzi* database based on similarity analysis, suggesting a high degree of conservation related to other eukaryotes (Table 12.1). A nuclear protein, named TcSof1, probably involved in ribosomal RNA processing, displayed a nuclear localization and is expressed during metacyclogenesis (Nardelli et al., 2007). Interesting TcSoft1 orthologue was not found in Esmeraldo genome, suggesting that strain-specific mechanisms might control the expression of key components of nucleolar RNA processing.

12.2.6. Nuclear envelope

The NE of *T. cruzi* appears similar to most of eukaryotic cells with membrane pores (Spadiliero et al., 2002). However, as in lower eukaryotes, *T. cruzi* lacks conserved lamin proteins. Instead, it contains a protein called TcNup that resembles a similar protein in *T. brucei.* TcNup was shown to behave like a lamin protein and to interact with specific regions of *T. cruzi* genome, probably anchoring chromosomes to the NE (Picchi et al., 2011). In fact, few of NE proteins were annotated, probably because they are quite different as compared to higher eukaryotes (Table 12.1).

Components involved in the nuclear RNA export and protein import in *T. cruzi* have not been characterized, although some are annotated in database (Table 12.1). However, RNA binding proteins, some of them involved in RNA export to the cytoplasm, have been identified (Kramer et al., 2010), particularly TcUB1 and TcUB2, found to depend on the metabolic status of the parasite (Cassola and Frasch, 2009). The nuclear localization signals in *T. cruzi* are complex, probably unique. Recent studies showed that it depends on unusual stretches of basic amino acids (Westergaard et al., 2010).

12.2.7. Transcription machineries

Multiple RNA polymerases are detected in *T. cruzi* (Hodo and Hatcher, 1986). The parasite RNA polymerase II (TcRNA Pol II) is inhibited by low (<10 μg/ml) α-amanitin concentrations and transcribes mRNAs as typical for most eukaryotes. All 12 canonical subunits of the RNA Pol II core enzyme have also been detected *in silico* in trypanosomes (Kelly et al., 2005). The most important difference is that the largest subunit, known to control transcription initiation, splicing and termination, is unusual in trypanosomes and lacks the typical carboxy-terminal repeats (Smith et al., 1989), and perhaps this explain the unusual characteristics of transcription regulation in most trypanosomes. Active RNA polymerase could be phosphorylated at its unusual C-terminus that is divergent among trypanosomes (Ejchel et al., 2003). However, the enzymes and phosphorylation sites in the carboxy-terminal domain as well as possible interacting molecules that could be involved in the transcription regulation are currently unknown in *T. cruzi.*

The *T. cruzi* RNA Pol II also transcribes the SL RNA, which donates a 35- to 39-nucleotide sequence to the 5′-end of pre-mRNA in a *trans*-splicing reaction (McCarthy-Burke et al., 1989). The transcription promoter for the SL RNA gene arrays was identified (Nunes et al., 1997) and shown to vary among the parasite isolates (Thomas et al., 2005). A detailed characterization of protein–protein interactions by yeast two-hybrid assay identified an enzymatic complex possibly involved in the pre-initiation of SL RNA transcription (Cribb and Serra, 2009). It is particularly interesting that a TATA-box binding protein is present in *T. cruzi* (TcTBP) in the absence of typical TATA promoters. Transcription initiation in this case might be stabilized by the presence of transcription factors such as the TFIIa-like protein.

Immunofluorescence analysis of the distribution of RNA Pol II in the nucleus showed a predominant localization of the enzyme near the nucleolus, which contains transcriptional activity of SL RNA genes. This transcriptional site was called SL body (Dossin and Schenkman, 2005). Remaining transcriptional activity involved in other genes appears more dispersed in regions less stained for DNA, forming discrete and smaller transcriptional machineries (Fig. 12.2). Upon transcription inhibition, or when transcription is reduced after the differentiation of epimastigotes in metacyclics, the SL body disappears (Ferreira et al., 2008). In the first case, the enzyme only disperses in the nucleoplasm, while during the differentiation, the amount of enzyme is reduced. As *T. cruzi* lacks an individual control of transcription initiation for each gene, a general mechanism might regulate the amount of enzyme and the activity of the RNA Pol II at the different life stages of the parasite.

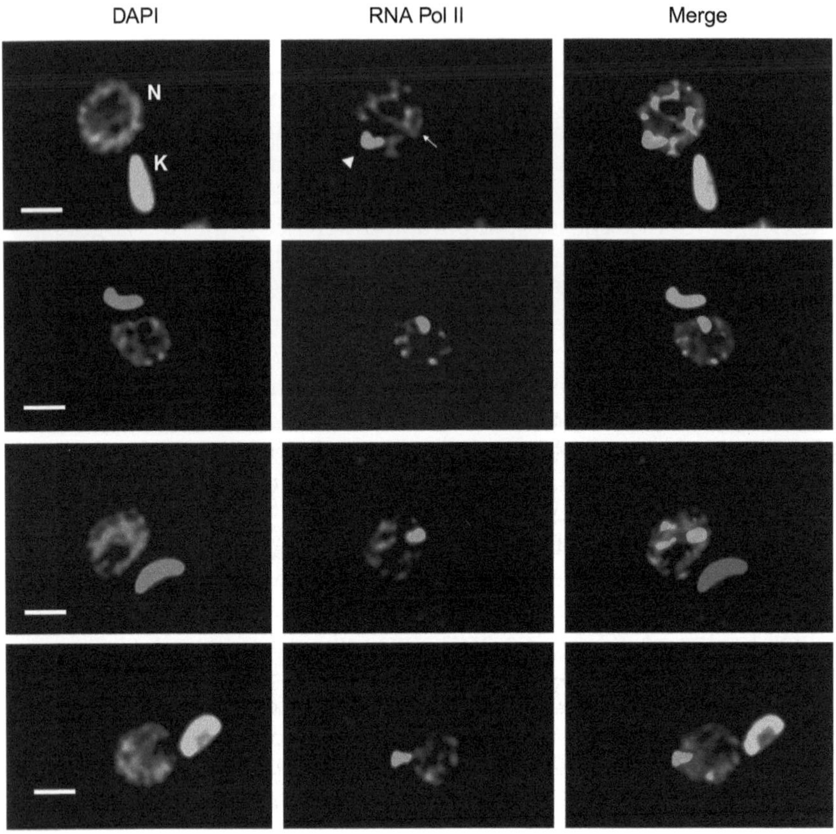

FIGURE 12.2 *Localization of the RNA Pol II in the nucleus of T. cruzi epimastigotes.* The image shows the DAPI (blue) and RNA Pol II staining (green) and the merged images of epimastigotes as described in Nardelli et al. (2009). Bars = 2 μm. The arrowhead indicates the position that corresponds to the SL transcription site and the arrows, other transcription site. (See Color Section.)

The fine structure of the promoter for RNA Pol I has been characterized (Figueroa-Angulo et al., 2006), and the ribosomal RNA genes have been found to diverge among isolates (Brisse et al., 2001; Kawashita et al., 2001). However, the mechanisms involved in the control of ribosomal gene transcription remain to be understood in *T. cruzi*.

Much less is known regarding the transcription of small RNA, by RNA Pol III, such as tRNAs in *T. cruzi*. *In silico* analysis revealed a low number of tRNA genes in trypanosomes, with low synteny among the species, suggesting unique features for each one and possible unexpected features for the RNA Pol III transcription (Padilla-Mejia et al., 2009).

12.2.8. Replication machinery

In eukaryotes, pre-replication protein complexes populate DNA replication sites at the beginning of the G1 phase of the cell cycle. When cells start S phase, pre-replication origins are removed allowing the assembly of replicating enzymes. *T. cruzi* contains most of the typical DNA pre-replication proteins, except for the presence of the origin replication complex (Orc) formed by six different subunits and named Orc1–Orc6. In the parasite, a single protein replaces the hexamer and was named TcOrc1/Cdc6 protein (Godoy et al., 2009). TcOrc1/Cd6 is able to interact with not yet identified replication origins displaying a DNA-dependent ATPase activity. Moreover, it complements yeast mutants lacking the Cdc6 protein, required for the origin firing. An analogous Orc1/Cdc6 protein is found in Archaea, indicating a similar phylogenetic origin or a convergent evolution within these organisms. Recently, it was shown that replication origins containing Orc1/Cdc6 move the periphery. Then, the proliferating cellular nuclear antigen (PCNA), a protein that increases DNA polymerase processivity, is captured by the DNA replication sites (Calderano et al., 2011). PCNA then localizes near the NE, as also seen by bromodeoxy-uridine incorporation (Elias et al., 2002). This localization is unique and might indicate a peculiar characteristic of trypanosomes, although fixed replication machineries are proposed for eukaryotes in general. By fluorescent *in situ* hybridization analysis, it was found that *T. cruzi* chromosomes are also in variable locations inside the nucleus depending on the cell cycle and parasite stage (Elias et al., 2002). At G2, for example, markers corresponding to satellite sequences are sequestered near the NE, dispersing after mitosis. This variable chromosome distribution seems to reflect movements towards the fixed replication machinery close to the NE, allowing all chromosome regions to replicate.

12.3. THE NUCLEUS UNDER STRESS

The nuclear structure of *T. cruzi* changes considerable during the transformation from replicative to infective stages and vice versa. It is conceivable that these alterations arise as consequence of variations on DNA replication and DNA transcription state. As *T. cruzi* finds variable environmental conditions, it should support different types of stresses. Therefore, it is important to understand how the nuclear structure varies upon extreme conditions.

12.3.1. DNA damage

T. cruzi nuclear structure changes significantly after DNA damage induced by gamma irradiation, known to cause double-strand DNA breaks. In gamma-irradiated epimastigotes, the dense chromatin seen in the nuclear periphery disappears and an enlarged nucleolus is detected by electron microscopy (Nardelli et al., 2009). DNA repair is robust in *T. cruzi*. It occurs by homologous recombination with the participation of TcRAD51, a protein involved in recognizing the breaks to promote the repair, ensuing parasite survival upon large doses of irradiation (Regis-da-Silva et al., 2006). Non-homologous end-joining enzymes are not found in the genome (Machado et al., 2006). Similar nuclear reorganization is observed in cells treated with hydroxyurea that stops replication but also causes double strand DNA breaks (Elias et al., 2002). These chromatin modifications correlate with an increase of histone H4 acetylation in the lysines 10 and 14, localized in normal cells in less dense chromatin, suggesting that chromatin modifications and nuclear remodelling are involved in DNA repair. Trypanosomes are devoid of histone H2AX, a histone variant that is phosphorylated upon DNA damage, signalling for DNA repair in most eukaryotes. Therefore, other signalling mechanisms and chromatin modifications might occur in *T. cruzi* after DNA damage. For example, UV irradiation has shown to cause increased expression of TcBRD2 that binds to acetylated histones (Villanova et al., 2009), suggesting that chromatin reorganization occurs after formation of thymine dimers modification. In *T. cruzi*, the oxidative damage induced by hydrogen peroxide was found to cause extensive poly(ADP-ribosyl) ation of the chromatin, which could also signals for DNA repair (Fernandez Villamil et al., 2008).

12.3.2. Nuclear responses to environmental stress

Oxidative stress affects *T. cruzi* by forming DNA adducts that have to be repaired. In addition, reactive oxygen species (ROS) produced by the interaction with hosts, or generated by the parasite metabolism itself, should promote a series of damages and would require detoxification (Piacenza et al., 2009). The involvement of nuclear reorganization in the response to ROS has not been directly examined, but the effect of arsenite, a potent oxidant, was shown to cause extensive relocalization of RNA binding proteins (Cassola and Frasch, 2009), supporting the notion that the nucleus organization is related to responses against oxidative damage independently of DNA damage.

Different *T. cruzi* isolates show distinct amounts of DNA in the nucleus indicating that during evolution, pieces of chromosomes have been lost or amplified. The large number of repetitive elements suggests chromosome instability, although no variations are seen in short period of times. The presence of hybrid strains point out that recombination events have occurred during evolution. Short-term exchange of DNA material and possible alterations in ploidy might occur during *T. cruzi* life cycle as this can be observed in cultured forms (Lewis et al., 2009). Earlier studies have detected differences in the nuclear and kinetoplast DNA content depending on the parasite isolate, stage, temperature of growth (Nozaki and Dvorak, 1991), after environmental stresses (Nozaki and Dvorak, 1993), and in drug-resistant isolates, which show enlarged nucleus (Nozaki et al., 1996). Therefore, the large genome plasticity in response to environmental changes must involve nuclear structure variations in *T. cruzi* and should be further studied.

12.4. CONCLUSION AND PERSPECTIVES

The nuclear structure has become a new discipline that contributes to our understanding of several cellular and molecular events in eukaryotes. The transfer of information from DNA to the final cell proteome can now be visualized under a 3D perspective, providing a more comprehensive view of how a eukaryotic cell works. The extension of this knowledge to a single cell parasite such as the *T. cruzi* that has to adapt to different host environments to cause a disease is, therefore, an essential step in understanding the basic mechanisms underlying the host–parasite interaction. It can also provide additional approaches to find new therapies and diagnosis for Chagas' disease. Compared to other trypanosomes and to other eukaryotes, the knowledge of the *T. cruzi* nucleus organization is still limited, mainly due to its complexity and because the field is still relatively unexplored. The main differential characteristics are illustrated in Table 12.2. Some of the concepts observed in other systems are applicable in understanding *T. cruzi* biology, but it is expected that particular and relevant aspects would be unique to *T. cruzi*. The fact that *T. cruzi* dividing in the mammalian cell cytosol and in the gut of the insect vector would require specific responses is particularly relevant, and its nucleus seems to play an important role in these responses. It is also noteworthy how a functional chromosome dynamics is maintained with a genome containing a large proportion of repetitive elements. The genomic stability should be largely influenced by the chromatin organization and robustness of DNA repair mechanisms. These processes should be linked to the control of gene expression during cellular differentiation. For example, it remains to be understood how the parasite decreases transcription and replication under stress. These questions will be better answered considering a structurally organized genome.

TABLE 12.2 Comparative features of nucleus structure between *T. cruzi* and mammalian cells

Characteristics	*T. cruzi*	Mammalian cells
Nucleus diameter	2 μm	10–20 μm
Genome size	$40–80 \times 10^6$ bp	2.9×10^9 bp
Chromosome number	40–64	46
Histones	H1, H2A, H2B, H3, H4	H1, H2A, H2B, H3, H4
Linker histone H1 variants	3	10
Core histone variants	5	>60
Described core histone acetylation and methylations	H4: A1m1, K4Ac, K10Ac, K14Ac, K18m1, R53m2, K57Ac	H4: K12ac, K16ac, K20me1, K20me3, K5ac, K8ac, K9ac, R3me2
	H3: K76m3	H3: K14ac, K18ac, K23ac, K27ac, K27me1, K27me2, K27me3, K36ac, K36me1, K36me3, K4ac, K4me1, K4me2, K4me3, K79me1, K79me2, K79me3, K9ac, K9me1, K9me2, H3K9me3, R2me1, R2me2
	H2A: unknown	H2A: K5ac, K9ac
	H2B: unknown	H2B: K120ac, K12ac, BK20ac, K5ac, K5me1
Histone acetylases	Present	Present
Histone deacetylase	Present (no inhibitors described)	Present (inhibitors are potential anti-cancer drugs)
Histone methyl-transferase	Present	Present

DNA modifications	Base J (β-D-glucopyranosyloxymethyluracil), controls gene expression	Methyl-cytidine controls gene expression
Transcription machinery	RNA Pol II lacks repeats at the CTD. Its regulatory role is unknown Concentrated on SL body as a major transcription factory	RNA Pol II CTD regulates transcription initiation, splicing and polyadenylation Many transcription factories
Replication machinery	Replication pre-initiation has partial characteristics of Archea (Orc1/Cdc6)	Replication pre-initiation is determined by the presence of Orc1-6 and regulated by Cdc6 protein
Nuclear lamina	Composed by divergent structural proteins	Composed of lamins
DNA repair mechanisms	Robust homologous recombination, absence of non-homologous end joining repair of double strand breaks. Robust anti-oxidative responses	Less robust homologous recombination, presence of non-homologous end joining repair of double strand breaks

ACKNOWLEDGEMENTS

This work was supported by grants from Fundação de Amparo à Pesquisa do Estado de São Paulo (FAPESP), Conselho Nacional de Desenvolvimento Científico e Tecnológico (CNPq), Brazil and US National Institutes of Health grant AI-068647. We also thank Roberto Docampo and Silvia Moreno for hosting S. S. in their laboratories.

REFERENCES

Albrethsen, J., Knol, J.C., Jimenez, C.R., 2009. Unravelling the nuclear matrix proteome. J. Proteomics 72, 71–81.

Astolfi-Filho, S., de Sá, C.M., Gander, E.S., 1980. On the chromatin structure of *Trypanosoma cruzi*. Mol. Biochem. Parasitol. 1, 45–53.

Berger, S.L., 2007. The complex language of chromatin regulation during transcription. Nature (London) 447, 407–412.

Bianchi, M.E., Agresti, A., 2005. HMG proteins: dynamic players in gene regulation and differentiation. Curr. Opin. Genet. Dev. 15, 496–506.

Boisvert, F.M., van Koningsbruggen, S., Navascues, J., Lamond, A.I., 2007. The multifunctional nucleolus. Nat. Rev. Mol. Cell Biol. 8, 574–585.

Branco, M.R., Pombo, A., 2006. Intermingling of chromosome territories in interphase suggests role in translocations and transcription-dependent associations. PLoS Biol. 4, e138.

Brisse, S., Verhoef, J., Tibayrenc, M., 2001. Characterisation of large and small subunit rRNA and mini-exon genes further supports the distinction of six *Trypanosoma cruzi* lineages. Int. J. Parasitol. 31, 1218–1226.

Calderano, S.G., de Melo, P.D., Motta, M.C.M., Mortara, R.M., Schenkman, S., Elias, M.C., 2011. Trypanosoma cruzi DNA replication includes the sequential recruitment of pre-replication and replication machineries close to nuclear periphery. Nucleus 2, 136–145.

Campos, E.I., Reinberg, D., 2009. Histones: annotating chromatin. Annu. Rev. Genet. 43, 559–599.

Cano, M.I., Gruber, A., Vazquez, M., Cortes, A., Levin, M.J., Gonzalez, A., et al., 1995. Molecular karyotype of clone CL Brener chosen for the *Trypanosoma cruzi* genome project. Mol. Biochem. Parasitol. 71, 273–278.

Cassola, A., Frasch, A.C., 2009. An RNA recognition motif mediates the nucleocytoplasmic transport of a trypanosome RNA-binding protein. J. Biol. Chem. 284, 35015–35028.

Chagin, V.O., Stear, J.H., Cardoso, M.C., 2010. Organization of DNA replication. Cold Spring Harb. Perspect. Biol. 2, a000737.

Chakalova, L., Fraser, P., 2010. Organization of transcription. Cold Spring Harb. Perspect. Biol. 2, a000729.

Cribb, P., Serra, E., 2009. One- and two-hybrid analysis of the interactions between components of the *Trypanosoma cruzi* spliced leader RNA gene promoter binding complex. Int. J. Parasitol. 39, 525–532.

da Cunha, J.P.C., Nakayasu, E.S., Elias, M.C., Pimenta, D.C., Tellez-Inon, M.T., Rojas, F., et al., 2005. *Trypanosoma cruzi* histone H1 is phosphorylated in a typical cyclin dependent kinase site accordingly to the cell cycle. Mol. Biochem. Parasitol. 140, 75–86.

da Cunha, J.P.C., Nakayasu, E.S., de Almeida, I.C., Schenkman, S., 2006. Post-translational modifications of *Trypanosoma cruzi* histone H4. Mol. Biochem. Parasitol. 150, 268–277.

de Souza, W., 2002. Basic cell biology of *Trypanosoma cruzi*. Curr. Pharm. Des. 8, 269–285.

de Souza, W., Meyer, H., 1974. On the fine structure of the nucleus in *Trypanosoma cruzi* in tissue culture forms. Spindle fibers in the dividing nucleus. J. Protozool. 21, 48–52.

Dechat, T., Adam, S.A., Taimen, P., Shimi, T., Goldman, R.D., 2010. Nuclear lamins. Cold Spring Harb. Perspect. Biol. 2, a000547.

Dossin, F.M., Schenkman, S., 2005. Actively transcribing RNA polymerase II concentrates on spliced leader genes in the nucleus of *Trypanosoma cruzi*. Eukaryot. Cell 4, 960–970.

Ejchel, T.F., Ramirez, M.I., Vargas, N., Nascimento, E.B., Zingales, B., Schenkman, S., 2003. The largest subunit of the RNA polymerase II of *Trypanosoma cruzi* lacks the repeats in the carboxy-terminal domain and is encoded by several genes. Parasitol. Int. 52, 243–249.

Ekanayake, D.K., Cipriano, M.J., Sabatini, R., 2007. Telomeric co-localization of the modified base J and contingency genes in the protozoan parasite *Trypanosoma cruzi*. Nucleic Acids Res. 35, 6367–6377.

El Sayed, N.M., Myler, P.J., Bartholomeu, D.C., Nilsson, D., Aggarwal, G., Tran, A.N., et al., 2005. The genome sequence of *Trypanosoma cruzi*, etiologic agent of Chagas disease. Science 309, 409–415.

Elias, M.C., Marques-Porto, R., Freymuller, E., Schenkman, S., 2001. Transcription rate modulation through the *Trypanosoma cruzi* life cycle occurs in parallel with changes in nuclear organisation. Mol. Biochem. Parasitol. 112, 79–90.

Elias, M.C., Faria, M., Mortara, R.A., Motta, M.C.M., de Souza, W., Thiry, M., et al., 2002. Chromosome localization changes in the *Trypanosoma cruzi* nucleus. Eukaryot. Cell 1, 944–953.

Elias, M.C., Vargas, N.S., Zingales, B., Schenkman, S., 2003. Organization of satellite DNA in the genome of *Trypanosoma cruzi*. Mol. Biochem. Parasitol. 129, 1–9.

Elias, M.C., Vargas, N., Tomazi, L., Pedroso, A., Zingales, B., Schenkman, S., et al., 2005. Comparative analysis of genomic sequences suggests that *Trypanosoma cruzi* CL Brener contains two sets of non-intercalated repeats of satellite DNA that correspond to *T. cruzi* I and *T. cruzi* II types. Mol. Biochem. Parasitol. 140, 221–227.

Elias, M.C., da Cunha, J.P., de Faria, F.P., Mortara, R.A., Freymuller, E., Schenkman, S., 2007. Morphological events during the *Trypanosoma cruzi* cell cycle. Protist 158, 147–157.

Elias, M.C., Nardelli, S.C., Schenkman, S., 2009. Chromatin and nuclear organization in *Trypanosoma cruzi*. Future Microbiol. 4, 1065–1074.

Fernandez Villamil, S.H., Baltanas, R., Alonso, G.D., Vilchez Larrea, S.C., Torres, H.N., Flawia, M.M., 2008. TcPARP: a DNA damage-dependent poly(ADP-ribose) polymerase from *Trypanosoma cruzi*. Int. J. Parasitol. 38, 277–287.

Ferreira, L.R., Dossin Fde, M., Ramos, T.C., Freymuller, E., Schenkman, S., 2008. Active transcription and ultrastructural changes during *Trypanosoma cruzi* metacyclogenesis. An. Acad. Bras. Ciênc. 80, 157–166.

Figueiredo, L.M., Cross, G.A., Janzen, C.J., 2009. Epigenetic regulation in African trypanosomes: a new kid on the block. Nat. Rev. Microbiol. 7, 504–513.

Figueroa-Angulo, E., Maria Cevallos, A., Zentella, A., Lopez-Villasenor, I., Hernandez, R., 2006. Potential regulatory elements in the *Trypanosoma cruzi* rRNA gene promoter. Biochim. Biophys. Acta 1759, 497–501.

Freitas-Junior, L.H., Porto, R.M., Pirrit, L.A., Schenkman, S., Scherf, A., 1999. Identification of the telomere in *Trypanosoma cruzi* reveals highly heterogeneous telomere lengths in different parasite strains. Nucleic Acids Res. 27, 2451–2456.

Galanti, N., Dvorak, J.A., Grenet, J., McDaniel, J.P., 1994. Hydroxyurea-induced synchrony of DNA replication in the Kinetoplastida. Exp. Cell Res. 214, 225–230.

Galindo, M., Sabaj, V., Espinoza, I., Toro, G.C., Bua, J., Grenet, J., et al., 2007. Chromosomal size conservation through the cell cycle supports karyotype stability in *Trypanosoma cruzi*. FEBS Lett. 581, 2022–2026.

Gaunt, M.W., Yeo, M., Frame, I.A., Stothard, J.R., Carrasco, H.J., Taylor, M.C., et al., 2003. Mechanism of genetic exchange in American trypanosomes. Nature (London) 421, 936–939.

Gibson, W.C., Miles, M.A., 1986. The karyotype and ploidy of *Trypanosoma cruzi*. EMBO J. 5, 1299–1305.

Gluenz, E., Taylor, M.C., Kelly, J.M., 2007. The *Trypanosoma cruzi* metacyclic-specific protein Met-III associates with the nucleolus and contains independent amino and carboxyl terminal targeting elements. Int. J. Parasitol. 37, 617–625.

Godoy, P.D., Nogueira-Junior, L.A., Paes, L.S., Cornejo, A., Martins, R.M., Silber, A.M., et al., 2009. Trypanosome prereplication machinery contains a single functional orc1/cdc6 protein, which is typical of archaea. Eukaryot. Cell 8, 1592–1603.

Gomes, N.M., Shay, J.W., Wright, W.E., 2010. Telomere biology in Metazoa. FEBS Lett. 584, 3741–3751.

Gomez, E.B., Kornblihtt, A.R., Tellez-Inon, M.T., 1998. Cloning of a cdc2-related protein kinase from *Trypanosoma cruzi* that interacts with mammalian cyclins. Mol. Biochem. Parasitol. 91, 337–351.

Gomez, E.B., Santori, M.I., Laria, S., Engel, J.C., Swindle, J., Eisen, H., et al., 2001. Characterization of the *Trypanosoma cruzi* Cdc2p-related protein kinase 1 and identification of three novel associating cyclins. Mol. Biochem. Parasitol. 113, 97–108.

Grewal, S.I., Jia, S., 2007. Heterochromatin revisited. Nat. Rev. Genet. 8, 35–46.

Gutiyama, L.M., da Cunha, J.P., Schenkman, S., 2008. Histone H1 of *Trypanosoma cruzi* is concentrated in the nucleolus region and disperses upon phosphorylation during progression to mitosis. Eukaryot. Cell 7, 560–568.

Hammarton, T.C., Clark, J., Douglas, F., Boshart, M., Mottram, J.C., 2003. Stage-specific differences in cell cycle control in *Trypanosoma brucei* revealed by RNA interference of a mitotic cyclin. J. Biol. Chem. 278, 22877–22886.

Hecker, H., Gander, E.S., 1985. The compaction pattern of the chromatin of trypanosomes. Biol. Cell 53, 199–208.

Hecker, H., Betschart, B., Bender, K., Burri, M., Schlimme, W., 1994. The chromatin of trypanosomes. Int. J. Parasitol. 24, 809–819.

Henriksson, J., Dujardin, J.C., Barnabe, C., Brisse, S., Timperman, G., Venegas, J., et al., 2002. Chromosomal size variation in *Trypanosoma cruzi* is mainly progressive and is evolutionarily informative. Parasitology 124, 277–286.

Hetzer, M.W., 2010. The nuclear envelope. Cold Spring Harb. Perspect. Biol. 2, a000539.

Hocine, S., Singer, R.H., Grunwald, D., 2010. RNA processing and export. Cold Spring Harb. Perspect. Biol. 2, a000752.

Hodo, H.G., Hatcher, F.M., 1986. Multiple DNA-dependent RNA polymerases in *Trypanosoma cruzi*. Mol. Biochem. Parasitol. 19, 77–81.

Horn, D., 2007. Introducing histone modification in trypanosomes. Trends Parasitol. 23, 239–242.

Ienne, S., Pedroso, A., Carmona, E.F.R., Briones, M.R., Zingales, B., 2010. Network genealogy of 195-bp satellite DNA supports the superimposed hybridization hypothesis of *Trypanosoma cruzi* evolutionary pattern. Infect. Genet. Evol. 10, 601–606.

Kasinsky, H.E., Lewis, J.D., Dacks, J.B., Ausio, J., 2001. Origin of H1 linker histones. FASEB J. 15, 34–42.

Kawashita, S.Y., Sanson, G.F., Fernandes, O., Zingales, B., Briones, M.R., 2001. Maximum-likelihood divergence date estimates based on rRNA gene sequences suggest two scenarios of *Trypanosoma cruzi* intraspecific evolution. Mol. Biol. Evol. 18, 2250–2259.

Kelly, S., Wickstead, B., Gull, K., 2005. An in silico analysis of trypanosomatid RNA polymerases: insights into their unusual transcription. Biochem. Soc. Trans. 33, 1435–1437.

Kim, D., Chiurillo, M.A., El-Sayed, N., Jones, K., Santos, M.R., Porcile, P.E., et al., 2005. Telomere and subtelomere of *Trypanosoma cruzi* chromosomes are enriched in (pseudo) genes of retrotransposon hot spot and trans-sialidase-like gene families: the origins of *T. cruzi* telomeres. Gene 346, 153–161.

Kramer, S., Kimblin, N.C., Carrington, M., 2010. Genome-wide in silico screen for CCCH-type zinc finger proteins of *Trypanosoma brucei*, Trypanosoma cruzi and Leishmania major. BMC Genomics 11, 283.

Lewis, M.D., Llewellyn, M.S., Gaunt, M.W., Yeo, M., Carrasco, H.J., Miles, M.A., 2009. Flow cytometric analysis and microsatellite genotyping reveal extensive DNA content variation in *Trypanosoma cruzi* populations and expose contrasts between natural and experimental hybrids. Int. J. Parasitol. 39, 1305–1317.

Lopez-Velazquez, G., Hernandez, R., Lopez-Villasenor, I., Reyes-Vivas, H., Segura-Valdez Mdc, L., Jimenez-Garcia, L.F., 2005. Electron microscopy analysis of the nucleolus of *Trypanosoma cruzi*. Microsc. Microanal. 11, 293–299.

Machado, C.R., Augusto-Pinto, L., McCulloch, R., Teixeira, S.M., 2006. DNA metabolism and genetic diversity in Trypanosomes. Mutat. Res. 612, 40–57.

Mandava, V., Fernandez, J.P., Deng, H., Janzen, C.J., Hake, S.B., Cross, G.A., 2007. Histone modifications in *Trypanosoma brucei*. Mol. Biochem. Parasitol. 156, 41–50.

Marques Porto, R., Amino, R., Elias, M.C., Faria, M., Schenkman, S., 2002. Histone H1 is phosphorylated in non-replicating and infective forms of *Trypanosoma cruzi*. Mol. Biochem. Parasitol. 119, 265–271.

McCarthy-Burke, C., Taylor, Z.A., Buck, G.A., 1989. Characterization of the spliced leader genes and transcripts in *Trypanosoma cruzi*. Gene 82, 177–189.

Mehta, G.D., Agarwal, M.P., Ghosh, S.K., 2010. Centromere identity: a challenge to be faced. Mol. Genet. Genomics 284, 75–94.

Munoz, D.P., Collins, K., 2004. Biochemical properties of *Trypanosoma cruzi* telomerase. Nucleic Acids Res. 32, 5214–5222.

Nardelli, S.C., Avila, A.R., Freund, A., Motta, M.C., Manhaes, L., de Jesus, T.C., et al., 2007. Small-subunit rRNA processome proteins are translationally regulated during differentiation of *Trypanosoma cruzi*. Eukaryot. Cell 6, 337–345.

Nardelli, S.C., da Cunha, J.P., Motta, M.C., Schenkman, S., 2009. Distinct acetylation of *Trypanosoma cruzi* histone H4 during cell cycle, parasite differentiation, and after DNA damage. Chromosoma 118, 487–499.

Nepomuceno-Mejia, T., Lara-Martinez, R., Cevallos, A.M., Lopez-Villasenor, I., Jimenez-Garcia, L.F., Hernandez, R., 2010. The *Trypanosoma cruzi* nucleolus: a morphometrical analysis of cultured epimastigotes in the exponential and stationary phases. FEMS Microbiol. Lett. 313, 41–46.

Nozaki, T., Dvorak, J.A., 1991. *Trypanosoma cruzi*: flow cytometric analysis of developmental stage differences in DNA. J. Protozool. 38, 234–243.

Nozaki, T., Dvorak, J.A., 1993. Intraspecific diversity in the response of *Trypanosoma cruzi* to environmental stress. J. Parasitol. 79, 451–454.

Nozaki, T., Engel, J.C., Dvorak, J.A., 1996. Cellular and molecular biological analyses of nifurtimox resistance in *Trypanosoma cruzi*. Am. J. Trop. Med. Hyg. 55, 111–117.

Nunes, L.R., Carvalho, M.R., Shakarian, A.M., Buck, G.A., 1997. The transcription promoter of the spliced leader gene from *Trypanosoma cruzi*. Gene 188, 157–168.

Obado, S.O., Bot, C., Nilsson, D., Andersson, B., Kelly, J.M., 2007. Repetitive DNA is associated with centromeric domains in *Trypanosoma brucei* but not *Trypanosoma cruzi*. Genome Biol. 8, R37.

Padilla-Mejia, N.E., Florencio-Martinez, L.E., Figueroa-Angulo, E.E., Manning-Cela, R.G., Hernandez-Rivas, R., Myler, P.J., et al., 2009. Gene organization and sequence analyses of transfer RNA genes in Trypanosomatid parasites. BMC Genomics 10, 232.

Pena, S.D., Machado, C.R., Macedo, A.M., 2009. *Trypanosoma cruzi*: ancestral genomes and population structure. Mem. Inst. Oswaldo Cruz 104 (Suppl. 1), 108–114.
Peterson, C.L., Laniel, M.A., 2004. Histones and histone modifications. Curr. Biol. 14, 546–551.
Piacenza, L., Alvarez, M.N., Peluffo, G., Radi, R., 2009. Fighting the oxidative assault: the *Trypanosoma cruzi* journey to infection. Curr. Opin. Microbiol. 12, 415–421.
Picchi, G.F., Ferreira, A.M., Souza, F.S., Lourenco, E.E., Arauco, P.R., Lorusso, A., et al., 2011. *Trypanosoma cruzi*: identification of DNA targets of the nuclear periphery coiled-coil protein TcNUP-1. Exp. Parasitol. 127, 147–152.
Raghuram, N., Carrero, G., Th'ng, J., Hendzel, M.J., 2009. Molecular dynamics of histone H1. Biochem. Cell Biol. 87, 189–206.
Ramirez, M.I., Yamauchi, L.M., de Freitas, L.H., Uemura, H., Schenkman, S., 2000. The use of the green fluorescent protein to monitor and improve transfection in *Trypanosoma cruzi*. Mol. Biochem. Parasitol. 111, 235–240.
Recinos, R.F., Kirchhoff, L.V., Donelson, J.E., 2001. Cell cycle expression of histone genes in *Trypanosoma cruzi*. Mol. Biochem. Parasitol. 113, 215–222.
Regis-da-Silva, C.G., Freitas, J.M., Passos-Silva, D.G., Furtado, C., Augusto-Pinto, L., Pereira, M.T., et al., 2006. Characterization of the *Trypanosoma cruzi* Rad51 gene and its role in recombination events associated with the parasite resistance to ionizing radiation. Mol. Biochem. Parasitol. 149, 191–200.
Respuela, P., Ferella, M., Rada-Iglesias, A., Aslund, L., 2008. Histone acetylation and methylation at sites initiating divergent polycistronic transcription in *Trypanosoma cruzi*. J. Biol. Chem. 283, 15884–15892.
Santori, M.I., Laria, S., Gomez, E.B., Espinosa, I., Galanti, N., Tellez-Inon, M.T., 2002. Evidence for CRK3 participation in the cell division cycle of *Trypanosoma cruzi*. Mol. Biochem. Parasitol. 121, 225–232.
Siegel, T.N., Hekstra, D.R., Kemp, L.E., Figueiredo, L.M., Lowell, J.E., Fenyo, D., et al., 2009. Four histone variants mark the boundaries of polycistronic transcription units in *Trypanosoma brucei*. Genes Dev. 23, 1063–1076.
Sirri, V., Urcuqui-Inchima, S., Roussel, P., Hernandez-Verdun, D., 2008. Nucleolus: the fascinating nuclear body. Histochem. Cell Biol. 129, 13–31.
Smith, J.L., Levin, J.R., Ingles, C.J., Agabian, N., 1989. In trypanosomes the homolog of the largest subunit of RNA polymerase II is encoded by two genes and has a highly unusual C-terminal domain structure. Cell 56, 815–827.
Solari, A.J., 1995. Mitosis and genome partition in trypanosomes. Biocell 19, 65–84.
Souza, W., 2009. Structural organization of *Trypanosoma cruzi*. Mem. Inst. Oswaldo Cruz 104 (Suppl. 1), 89–100.
Spadiliero, B., Nicolini, C., Mascetti, G., Henriquez, D., Vergani, L., 2002. Chromatin of *Trypanosoma cruzi*: in situ analysis revealed its unusual structure and nuclear organization. J. Cell. Biochem. 85, 798–808.
Spector, D.L., Lamond, A.I., 2010. Nuclear speckles. Cold Spring Harb. Perspect. Biol. 2, a000646.
Strahl, B.D., Allis, C.D., 2000. The language of covalent histone modifications. Nature (London) 403, 41–45.
Stros, M., 2010. HMGB proteins: interactions with DNA and chromatin. Biochim. Biophys. Acta 1799, 101–113.
Taverna, S.D., Li, H., Ruthenburg, A.J., Allis, C.D., Patel, D.J., 2007. How chromatin-binding modules interpret histone modifications: lessons from professional pocket pickers. Nat. Struct. Mol. Biol. 14, 1025–1040.
Thomas, S., Westenberger, S.J., Campbell, D.A., Sturm, N.R., 2005. Intragenomic spliced leader RNA array analysis of kinetoplastids reveals unexpected transcribed region diversity in *Trypanosoma cruzi*. Gene 352, 100–108.

Toro, G.C., Galanti, N., 1988. H1 histone and histone variants in *Trypanosoma cruzi*. Exp. Cell Res. 174, 16–24.

Vickerman, K., Preston, T.M., 1970. Spindle microtubules in the dividing nuclei of trypanosomes. J. Cell Sci. 6, 365–383.

Villanova, G.V., Nardelli, S.C., Cribb, P., Magdaleno, A., Silber, A.M., Motta, M.C., et al., 2009. *Trypanosoma cruzi* bromodomain factor 2 (BDF2) binds to acetylated histones and is accumulated after UV irradiation. Int. J. Parasitol. 39, 665–673.

Weatherly, D.B., Boehlke, C., Tarleton, R.L., 2009. Chromosome level assembly of the hybrid *Trypanosoma cruzi* genome. BMC Genomics 10, 255.

Westergaard, G.G., Bercovich, N., Reinert, M.D., Vazquez, M.P., 2010. Analysis of a nuclear localization signal in the p14 splicing factor in *Trypanosoma cruzi*. Int. J. Parasitol. 40, 1029–1035.

Woodcock, C.L., Ghosh, R.P., 2010. Chromatin higher-order structure and dynamics. Cold Spring Harb. Perspect. Biol. 2, a000596.

Woodcock, C.L., Skoultchi, A.I., Fan, Y., 2006. Role of linker histone in chromatin structure and function: H1 stoichiometry and nucleosome repeat length. Chromosome Res. 14, 17–25.

CHAPTER 13

Aspects of *Trypanosoma cruzi* Stage Differentiation

Samuel Goldenberg and **Andrea Rodrigues Ávila**

Contents

Abstract

Trypanosoma cruzi alternates between different morphological and functional types during its life cycle. Since the discovery of this parasite at the beginning of the twentieth century, efforts have been made to determine the basis of its pathogenesis in the course of Chagas disease and its biochemical constituents. There has also been work to develop tools and strategies for prophylaxis of the important disease caused by these parasites which affects millions of people in Latin America. The identification of axenic conditions allowing *T. cruzi* growth and differentiation has led to the identification and characterization of stage-specific antigens as well as a better characterization of the biological properties and biochemical particularities of each individual developmental stage. The recent availability of genomic data should pave the way to new progress in our knowledge of the biology and pathogenesis of *T. cruzi*.

Instituto Carlos Chagas, ICC—Fiocruz-PR, Rua Prof. Algacyr Munhoz Mader, Curitiba, PR, Brazil

Advances in Parasitology, Volume 75
ISSN 0065-308X, DOI: 10.1016/B978-0-12-385863-4.00013-7

This review addresses the differentiation and major stage-specific antigens of *T. cruzi* and attempts to describe the complexity of the parasite and of the disease it causes.

13.1. INTRODUCTION

It is remarkable that Carlos Chagas, with the limited tools available more than 100 years ago, was able to describe, in a short period of time and so precisely, the cycle of *Trypanosoma cruzi* in nature and the disease that this parasite causes (Chagas, 1909). Although the nomenclature at that time was different from that we now use, his drawings show with accuracy the major developmental stages of the parasite: epimastigotes, trypomastigotes and amastigotes.

The developmental stages of *T. cruzi* alternate between non-infective (replicative) and infective forms (non-replicative). Blood trypomastigotes ingested by the triatomine invertebrate vector transform into epimastigotes in the stomach and then they multiply repeatedly along the digestive tract. At the posterior end of the intestine, epimastigotes adhere to the rectal cuticle and they transform into metacyclic trypomastigotes (metacyclogenesis) that are released in the excreta of the insect upon feeding on blood of the mammalian host. These are infective forms that penetrate mammalian host cells where they transform into amastigotes (amastigogenesis) that replicate within the vertebrate host cells. After several cycles of replication, the cells are lysed and the parasites are thereby released into the blood as blood trypomastigotes that will either infect new cells or be ingested by the triatomine vector and thus complete the cycle (comprehensive reviews by De Souza, 2002 and de Souza et al., 2010).

Most work investigating stage differentiation has focused on the metacyclogenesis process (Bonaldo et al., 1988; Contreras et al., 1985b; Krieger et al., 1999). This is mainly due to the availability of well-established axenic culture conditions that allow epimastigotes to be obtained (Camargo, 1964; Sullivan, 1982). The transformation of these forms into metacyclic trypomastigotes can even occur spontaneously upon prolonged incubation in growth media. The study of this differentiation step has been greatly facilitated by the availability of media that induce and support the transformation of epimastigotes into metacyclic trypomastigotes. More details about factors involved into this differentiation process are described below.

13.2. *TRYPANOSOMA CRUZI* DIFFERENTIATION

Most studies concerning the requirements and factors affecting *T. cruzi* differentiation focused on the metacyclogenesis process due to the availability of axenic culture conditions, as described above. There are several factors involved in triggering *T. cruzi* metacyclogenesis. The availability of nutrients is of great importance both within the host and under *in vitro* conditions. An early observation was that, in the particular case of the metacyclogenesis process, impoverishment of the medium stimulates the transformation of epimastigotes into metacyclic trypomastigotes (Contreras et al., 1985a,b; Sullivan, 1982). This is one of the reasons why spontaneous metacyclic trypomastigotes are found in late stationary phase cultures (Camargo, 1964). *T. cruzi* metabolism is primarily organized around the fast consumption of glucose, but the process does not go to completion and glucose is not fully metabolized (Cazzulo, 1992; Urbina, 1994). Upon carbohydrate exhaustion, the parasites fulfil their energy requirements by consuming amino acids (Cazzulo, 1984, 1994). The amino acids glutamic acid and proline are particularly important metabolites for energy production (Sylvester and Krassner, 1976); note that proline is the most abundant amino acid in triatomine hemolymph (Barrett, 1974) and it might have a role in potentiating the infectivity of metacyclic trypomastigotes (Martins et al., 2009). Further, epimastigote forms have been described during the intracellular differentiation of amastigotes into trypomastigotes (Almeida-de-Faria et al., 1999), and proline seems to make a major contribution to this process (Tonelli et al., 2004). It is important also to note that *T. cruzi* metacyclogenesis can occur under chemically defined conditions using proline and glucose as the sole carbon sources (Contreras et al., 1985b). Thus, there is no doubt that amino acid metabolism and, in particular, that of proline is important for *T. cruzi* energy production. This exploitation of amino acids for energy production might indicate that carbohydrates are scarce in the parasite's environment and also that environmental energy source availability and, in particular, nutritional stress may be a differentiation trigger for *T. cruzi*.

T. cruzi does not store carbohydrates for energy production and uses proteins and lipids as energy storage macromolecules. These molecules are stored in organelles named reservosomes which were first described in epimastigote forms (Figueiredo et al., 2004; Soares et al., 1992). These are large membrane-bound organelles found at the posterior end of epimastigotes and are abundant in these forms due to their endocytic activity. For some time, they were believed to be epimastigote-specific organelles (Figueiredo et al., 2004), but recent analysis has suggested that they may also exist in the other developmental stages, although with different sizes and shapes (Sant'Anna et al., 2008). A stereological study of reservosomes in the course of *T. cruzi* metacyclogenesis in chemically defined media revealed that these organelles decrease in volume during this process, probably due to the consumption of the proteins and lipids stored therein (Soares et al., 1989).

One of the pioneers in the field of Chagas disease (Dias, 1934) noted that in addition to energy requirements, the adhesion of epimastigotes is also necessary during *T. cruzi* metacyclogenesis. Indeed, studies using *in vitro* differentiation conditions showed that cell–substrate adhesion is necessary, though not sufficient, for the transformation of epimastigotes into metacyclic trypomastigotes (Bonaldo et al., 1988; Contreras et al., 1985a,b). Interestingly, a similar observation has been reported for metacyclogenesis within the triatomine vector: epimastigotes attach to the epithelium of the insect rectal gland and are released when they transform into metacyclic trypomastigotes (Boker and Schaub, 1984; Zeledon et al., 1984). The details of the mechanism by which epimastigote adhesion contributes to differentiation remain to be elucidated; however, mutations of Rho-family small GTPase proteins affect the progression of *T. cruzi* metacyclogenesis (de Melo et al., 2004), so the mechanism may involve cell signalling or cytoskeleton dynamics.

It has also been demonstrated that adhesion of epimastigotes to the substrate under *in vitro* differentiating conditions is triggered by nutritional stress (Bonaldo et al., 1988; Figueiredo et al., 2000). The observations that a nutritional stress stimulates the induction of *T. cruzi* metacyclogenesis and that differentiating cells adhere to a substrate prior to differentiation suggest that *T. cruzi* differentiation might be similar to the differentiation of some fungi (Kriebel and Parent, 2004; Strmecki et al., 2005) in which cAMP is a key signalling molecule involved in the induction of differentiation. Consequently, the role of cAMP in *T. cruzi* differentiation was investigated: an increase in the intracellular level of cAMP is accompanied by an increase in the transformation of epimastigotes into metacyclic trypomastigotes (Gonzales-Perdomo et al., 1988; Rangel-Aldao et al., 1988). Studies with agonists and antagonists of cAMP confirmed the involvement of this second messenger in the induction of *T. cruzi* differentiation and also implicated a protein kinase A (PKA; Gonzales-Perdomo et al., 1988). Indeed, blocking PKA results in parasite death demonstrating the importance of this enzyme in the *T. cruzi* life cycle (Bao et al., 2008). Signalling pathways and their role in *T. cruzi* biology constitute a vast field only recently addressed (Burleigh and Woosley, 2002).

It is important to remember that the various developmental stages of *T. cruzi* present distinct biological properties and morphological features (De Souza, 2002), as well as characteristic biochemical components (de Lederkremer and Agusti, 2009; Elias et al., 2009; Previato et al., 2004). For example, the differences in membrane fluidity at the various developmental stages are very likely related to their different functional and biological properties (Bronia et al., 1986; Esteves et al., 1989; Harrington et al., 2010). The adhesion phenomenon has also been widely described in trypomastigotes (Alves and Colli, 2007, 2008; Giordano et al., 1994; Katzin and Colli, 1983; Ouaissi et al., 1992), but the process is related to the invasion of host cells rather than to differentiation. It has been clearly established that the surface of the parasites contains specific antigens and presents a particular composition in terms of carbohydrates and glycolipids. Most of those surface factors, mainly stage-specific antigens including glycoproteins (GPs), display adhesion properties (Alves and Colli, 2007; de Souza et al., 2010).

13.3. STAGE-SPECIFIC ANTIGENS

Several groups have focused on the search for, and characterization of, *T. cruzi* stage-specific antigens. Such antigens are potential candidates for the development of vaccines (in the case of infective-form antigens), and some may serve as models for investigating the mechanisms involved in the regulation of gene expression or in *T. cruzi* stage-specific properties, such as the ability of trypomastigotes to resist complement-mediated lysis (Norris et al., 1991, 1997). We will briefly describe below the more thoroughly studied gene families that are stage-specifically expressed. Most of them encode surface antigens and are thought to mediate parasite–host interactions.

13.3.1. *Trans*-sialidases

T. cruzi trans-sialidases (TSs; Colli, 1993; Schenkman et al., 1991, 1992) are encoded by a family of genes containing a conserved region, which corresponds to the catalytic and amino-terminal domains of the enzyme. The genes are organized as tandem repeats (Dallagiovanna et al., 1996; Egima et al., 1996), and their expression is post-transcriptionally regulated (Abuin et al., 1999; Holetz et al., 2010; Jager et al., 2008). Members of the TS superfamily are expressed in epimastigotes, but the 3′-ends of the mRNAs differ between epimastigotes and trypomastigotes, although they are conserved within each gene family (Jager et al., 2008); in addition, the epimastigote TS mRNAs do not have the repeated portion of the trypomastigote TS (Briones et al., 1995). The TS enzymes have unique features, promoting both acquisition and the removal of sialic acid from host tissues (Schenkman et al., 1992). The TS family comprises several subfamilies that share a characteristic sialidase domain at their amino termini; however, they are functionally distinct (Cross and Takle, 1993). TS and sialic acid acceptors are essential for parasite survival in their host because trypanosomes are unable to synthesize sialic acid (Schenkman et al., 1994). In *T. cruzi*, surface sialylation is central to the parasite–host cell adhesion/invasion mechanism (Schenkman and Eichinger, 1993; Schenkman et al., 1993). There are various lines of evidence both for a direct role of TS as a virulence factor in animal pathogenesis (Belen Carrillo et al., 2000) and for TS being responsible for differences of infectivity between *T. cruzi* isolates (Risso et al., 2004). Interestingly, TS is more strongly expressed in cell-derived trypomastigotes than in metacyclic trypomastigotes, and this is responsible for the earlier exit of the cell-derived form from the parasitophorous vacuole to the cytoplasm and their subsequent differentiation into amastigotes (Rubin-de-Celis et al., 2006). Both the absence of TS in mammals and its role in *T. cruzi* infectivity validate this enzyme as a potential target for drugs to treat Chagas disease (Carvalho et al., 2010; Neres et al., 2008). In this sense, the determination of the crystal structure of TS was a significant step forward (Buschiazzo et al., 2002) because this provides a basis for designing new drugs.

13.3.2. Surface GPs

Metacyclic trypomastigotes, which establish the initial parasite–host cell interaction when triatomines feed on blood, express two major stage-specific Glycosylphosphatidylinositol (GPI)-anchored GPs, namely GP90 (Teixeira and Yoshida, 1986) and GP82 (Araya et al., 1994), which have no counterparts in bloodstream trypomastigotes. Proteomic analysis, using fractions rich in GPI-anchored and other membrane proteins from insect developmental stages of *T. cruzi*, confirmed that, unlike the non-infective proliferative epimastigote forms, the infective non-proliferative metacyclic trypomastigote forms express a large repertoire of surface GPs including GP90 and GP82. These GPs are involved in adhesion and invasion of host cells. This study revealed stage-specific protein profiles that appear to be related to the biology of each insect-derived *T. cruzi* developmental form (Cordero et al., 2009).

13.3.2.1. GP82

Antiserum raised against a recombinant polypeptide recognized a 82-kDa GP in metacyclic trypomastigotes, without any detectable reaction against amastigotes, epimastigotes or tissue culture-derived trypomastigotes (Araya et al., 1994). Thus, this GP, named GP82, is specifically expressed by metacyclic trypomastigotes. Several genes encoding GP82 have been found. Three subfamilies of gp82 were detected in the genome of *T. cruzi*, and they seem to be equally transcribed into mRNA in a stage-specific manner (Songthamwat et al., 2007). The accumulation of transcripts in metacyclic forms is a consequence of post-transcriptional mechanisms, and indeed, transcription also occurs in epimastigotes in which this antigen is not expressed (Gentil et al., 2009). Interestingly, investigations of *in vivo* metacyclogenesis show that as epimastigotes transform into metacyclic trypomastigotes, GP82 appears on the parasite surface and a coordinated mechanism links stabilization of GP82 mRNA and its translation (Cordero et al., 2009).

The biological role of this antigen has been studied, and the portion of GP82 required for mammalian cell attachment and invasion has been mapped to the central domain of the molecule (Manque et al., 2000; Santori et al., 1996). This GP is necessary but not sufficient for cell infection (Manque et al., 2003) and early studies demonstrated that it triggers signal transduction pathways that lead to intracellular calcium mobilization (Ruiz et al., 1998), an essential event for *T. cruzi* internalization (Burleigh and Andrews, 1998; Moreno et al., 1994; Tardieux et al., 1994). Cell invasion assays indicate that GP82 is involved in mediating the interaction between metacyclic trypomastigotes and gastric mucin, and in the penetration of epithelial cells during oral infection (Neira et al., 2003). More recently, it was confirmed that interaction with gastric mucin during oral infection by *T. cruzi* is mediated by GP82 and this may direct the parasites to stomach mucosal epithelium (Staquicini et al., 2010). By virtue of its role in parasite infectivity, GP82 has been tested as a vaccine candidate: following intranasal vaccination of mice, it induced protective immune responses against mucosal *T. cruzi* challenge (Eickhoff et al., 2010).

13.3.2.2. GP90

Data about GPs of 90 kDa related to *T. cruzi* stage-specific antigens were among the first to be described (Snary and Hudson, 1979). GP90 was found to be expressed exclusively by metacyclic trypomastigotes (Franco et al., 1993). This GP is encoded by a large gene family with more than 200 members sharing extensive sequence similarity (do Carmo et al., 2002). Interestingly, GP90 is differentially expressed in various *T. cruzi* strains (Ruiz et al., 1998), and when the expression of GP90 is specifically reduced, the ability of the parasite to invade host cells is significantly increased (Malaga and Yoshida, 2001). In the case of experimental oral infections, it was observed that *T. cruzi* strains expressing high GP90 levels invade cells poorly *in vitro* (Yoshida, 2009) and this molecule can be considered a down-modulator of *T. cruzi* infection *in vivo* (Cortez et al., 2006).

13.3.2.3. GP85/TS

Trypomastigotes of *T. cruzi* specifically express a set of surface GPs known, collectively, as Tc-85/TS (Alves and Colli, 2008). They form a population of heterogeneous GPI-anchored surface GPs with similar molecular masses but with different electric charges (Andrews et al., 1984; Katzin and Colli, 1983). The cloning and characterization of one member of the Tc-85 family led to the interesting hypothesis that several members of this superfamily might possess the capacity to adhere to various receptor molecules either located on the cell surface or belonging to components of the extracellular matrix (Giordano et al., 1994, 1999;

Velge et al., 1988). Studies of genes of this family demonstrated that their expression correlates with a virulent phenotype (Weston et al., 1999b). More recently, it was demonstrated that the peptide motif FLY (Magdesian et al., 2007; Tonelli et al., 2010b), common to all gp85/TS family members, interacts with the endothelium from different organs, but with significantly higher avidity for the heart vasculature (Tonelli et al., 2010a). This work also provided evidence that intermediate filaments in general might be involved in cell invasion by *T. cruzi* and tissue homing. In addition, various findings suggest that FLY facilitates *in vivo* infection by *T. cruzi* and cooperates with other factors to improve parasite survival to such an extent that it may influence the progression of Chagas disease (Tonelli et al., 2010b).

13.3.3. Mucin-like GPs

Mucin-like GPs are an important family of *T. cruzi* proteins (Tc-MUC) involved in incorporation of host-derived sialic acid transferred by TSs. They form a group of highly glycosylated GPI-anchored proteins rich in threonine, serine and proline residues and are produced in large amounts. They were first identified in epimastigotes (Alves and Colli, 1975), but their expression has been described in all developmental stages, although with different composition in terms of polypeptide sequence and GPI structure (see reviews Acosta-Serrano et al., 2001; Buscaglia et al., 2006; Schenkman et al., 1994). Tc-MUC genes account for at least 1% of the *T. cruzi* genome, although up to 25% of these genes are pseudogenes (El-Sayed et al., 2005).

The sequencing of the *T. cruzi* genome allowed the identification of a novel large multigene family corresponding to ~6% of the parasite's diploid genome. These genes encode polypeptides named mucin-associated surface proteins (MASPs) due to the clustering of the genes with genes encoding Tc-MUC and other surface protein families (Bartholomeu et al., 2009).

Two major groups of mucin-like molecules have been identified in *T. cruzi*. The GPs in the first group have an apparent molecular mass of 35–50 kDa and are produced by the parasite forms found in the insect vector (epimastigote and metacyclic trypomastigote; Mortara et al., 1992). The GPs in the second group are diverse in size (80–200 kDa) and are produced by cell-derived trypomastigotes in mammals (Almeida et al., 1994; Buscaglia et al., 2004). Metacyclic trypomastigote mucins trigger calcium mobilization in the host cell (Ruiz et al., 1998) and antibodies against metacyclic mucins inhibit cell invasion (Ruiz et al., 1993). Thus, Tc-MUC play an important role in the mechanisms leading to *T. cruzi* infection. In addition, mucins from cell-derived trypomastigotes are very probably involved in the resistance of the parasite to complement-mediated lysis (Tomlinson et al., 1992) and in the attachment to, and invasion of, mammal host cells by trypomastigotes (Schenkman et al., 1991). More detailed discussions of mucin-like proteins and their role in the mechanisms of parasite invasion and evasion from the host immune response are presented in other chapters of this issue. However, note that the GPI composition and polypeptide sequences are characteristic of each developmental stage indicating that the dynamics of the surface coat change as *T. cruzi* differentiates from one stage to another.

13.4. PROTEINASES AND DIFFERENTIATION

Proteinases are another category of stage-specific factors relevant to differentiation of, and invasion by, the parasite; they were detected in *T. cruzi* extracts in early studies (Itow and Camargo, 1977). *T. cruzi* is very rich in various classes of proteinases (Bastos et al., 2005; Burleigh et al., 1997; Caler et al., 1998; Cazzulo, 2002; Cuevas et al., 2003; da Silva-Lopez et al., 2008; Kosec et al., 2006; Lowndes et al., 1996; Pinho et al., 2009; Roberts et al., 1990; Santana et al., 1997), with a predominance of the cysteine proteinase cruzipain (Duschak and Couto, 2009) which will be discussed below in more detail. Inhibitors of individual classes of proteinases block *T. cruzi* differentiation (Bonaldo et al., 1991; Franke de Cazzulo et al., 1994). Interestingly, the transformation of trypomastigotes into amastigotes (Gonzalez et al., 1996) and the transformation of epimastigotes into metacyclic trypomastigotes (Cardoso et al., 2008) are blocked by proteasome inhibitors. This indicates that not only individual proteinases but also large proteolytic complexes are important for *T. cruzi* differentiation.

Cruzipain is the major cysteine proteinase of *T. cruzi* epimastigotes (Cazzulo et al., 1990, 1997; Duschak and Couto, 2009). The first evidence of its enzymatic activity was provided by analysis of proteinase activity in different forms of the parasite (Campetella et al., 1990). It was initially described as an antigen important for parasite infection and characterized as a GP (Campetella et al., 1992; Eakin et al., 1992; Murta et al., 1990). It was also characterized as an active cysteine proteinase present in epimastigotes and shown to be developmentally regulated. Its expression increases upon adhesion of epimastigotes prior to differentiation into metacyclic trypomastigotes (Bonaldo et al., 1991), implicating it in the metacyclogenesis process. Immunocytochemical analyses demonstrated that cruzipain is located in lysosomes of epimastigotes but that it is also present on the surface of epimastigotes and amastigote–trypomastigote transitional forms (Souto-Padron et al., 1990). Cruzipain is encoded by a large number of tandemly arranged genes on different chromosomes of several parasite isolates (Campetella et al., 1992). Analysis of diverse *T. cruzi* isolates showed highly heterogeneous profiles of surface cruzipain molecules (Fampa et al., 2010), reflecting polymorphisms of the GP (Martinez et al., 1998). This heterogeneity may have a role in the mechanisms of parasite evasion from the host immune response. Interestingly, isolates that express higher levels of surface cruzipain also display elevated levels of metacyclogenesis *in vitro* (Fampa et al., 2010), in agreement with previous results showing that overexpression of cruzipain resulted in elevated metacyclogenesis rates (Tomas et al., 1997).

The cruzipain genes are transcribed as a 1.8-kb transcript which is constitutively expressed throughout the parasite life cycle. Interestingly, the protein abundance and consequently the enzymatic activity are four to five times higher in the insect epimastigote stage than in the trypomastigote and amastigote stages (Hanke et al., 1996). Accordingly, it has been suggested that the developmental regulation of cruzipain expression is likely to be mostly translational and/or post-translational (Tomas and Kelly, 1996).

Inhibitors of this cruzipain impair host cell invasion and arrest *in vitro* intracellular development (Meirelles et al., 1992) revealing that cruzipain is important for the intracellular development of the parasite. *T. cruzi* metacyclogenesis is also inhibited by cysteine proteinase inhibitors (Bonaldo et al., 1991), suggesting that in addition to rendering amino acids available for energy production, it might have a functional role in *T. cruzi* differentiation. Because of its potential biological importance, cruzipain is considered a potential target for chemotherapy to treat Chagas disease (Cazzulo, 2002; Jose Cazzulo et al., 2001; Urbina, 2010). The crystallographic structure of this enzyme in the presence of inhibitors has been resolved (McGrath et al., 1995), and there is experimental evidence that cysteine proteinase inhibitors reduce parasitemia in cell culture with no adverse effect on mammalian cells (Meirelles et al., 1992). Interestingly, cruzipain has a natural inhibitor (chagasin) that is thought to control its activity *in vivo* (Figueiredo da Silva et al., 2007; Monteiro et al., 2001; Santos et al., 2005; Scharfstein and Lima, 2008). Irreversible inhibitors of cruzipain (peptidyl diazomethylketones, peptidyl fluoromethylketones, peptidyl vinyl sulphones) have been tested and were able to block the differentiation and in some cases kill the parasite (Scharfstein and Lima, 2008). Attempts by different groups to develop efficient inhibitors of cruzipain are underway (Beaulieu et al., 2010; McKerrow et al., 2009; Urbina, 2010).

13.5. STAGE-SPECIFIC GENE EXPRESSION

In addition to the work on stage-specific factors, several groups have also been investigating the mechanisms responsible for the modulation of gene expression during *T. cruzi* differentiation. It is now generally accepted that differential mRNA stability plays a major role in modulating gene expression in *T. cruzi* (Bartholomeu et al., 2002; Coughlin et al., 2000; da Silva et al., 2006; Gentil et al., 2009; Teixeira et al., 1999; Yamada-Ogatta et al., 2004). *T. cruzi* genes are organized and transcribed as polycistronic units, although genes are not necessarily clustered according to their cell-cycle expression. The regulation of the stability and translation of some mRNAs involves elements in their untranslated regions (UTR; Teixeira and daRocha, 2003). This is the case of amastin: steady-state mRNA levels are 68 times higher in amastigotes than in epimastigotes (Teixeira et al., 1995) due to a *cis*-element in the 3′-UTR responsible for amastin mRNA up regulation (Coughlin et al., 2000). A similar situation has been described for the gene encoding the surface antigen FL-160: the steady-state levels of the mRNA are almost 100 times higher in trypomastigotes than in epimastigotes, although mRNA transcription occurs at the same rate during the two stages (Weston et al., 1999a). There is recent data indicating that sequences located within the 3′-UTR and coding region of the α-tubulin gene are involved in transcript stability (da Silva et al., 2006). Some elements, consisting of AU-rich sequences, improve translational efficiency in addition to mRNA stability by interacting with specific RNA binding proteins (RBP; Di Noia et al., 2000; D'Orso and Frasch, 2001). Several genes potentially encoding RBPs (De Gaudenzi et al., 2005) have been identified by *in silico* analysis of the *T. cruzi* genome database (El-Sayed et al., 2005), and their functional characterization should provide important clues for the understanding of the mechanisms involved in the regulation of gene expression in *T. cruzi*.

Evidence supporting the existence of proteins specifically interacting with mRNAs in *T. cruzi*, forming mRNP complexes that stabilize non-translated mRNAs, have been provided by studies showing the presence of RNA not associated with polysomes that could be actively translated in a rabbit reticulocyte *in vitro* system after protein extraction (Goldenberg et al., 1985). The presence of stable non-translated mRNAs was further confirmed by Northern blot analysis of polysomal and total RNA probed with stage-specific genes (Avila et al., 2001; Yamada-Ogatta et al., 2004). These mRNP complexes are defined according to their function or the presence of specific proteins. As they are transported out from the nucleus, mRNPs are either translated (polysomal mRNPs) or sequestered to the cytoplasm where they are either degraded or stored as cytoplasmic-free mRNP. These free mRNPs then form microscopic foci, which may differ in function depending on the proteins associated or on the stimuli during their creation. The untranslated mRNAs assemble as P bodies, which are generally associated with mRNA degradation (Parker and Sheth, 2007), but can also form cytoplasmic granules known as stress granules (Anderson and Kedersha, 2008, 2009). Ribonomic analysis indicates that the mRNAs encoding several metacyclic trypomastigote stage-specific proteins are found in the epimastigote cytoplasm where they are associated with proteins characteristic of RNA granules (Holetz et al., 2010). The presence of RNP granules in *T. cruzi* is well documented (Cassola et al., 2007; Holetz et al., 2007). The use of functional genomics tools should improve our understanding of the mechanisms by which gene expression is regulated in *T. cruzi*.

13.6. CONCLUSION

It is very likely that the human disease caused by *T. cruzi*, first described 100 years ago, will be controlled within the next 100 years. It is conceivable that progress in both our knowledge of the parasite and social policies in the endemic countries will result in effective eradication of the disease by vector transmission control, better diagnostics of transfused blood or even development of a safe and reliable prophylaxis. Work based on holistic approaches, such as systems biology, should allow a better comprehension of *T. cruzi* differentiation, the function of stage-specific genes and how the parasites change their metabolism and surface constituents to face new environmental conditions. Notwithstanding all the progress made over the last 100 years, current and future investigations have some way to go to elucidate the fascinating natural history of this primitive unicellular organism with a complexity level never anticipated by Carlos Chagas when he first described *T. cruzi*.

REFERENCES

Abuin, G., Freitas-Junior, L.H., Colli, W., Alves, M.J., Schenkman, S., 1999. Expression of trans-sialidase and 85-kDa glycoprotein genes in *Trypanosoma cruzi* is differentially regulated at the post-transcriptional level by labile protein factors. J. Biol. Chem. 274, 13041–13047.

Acosta-Serrano, A., Almeida, I.C., Freitas-Junior, L.H., Yoshida, N., Schenkman, S., 2001. The mucin-like glycoprotein super-family of *Trypanosoma cruzi*: structure and biological roles. Mol. Biochem. Parasitol. 114, 143–150.

Almeida, I.C., Ferguson, M.A., Schenkman, S., Travassos, L.R., 1994. GPI-anchored glycoconjugates from *Trypanosoma cruzi* trypomastigotes are recognized by lytic anti-alpha-galactosyl antibodies isolated from patients with chronic Chagas' disease. Braz. J. Med. Biol. Res. 27, 443–447.

Almeida-de-Faria, M., Freymuller, E., Colli, W., Alves, M.J., 1999. *Trypanosoma cruzi*: characterization of an intracellular epimastigote-like form. Exp. Parasitol. 92, 263–274.

Alves, M.J., Colli, W., 1975. Glycoproteins from *Trypanosoma cruzi*: partial purification by gel chromatography. FEBS Lett. 52, 188–190.

Alves, M.J., Colli, W., 2007. *Trypanosoma cruzi*: adhesion to the host cell and intracellular survival. IUBMB Life 59, 274–279.

Alves, M.J., Colli, W., 2008. Role of the gp85/trans-sialidase superfamily of glycoproteins in the interaction of *Trypanosoma cruzi* with host structures. Subcell. Biochem. 47, 58–69.

Anderson, P., Kedersha, N., 2008. Stress granules: the Tao of RNA triage. Trends Biochem. Sci. 33, 141–150.

Anderson, P., Kedersha, N., 2009. RNA granules: post-transcriptional and epigenetic modulators of gene expression. Nat. Rev. Mol. Cell Biol. 10, 430–436.

Andrews, N.W., Katzin, A.M., Colli, W., 1984. Mapping of surface glycoproteins of Trypanosoma cruzi by two-dimensional electrophoresis. A correlation with the cell invasion capacity. Eur. J. Biochem. 140, 599–604.

Araya, J.E., Cano, M.I., Yoshida, N., da-Silveira, J.F., 1994. Cloning and characterization of a gene for the stage-specific 82-kDa surface antigen of metacyclic trypomastigotes of *Trypanosoma cruzi*. Mol. Biochem. Parasitol. 65, 161–169.

Avila, A.R., Yamada-Ogatta, S.F., da Silva Monteiro, V., Krieger, M.A., Nakamura, C.V., de Souza, W., et al., 2001. Cloning and characterization of the metacyclogenin gene, which is specifically expressed during *Trypanosoma cruzi* metacyclogenesis. Mol. Biochem. Parasitol. 117, 169–177.

Bao, Y., Weiss, L.M., Braunstein, V.L., Huang, H., 2008. Role of protein kinase A in *Trypanosoma cruzi*. Infect. Immun. 76, 4757–4763.

Barrett, F.M., 1974. Changes in the concentration of free amino acids in the haemolymph of Rhodnius prolixus during the fifth instar. Comp. Biochem. Physiol. B 48, 241–250.

Bartholomeu, D.C., Silva, R.A., Galvao, L.M., el-Sayed, N.M., Donelson, J.E., Teixeira, S.M., 2002. *Trypanosoma cruzi*: RNA structure and post-transcriptional control of tubulin gene expression. Exp. Parasitol. 102, 123–133.

Bartholomeu, D.C., Cerqueira, G.C., Leao, A.C., daRocha, W.D., Pais, F.S., Macedo, C., et al., 2009. Genomic organization and expression profile of the mucin-associated surface protein (masp) family of the human pathogen *Trypanosoma cruzi*. Nucleic Acids Res. 37, 3407–3417.

Bastos, I.M., Grellier, P., Martins, N.F., Cadavid-Restrepo, G., de Souza-Ault, M.R., Augustyns, K., et al., 2005. Molecular, functional and structural properties of the prolyl oligopeptidase of *Trypanosoma cruzi* (POP Tc80), which is required for parasite entry into mammalian cells. Biochem. J. 388, 29–38.

Beaulieu, C., Isabel, E., Fortier, A., Masse, F., Mellon, C., Methot, N., et al., 2010. Identification of potent and reversible cruzipain inhibitors for the treatment of Chagas disease. Bioorg. Med. Chem. Lett. 20, 7444–7449.

Belen Carrillo, M., Gao, W., Herrera, M., Alroy, J., Moore, J.B., Beverley, S.M., et al., 2000. Heterologous expression of *Trypanosoma cruzi* trans-sialidase in Leishmania major enhances virulence. Infect. Immun. 68, 2728–2734.

Boker, C.A., Schaub, G.A., 1984. Scanning electron microscopic studies of *Trypanosoma cruzi* in the rectum of its vector Triatoma infestans. Z. Parasitenkd. 70, 459–469.

Bonaldo, M.C., Souto-Padron, T., De Souza, W., Goldenberg, S., 1988. Cell-substrate adhesion during *Trypanosoma cruzi* differentiation. J. Cell Biol. 106, 1349–1358.

Bonaldo, M.C., d'Escoffier, L.N., Salles, J.M., Goldenberg, S., 1991. Characterization and expression of proteases during *Trypanosoma cruzi* metacyclogenesis. Exp. Parasitol. 73, 44–51.

Briones, M.R., Egima, C.M., Schenkman, S., 1995. *Trypanosoma cruzi* trans-sialidase gene lacking C-terminal repeats and expressed in epimastigote forms. Mol. Biochem. Parasitol. 70, 9–17.

Bronia, D.H., Aguerri, A.M., Bertetto, S.T., 1986. *Trypanosoma cruzi*: changes in lipid composition during aging in culture. Exp. Parasitol. 61, 151–159.

Burleigh, B.A., Andrews, N.W., 1998. Signaling and host cell invasion by *Trypanosoma cruzi*. Curr. Opin. Microbiol. 1, 461–465.

Burleigh, B.A., Caler, E.V., Webster, P., Andrews, N.W., 1997. A cytosolic serine endopeptidase from *Trypanosoma cruzi* is required for the generation of Ca2+ signaling in mammalian cells. J. Cell Biol. 136, 609–620.
Burleigh, B.A., Woolsey, A.M., 2002. Cell signalling and *Trypanosoma cruzi* invasion. Cell Microbiol. 4 (11), 701–711.
Buscaglia, C.A., Campo, V.A., Di Noia, J.M., Torrecilhas, A.C., De Marchi, C.R., Ferguson, M.A., et al., 2004. The surface coat of the mammal-dwelling infective trypomastigote stage of *Trypanosoma cruzi* is formed by highly diverse immunogenic mucins. J. Biol. Chem. 279, 15860–15869.
Buscaglia, C.A., Campo, V.A., Frasch, A.C., Di Noia, J.M., 2006. *Trypanosoma cruzi* surface mucins: host-dependent coat diversity. Nat. Rev. Microbiol. 4, 229–236.
Buschiazzo, A., Amaya, M.F., Cremona, M.L., Frasch, A.C., Alzari, P.M., 2002. The crystal structure and mode of action of trans-sialidase, a key enzyme in *Trypanosoma cruzi* pathogenesis. Mol. Cell 10, 757–768.
Caler, E.V., Vaena de Avalos, S., Haynes, P.A., Andrews, N.W., Burleigh, B.A., 1998. Oligopeptidase B-dependent signaling mediates host cell invasion by *Trypanosoma cruzi*. EMBO J. 17, 4975–4986.
Camargo, E.P., 1964. Growth and differentiation in *Trypanosoma cruzi* I. Origin of metacyclic trypanosomes in liquid media. Rev. Inst. Med. Trop. São Paulo 6, 93–100.
Campetella, O., Martinez, J., Cazzulo, J.J., 1990. A major cysteine proteinase is developmentally regulated in *Trypanosoma cruzi*. FEMS Microbiol. Lett. 55, 145–149.
Campetella, O., Henriksson, J., Aslund, L., Frasch, A.C., Pettersson, U., Cazzulo, J.J., 1992. The major cysteine proteinase (cruzipain) from *Trypanosoma cruzi* is encoded by multiple polymorphic tandemly organized genes located on different chromosomes. Mol. Biochem. Parasitol. 50, 225–234.
Cardoso, J., Soares, M.J., Menna-Barreto, R.F., Le Bloas, R., Sotomaior, V., Goldenberg, S., et al., 2008. Inhibition of proteasome activity blocks *Trypanosoma cruzi* growth and metacyclogenesis. Parasitol. Res. 103, 941–951.
Carvalho, S.T., Sola-Penna, M., Oliveira, I.A., Pita, S., Goncalves, A.S., Neves, B.C., et al., 2010. A new class of mechanism-based inhibitors for *Trypanosoma cruzi* trans-sialidase and their influence on parasite virulence. Glycobiology 20, 1034–1045.
Cassola, A., De Gaudenzi, J.G., Frasch, A.C., 2007. Recruitment of mRNAs to cytoplasmic ribonucleoprotein granules in trypanosomes. Mol. Microbiol. 65, 655–670.
Cazzulo, J.J., 1984. Protein and amino acid catabolism in *Trypanosoma cruzi*. Comp. Biochem. Physiol. B 79, 309–320.
Cazzulo, J.J., 1992. Aerobic fermentation of glucose by trypanosomatids. FASEB J. 6, 3153–3161.
Cazzulo, J.J., 1994. Intermediate metabolism in *Trypanosoma cruzi*. J. Bioenerg. Biomembr. 26, 157–165.
Cazzulo, J.J., 2002. Proteinases of *Trypanosoma cruzi*: potential targets for the chemotherapy of Chagas disease. Curr. Top. Med. Chem. 2, 1261–1271.
Cazzulo, J.J., Cazzulo Franke, M.C., Martinez, J., Franke de Cazzulo, B.M., 1990. Some kinetic properties of a cysteine proteinase (cruzipain) from *Trypanosoma cruzi*. Biochim. Biophys. Acta 1037, 186–191.
Cazzulo, J.J., Stoka, V., Turk, V., 1997. Cruzipain, the major cysteine proteinase from the protozoan parasite *Trypanosoma cruzi*. Biol. Chem. 378, 1–10.
Chagas, C., 1909. Nova tripanosomiase humana. Estudo sobre a morfolojia e o cyclo evolutivo do Schizotrypanum cruzi n.gen., n.sp., ajente etiolojico de nova entidade morbida no homem. Mem. Inst. Oswaldo Cruz 1, 159–218.
Colli, W., 1993. Trans-sialidase: a unique enzyme activity discovered in the protozoan *Trypanosoma cruzi*. FASEB J. 7, 1257–1264.

Contreras, V.T., Morel, C.M., Goldenberg, S., 1985a. Stage specific gene expression precedes morphological changes during *Trypanosoma cruzi* metacyclogenesis. Mol. Biochem. Parasitol. 14, 83–96.

Contreras, V.T., Salles, J.M., Thomas, N., Morel, C.M., Goldenberg, S., 1985b. In vitro differentiation of *Trypanosoma cruzi* under chemically defined conditions. Mol. Biochem. Parasitol. 16, 315–327.

Cordero, E.M., Nakayasu, E.S., Gentil, L.G., Yoshida, N., Almeida, I.C., da Silveira, J.F., 2009. Proteomic analysis of detergent-solubilized membrane proteins from insect-developmental forms of *Trypanosoma cruzi*. J. Proteome Res. 8, 3642–3652.

Cortez, M., Silva, M.R., Neira, I., Ferreira, D., Sasso, G.R., Luquetti, A.O., et al., 2006. *Trypanosoma cruzi* surface molecule gp90 downregulates invasion of gastric mucosal epithelium in orally infected mice. Microbes Infect. 8, 36–44.

Coughlin, B.C., Teixeira, S.M., Kirchhoff, L.V., Donelson, J.E., 2000. Amastin mRNA abundance in *Trypanosoma cruzi* is controlled by a 3′-untranslated region position-dependent cis-element and an untranslated region-binding protein. J. Biol. Chem. 275, 12051–12060.

Cross, G.A., Takle, G.B., 1993. The surface trans-sialidase family of *Trypanosoma cruzi*. Annu. Rev. Microbiol. 47, 385–411.

Cuevas, I.C., Cazzulo, J.J., Sanchez, D.O., 2003. gp63 homologues in *Trypanosoma cruzi*: surface antigens with metalloprotease activity and a possible role in host cell infection. Infect. Immun. 71, 5739–5749.

da Silva, R.A., Bartholomeu, D.C., Teixeira, S.M., 2006. Control mechanisms of tubulin gene expression in *Trypanosoma cruzi*. Int. J. Parasitol. 36, 87–96.

da Silva-Lopez, R.E., Morgado-Diaz, J.A., dos Santos, P.T., Giovanni-De-Simone, S., 2008. Purification and subcellular localization of a secreted 75 kDa *Trypanosoma cruzi* serine oligopeptidase. Acta Trop. 107, 159–167.

Dallagiovanna, B., Gamarro, F., Castanys, S., 1996. Organization of trans-sialidase genes in *Trypanosoma cruzi*. Mol. Biochem. Parasitol. 77, 115–125.

De Gaudenzi, J., Frasch, A.C., Clayton, C., 2005. RNA-binding domain proteins in kinetoplastids: a comparative analysis. Eukaryot. Cell 4 (12), 2106–2114.

de Lederkremer, R.M., Agusti, R., 2009. Glycobiology of *Trypanosoma cruzi*. Adv. Carbohydr. Chem. Biochem. 62, 311–366.

de Melo, L.D., Nepomuceno-Silva, J.L., Sant'Anna, C., Eisele, N., Ferraro, R.B., Meyer-Fernandes, J.R., et al., 2004. TcRho1 of *Trypanosoma cruzi*: role in metacyclogenesis and cellular localization. Biochem. Biophys. Res. Commun. 323, 1009–1016.

De Souza, W., 2002. Basic cell biology of *Trypanosoma cruzi*. Curr. Pharm. Des. 8, 269–285.

de Souza, W., de Carvalho, T.M., Barrias, E.S., 2010. Review on *Trypanosoma cruzi*: host cell interaction. Int. J. Cell Biol. 2010, 1–19.

Di Noia, J.M., D'Orso, I., Sanchez, D.O., Frasch, A.C., 2000. AU-rich elements in the 3′-untranslated region of a new mucin-type gene family of *Trypanosoma cruzi* confers mRNA instability and modulates translation efficiency. J. Biol. Chem. 275, 10218–10227.

Dias, F., 1934. Estudos sobre o Schizotrypanum cruzi. Mem. Inst. Oswaldo Cruz 28, 1–110.

do Carmo, M.S., dos Santos, M.R., Cano, M.I., Araya, J.E., Yoshida, N., da Silveira, J.F., 2002. Expression and genome-wide distribution of the gene family encoding a 90 kDa surface glycoprotein of metacyclic trypomastigotes of *Trypanosoma cruzi*. Mol. Biochem. Parasitol. 125, 201–206.

D'Orso, I., Frasch, A.C., 2001. TcUBP-1, a developmentally regulated U-rich RNA-binding protein involved in selective mRNA destabilization in trypanosomes. J. Biol. Chem. 276, 34801–34809.

Duschak, V.G., Couto, A.S., 2009. Cruzipain, the major cysteine protease of *Trypanosoma cruzi*: a sulfated glycoprotein antigen as relevant candidate for vaccine development and drug target. A review. Curr. Med. Chem. 16, 3174–3202.

Eakin, A.E., Mills, A.A., Harth, G., McKerrow, J.H., Craik, C.S., 1992. The sequence, organization, and expression of the major cysteine protease (cruzain) from *Trypanosoma cruzi*. J. Biol. Chem. 267, 7411–7420.
Egima, C.M., Briones, M.R., Freitas Junior, L.H., Schenkman, R.P., Uemura, H., Schenkman, S., 1996. Organization of trans-sialidase genes in *Trypanosoma cruzi*. Mol. Biochem. Parasitol. 77, 115–125.
Eickhoff, C.S., Giddings, O.K., Yoshida, N., Hoft, D.F., 2010. Immune responses to gp82 provide protection against mucosal *Trypanosoma cruzi* infection. Mem. Inst. Oswaldo Cruz 105, 687–691.
Elias, M.C., Nardelli, S.C., Schenkman, S., 2009. Chromatin and nuclear organization in *Trypanosoma cruzi*. Future Microbiol. 4, 1065–1074.
El-Sayed, N.M., Myler, P.J., Bartholomeu, D.C., Nilsson, D., Aggarwal, G., Tran, A.N., et al., 2005. The genome sequence of *Trypanosoma cruzi*, etiologic agent of Chagas disease. Science 309, 409–415.
Esteves, M.G., Gonzales-Perdomo, M., Alviano, C.S., Angluster, J., Goldenberg, S., 1989. Changes in fatty acid composition associated with differentiation of *Trypanosoma cruzi*. FEMS Microbiol. Lett. 50, 31–34.
Fampa, P., Santos, A.L., Ramirez, M.I., 2010. *Trypanosoma cruzi*: ubiquity expression of surface cruzipain molecules in TCI and TCII field isolates. Parasitol. Res. 107, 443–447.
Figueiredo da Silva, A.A., de Carvalho Vieira, L., Krieger, M.A., Goldenberg, S., Zanchin, N.I., Guimaraes, B.G., 2007. Crystal structure of chagasin, the endogenous cysteine-protease inhibitor from *Trypanosoma cruzi*. J. Struct. Biol. 157, 416–423.
Figueiredo, R.C., Rosa, D.S., Soares, M.J., 2000. Differentiation of *Trypanosoma cruzi* epimastigotes: metacyclogenesis and adhesion to substrate are triggered by nutritional stress. J. Parasitol. 86, 1213–1218.
Figueiredo, R.C., Rosa, D.S., Gomes, Y.M., Nakasawa, M., Soares, M.J., 2004. Reservosome: an endocytic compartment in epimastigote forms of the protozoan *Trypanosoma cruzi* (Kinetoplastida: Trypanosomatidae). Correlation between endocytosis of nutrients and cell differentiation. Parasitology 129, 431–438.
Franco, F.R., Paranhos-Bacalla, G.S., Yamauchi, L.M., Yoshida, N., da-Silveira, J.F., 1993. Characterization of a cDNA clone encoding the carboxy-terminal domain of a 90-kilodalton surface antigen of *Trypanosoma cruzi* metacyclic trypomastigotes. Infect. Immun. 61, 4196–4201.
Franke de Cazzulo, B.M., Martinez, J., North, M.J., Coombs, G.H., Cazzulo, J.J., 1994. Effects of proteinase inhibitors on the growth and differentiation of *Trypanosoma cruzi*. FEMS Microbiol. Lett. 124, 81–86.
Gentil, L.G., Cordero, E.M., do Carmo, M.S., dos Santos, M.R., da Silveira, J.F., 2009. Post-transcriptional mechanisms involved in the control of expression of the stage-specific GP82 surface glycoprotein in *Trypanosoma cruzi*. Acta Trop. 109, 152–158.
Giordano, R., Chammas, R., Veiga, S.S., Colli, W., Alves, M.J., 1994. *Trypanosoma cruzi* binds to laminin in a carbohydrate-independent way. Braz. J. Med. Biol. Res. 27, 2315–2318.
Giordano, R., Fouts, D.L., Tewari, D., Colli, W., Manning, J.E., Alves, M.J., 1999. Cloning of a surface membrane glycoprotein specific for the infective form of *Trypanosoma cruzi* having adhesive properties to laminin. J. Biol. Chem. 274, 3461–3468.
Goldenberg, S., Salles, J.M., Contreras, V.T., Lima Franco, M.P., Katzin, A.M., Colli, W., et al., 1985. Characterization of messenger RNA from epimastigotes and metacyclic trypomastigotes of *Trypanosoma cruzi*. FEBS Lett. 180, 265–270.
Gonzales-Perdomo, M., Romero, P., Goldenberg, S., 1988. Cyclic AMP and adenylate cyclase activators stimulate *Trypanosoma cruzi* differentiation. Exp. Parasitol. 66, 205–212.
Gonzalez, J., Ramalho-Pinto, F.J., Frevert, U., Ghiso, J., Tomlinson, S., Scharfstein, J., et al., 1996. Proteasome activity is required for the stage-specific transformation of a protozoan parasite. J. Exp. Med. 184, 1909–1918.

Hanke, J., Sánchez, D.O., Henriksson, J., Aslund, L., Pettersson, U., Frasch, A.C., et al., 1996. Stage-regulated expression of cruzipain, the major cysteine protease of *Trypanosoma cruzi* is independent of the level of RNA1. Mol. Biochem. Parasitol. 76, 91–103.

Harrington, J.M., Widener, J., Stephens, N., Johnson, T., Francia, M., Capewell, P., et al., 2010. The plasma membrane of bloodstream-form African trypanosomes confers susceptibility and specificity to killing by hydrophobic peptides. J. Biol. Chem. 285, 28659–28666.

Holetz, F.B., Correa, A., Avila, A.R., Nakamura, C.V., Krieger, M.A., Goldenberg, S., 2007. Evidence of P-body-like structures in *Trypanosoma cruzi*. Biochem. Biophys. Res. Commun. 356, 1062–1067.

Holetz, F., Alves, L., Probst, C., Dallagiovanna, B., Marchini, F., Manque, P., et al., 2010. Protein and mRNA content of TcDHH1-containing mRNPs in *Trypanosoma cruzi*. FEBS J. 277, 3415–3426.

Itow, S., Camargo, E.P., 1977. Proteolytic activities in cell extracts of *Trypanosoma cruzi*. J. Protozool. 24, 591–595.

Jager, A.V., Muia, R.P., Campetella, O., 2008. Stage-specific expression of *Trypanosoma cruzi* trans-sialidase involves highly conserved 3′ untranslated regions. FEMS Microbiol. Lett. 283, 182–188.

Jose Cazzulo, J., Stoka, V., Turk, V., 2001. The major cysteine proteinase of *Trypanosoma cruzi*: a valid target for chemotherapy of Chagas disease. Curr. Pharm. Des. 7, 1143–1156.

Katzin, A.M., Colli, W., 1983. Lectin receptors in *Trypanosoma cruzi*. An N-acetyl-D-glucosamine-containing surface glycoprotein specific for the trypomastigote stage.. Biochim. Biophys. Acta 727, 403–411.

Kosec, G., Alvarez, V.E., Aguero, F., Sanchez, D., Dolinar, M., Turk, B., et al., 2006. Metacaspases of *Trypanosoma cruzi*: possible candidates for programmed cell death mediators. Mol. Biochem. Parasitol. 145, 18–28.

Kriebel, P.W., Parent, C.A., 2004. Adenylyl cyclase expression and regulation during the differentiation of Dictyostelium discoideum. IUBMB Life 56, 541–546.

Krieger, M.A., Avila, A.R., Ogatta, S.F., Plazanet-Menut, C., Goldenberg, S., 1999. Differential gene expression during *Trypanosoma cruzi* metacyclogenesis. Mem. Inst. Oswaldo Cruz 94 (Suppl 1), 165–168.

Lowndes, C.M., Bonaldo, M.C., Thomaz, N., Goldenberg, S., 1996. Heterogeneity of metalloprotease expression in *Trypanosoma cruzi*. Parasitology 112, 393–399.

Magdesian, M.H., Tonelli, R.R., Fessel, M.R., Silveira, M.S., Schumacher, R.I., Linden, R., et al., 2007. A conserved domain of the gp85/trans-sialidase family activates host cell extracellular signal-regulated kinase and facilitates *Trypanosoma cruzi* infection. Exp. Cell Res. 313, 210–218.

Malaga, S., Yoshida, N., 2001. Targeted reduction in expression of *Trypanosoma cruzi* surface glycoprotein gp90 increases parasite infectivity. Infect. Immun. 69, 353–359.

Manque, P.M., Eichinger, D., Juliano, M.A., Juliano, L., Araya, J.E., Yoshida, N., 2000. Characterization of the cell adhesion site of *Trypanosoma cruzi* metacyclic stage surface glycoprotein gp82. Infect. Immun. 68, 478–484.

Manque, P.M., Neira, I., Atayde, V.D., Cordero, E., Ferreira, A.T., da Silveira, J.F., et al., 2003. Cell adhesion and Ca2+ signaling activity in stably transfected *Trypanosoma cruzi* epimastigotes expressing the metacyclic stage-specific surface molecule gp82. Infect. Immun. 71, 1561–1565.

Martinez, J., Henriksson, J., Ridaker, M., Pettersson, U., Cazzulo, J.J., 1998. Polymorphisms of the genes encoding cruzipain, the major cysteine proteinase of *Trypanosoma cruzi*, in the region encoding the C-terminal domain. FEMS Microbiol. Lett. 159, 35–39.

Martins, R.M., Covarrubias, C., Rojas, R.G., Silber, A.M., Yoshida, N., 2009. Use of L-proline and ATP production by *Trypanosoma cruzi* metacyclic forms as requirements for host cell invasion. Infect. Immun. 77, 3023–3032.

McGrath, M.E., Eakin, A.E., Engel, J.C., McKerrow, J.H., Craik, C.S., Fletterick, R.J., 1995. The crystal structure of cruzain: a therapeutic target for Chagas' disease. J. Mol. Biol. 247, 251–259.

McKerrow, J.H., Doyle, P.S., Engel, J.C., Podust, L.M., Robertson, S.A., Ferreira, R., et al., 2009. Two approaches to discovering and developing new drugs for Chagas disease. Mem. Inst. Oswaldo Cruz 104 (Suppl. 1), 263–269.

Meirelles, M.N., Juliano, L., Carmona, E., Silva, S.G., Costa, E.M., Murta, A.C., et al., 1992. Inhibitors of the major cysteinyl proteinase (GP57/51) impair host cell invasion and arrest the intracellular development of *Trypanosoma cruzi* in vitro. Mol. Biochem. Parasitol. 52, 175–184.

Monteiro, A.C., Abrahamson, M., Lima, A.P., Vannier-Santos, M.A., Scharfstein, J., 2001. Identification, characterization and localization of chagasin, a tight-binding cysteine protease inhibitor in *Trypanosoma cruzi*. J. Cell Sci. 114, 3933–3942.

Moreno, S.N., Silva, J., Vercesi, A.E., Docampo, R., 1994. Cytosolic-free calcium elevation in *Trypanosoma cruzi* is required for cell invasion. J. Exp. Med. 180, 1535–1540.

Mortara, R.A., da-Silva, S., Araguth, M.F., Blanco, S.A., Yoshida, N., 1992. Polymorphism of the 35- and 50-kilodalton surface glycoconjugates of *Trypanosoma cruzi* metacyclic trypomastigotes. Infect. Immun. 60, 4673–4678.

Murta, A.C.M., Persechini, P., Souto-Padron, T., De Souza, W., Guimarães, J.A., Scharfstein, J., 1990. Structural and functional identification of Gp57/51 antigen of *Trypanosoma cruzi* as a cysteine proteinase. Mol. Biochem. Parasitol. 43, 27–38.

Neira, I., Silva, F.A., Cortez, M., Yoshida, N., 2003. Involvement of *Trypanosoma cruzi* metacyclic trypomastigote surface molecule gp82 in adhesion to gastric mucin and invasion of epithelial cells. Infect. Immun. 71, 557–561.

Neres, J., Bryce, R.A., Douglas, K.T., 2008. Rational drug design in parasitology: trans-sialidase as a case study for Chagas disease. Drug Discov. Today 13, 110–117.

Norris, K.A., Bradt, B., Cooper, N.R., So, M., 1991. Characterization of a *Trypanosoma cruzi* C3 binding protein with functional and genetic similarities to the human complement regulatory protein, decay-accelerating factor. J. Immunol. 147, 2240–2247.

Norris, K.A., Schrimpf, J.E., Szabo, M.J., 1997. Identification of the gene family encoding the 160-kilodalton *Trypanosoma cruzi* complement regulatory protein. Infect. Immun. 65, 349–357.

Ouaissi, A., Cornette, J., Schöneck, R., Plumas-Marty, B., Taibi, A., Loyens, M., et al., 1992. Fibronectin cleavage fragments provide a growth factor-like activity for the differentiation of *Trypanosoma cruzi* trypomastigotes to amastigotes. Eur. J. Cell Biol. 59, 68–79.

Parker, R., Sheth, U., 2007. P bodies and the control of mRNA translation and degradation. Mol. Cell 25, 635–646.

Pinho, R.T., Beltramini, L.M., Alves, C.R., De-Simone, S.G., 2009. *Trypanosoma cruzi*: isolation and characterization of aspartyl proteases. Exp. Parasitol. 122, 128–133.

Previato, J.O., Wait, R., Jones, C., DosReis, G.A., Todeschini, A.R., Heise, N., et al., 2004. Glycoinositolphospholipid from *Trypanosoma cruzi*: structure, biosynthesis and immunobiology. Adv. Parasitol. 56, 1–41.

Rangel-Aldao, R., Triana, F., Fernandez, V., Comach, G., Abate, T., Montoreano, R., 1988. Cyclic AMP as an inducer of the cell differentiation of *Trypanosoma cruzi*. Biochem. Int. 17, 337–344.

Risso, M.G., Garbarino, G.B., Mocetti, E., Campetella, O., Gonzalez Cappa, S.M., Buscaglia, C.A., et al., 2004. Differential expression of a virulence factor, the trans-sialidase, by the main *Trypanosoma cruzi* phylogenetic lineages. J. Infect. Dis. 189, 2250–2259.

Roberts, H., Healy, N., Shaw, E., Ashall, F., 1990. Substrate specificity and inhibitor sensitivity of a *Trypanosoma cruzi* alkaline peptidase. Biochem. Soc. Trans. 18, 866–867.

Rubin-de-Celis, S.S., Uemura, H., Yoshida, N., Schenkman, S., 2006. Expression of trypomastigote trans-sialidase in metacyclic forms of *Trypanosoma cruzi* increases parasite escape from its parasitophorous vacuole. Cell. Microbiol. 8, 1888–1898.

Ruiz, R.C., Rigoni, V.L., Gonzalez, J., Yoshida, N., 1993. The 35/50 kDa surface antigen of *Trypanosoma cruzi* metacyclic trypomastigotes, an adhesion molecule involved in host cell invasion. Parasite Immunol. 15, 121–125.

Ruiz, R.C., Favoreto, S., Jr., Dorta, M.L., Oshiro, M.E., Ferreira, A.T., Manque, P.M., et al., 1998. Infectivity of *Trypanosoma cruzi* strains is associated with differential expression of surface glycoproteins with differential Ca2+ signalling activity. Biochem. J. 330 (Pt. 1), 505–511.

Santana, J.M., Grellier, P., Schrevel, J., Teixeira, A.R., 1997. A *Trypanosoma cruzi*-secreted 80 kDa proteinase with specificity for human collagen types I and IV. Biochem. J. 325 (Pt 1), 129–137.

Sant'Anna, C., Parussini, F., Lourenco, D., de Souza, W., Cazzulo, J.J., Cunha-e-Silva, N.L., 2008. All *Trypanosoma cruzi* developmental forms present lysosome-related organelles. Histochem. Cell Biol. 130, 1187–1198.

Santori, F.R., Dorta, M.L., Juliano, L., Juliano, M.A., da Silveira, J.F., Ruiz, R.C., et al., 1996. Identification of a domain of *Trypanosoma cruzi* metacyclic trypomastigote surface molecule gp82 required for attachment and invasion of mammalian cells. Mol. Biochem. Parasitol. 78, 209–216.

Santos, C.C., Sant'anna, C., Terres, A., Cunha-e-Silva, N.L., Scharfstein, J., Lima, A.P.P., 2005. Chagasin, the endogenous cysteine-protease inhibitor of *Trypanosoma cruzi*, modulates parasite differentiation and invasion of mammalian cells. J. Cell Sci. 118, 901–915.

Scharfstein, J., Lima, A.P., 2008. Roles of naturally occurring protease inhibitors in the modulation of host cell signaling and cellular invasion by *Trypanosoma cruzi*. Subcell. Biochem. 47, 140–154.

Schenkman, S., Eichinger, D., 1993. *Trypanosoma cruzi* trans-sialidase and cell invasion. Parasitol. Today 9, 218–222.

Schenkman, S., Jiang, M.S., Hart, G.W., Nussenzweig, V., 1991. A novel cell surface trans-sialidase of *Trypanosoma cruzi* generates a stage-specific epitope required for invasion of mammalian cells. Cell 65, 1117–1125.

Schenkman, S., Pontes de Carvalho, L., Nussenzweig, V., 1992. *Trypanosoma cruzi* trans-sialidase and neuraminidase activities can be mediated by the same enzymes. J. Exp. Med. 175, 567–575.

Schenkman, R.P., Vandekerckhove, F., Schenkman, S., 1993. Mammalian cell sialic acid enhances invasion by *Trypanosoma cruzi*. Infect. Immun. 61, 898–902.

Schenkman, S., Eichinger, D., Pereira, M.E., Nussenzweig, V., 1994. Structural and functional properties of Trypanosoma trans-sialidase. Annu. Rev. Microbiol. 48, 499–523.

Snary, D., Hudson, L., 1979. *Trypanosoma cruzi* cell surface proteins: identification of one major glycoprotein. FEBS Lett. 100, 166–170.

Soares, M.J., Souto-Padrón, T., Bonaldo, M.C., Goldenberg, S., de Souza, W., 1989. A stereological study of the differentiation process in *Trypanosoma cruzi*. Parasitol. Res. 75, 522–527.

Soares, M.J., Souto-Padron, T., De Souza, W., 1992. Identification of a large pre-lysosomal compartment in the pathogenic protozoon *Trypanosoma cruzi*. J. Cell Sci. 102 (Pt. 1), 157–167.

Songthamwat, D., Kajihara, K., Kikuchi, M., Uemura, H., Tran, S.P., Yanagi, T., et al., 2007. Structure and expression of three gp82 gene subfamilies of *Trypanosoma cruzi*. Parasitol. Int. 56, 273–280.

Souto-Padron, T., Campetella, O.E., Cazzulo, J.J., de Souza, W., 1990. Cysteine proteinase in *Trypanosoma cruzi*: immunocytochemical localization and involvement in parasite-host cell interaction. J. Cell Sci. 96 (Pt. 3), 485–490.

Staquicini, D.I., Martins, R.M., Macedo, S., Sasso, G.R., Atayde, V.D., Juliano, M.A., et al., 2010. Role of GP82 in the selective binding to gastric mucin during oral infection with *Trypanosoma cruzi*. PLoS Negl. Trop. Dis. 4, e613.

Strmecki, L., Greene, D.M., Pears, C.J., 2005. Developmental decisions in Dictyostelium discoideum. Dev. Biol. 284, 25–36.

Sullivan, J.J., 1982. Metacyclogenesis of *Trypanosoma cruzi* in vitro: a simplified procedure. Trans. R. Soc. Trop. Med. Hyg. 76, 300–303.

Sylvester, D., Krassner, S.M., 1976. Proline metabolism in *Trypanosoma cruzi* epimastigotes. Comp. Biochem. Physiol. B 55, 443–447.

Tardieux, I., Nathanson, M.H., Andrews, N.W., 1994. Role in host cell invasion of *Trypanosoma cruzi*-induced cytosolic-free Ca2+ transients. J. Exp. Med. 179, 1017–1022.

Teixeira, S.M., daRocha, W.D., 2003. Control of gene expression and genetic manipulation in the Trypanosomatidae. Genet. Mol. Res. 2, 148–158.

Teixeira, M.M., Yoshida, N., 1986. Stage-specific surface antigens of metacyclic trypomastigotes of *Trypanosoma cruzi* identified by monoclonal antibodies. Mol. Biochem. Parasitol. 18, 271–282.

Teixeira, S.M., Kirchhoff, L.V., Donelson, J.E., 1995. Post-transcriptional elements regulating expression of mRNAs from the amastin/tuzin gene cluster of *Trypanosoma cruzi*. J. Biol. Chem. 270, 22586–22594.

Teixeira, S.M., Kirchhoff, L.V., Donelson, J.E., 1999. *Trypanosoma cruzi*: suppression of tuzin gene expression by its 5′-UTR and spliced leader addition site. Exp. Parasitol. 93, 143–151.

Tomas, A.M., Kelly, J.M., 1996. Stage-regulated expression of cruzipain, the major cysteine protease of *Trypanosoma cruzi* is independent of the level of RNA1. Mol. Biochem. Parasitol. 76, 91–103.

Tomas, A.M., Miles, M.A., Kelly, J.M., 1997. Overexpression of cruzipain, the major cysteine proteinase of *Trypanosoma cruzi*, is associated with enhanced metacyclogenesis. Eur. J. Biochem. 244, 596–603.

Tomlinson, S., Pontes de Carvalho, L., Vandekerckhove, F., Nussenzweig, V., 1992. Resialylation of sialidase-treated sheep and human erythrocytes by *Trypanosoma cruzi* trans-sialidase: restoration of complement resistance of desialylated sheep erythrocytes. Glycobiology 2, 549–551.

Tonelli, R.R., Silber, A.M., Almeida-de-Faria, M., Hirata, I.Y., Colli, W., Alves, M.J., 2004. L-proline is essential for the intracellular differentiation of *Trypanosoma cruzi*. Cell. Microbiol. 6, 733–741.

Tonelli, R.R., Giordano, R.J., Barbu, E.M., Torrecilhas, A.C., Kobayashi, G.S., Langley, R.R., et al., 2010a. Role of the gp85/trans-sialidases in *Trypanosoma cruzi* tissue tropism: preferential binding of a conserved peptide motif to the vasculature in vivo. PLoS Negl. Trop. Dis. 4, e864.

Tonelli, R.R., Torrecilhas, A.C., Jacysyn, J.F., Juliano, M.A., Colli, W., Alves, M.J., 2010b. In vivo infection by *Trypanosoma cruzi*: the conserved FLY domain of the gp85/trans-sialidase family potentiates host infection. Parasitology 138 (4), 481–492.

Urbina, J.A., 1994. Intermediary metabolism of *Trypanosoma cruzi*. Parasitol. Today 10, 107–110.

Urbina, J.A., 2010. Specific chemotherapy of Chagas disease: relevance, current limitations and new approaches. Acta Trop. 115, 55–68.

Velge, P., Ouaissi, M.A., Cornette, J., Afchain, D., Capron, A., 1988. Identification and isolation of *Trypanosoma cruzi* trypomastigote collagen-binding proteins: possible role in cell-parasite interaction. Parasitology 97 (Pt. 2), 255–268.

Weston, D., La Flamme, A.C., Van Voorhis, W.C., 1999a. Expression of *Trypanosoma cruzi* surface antigen FL-160 is controlled by elements in the 3′ untranslated, the 3′ intergenic, and the coding regions. Mol. Biochem. Parasitol. 102, 53–66.

Weston, D., Patel, B., Van Voorhis, W.C., 1999b. Virulence in *Trypanosoma cruzi* infection correlates with the expression of a distinct family of sialidase superfamily genes. Mol. Biochem. Parasitol. 98, 105–116.

Yamada-Ogatta, S.F., Motta, M.C., Toma, H.K., Monteiro-Goes, V., Avila, A.R., Muniz, B.D., et al., 2004. *Trypanosoma cruzi*: cloning and characterization of two genes whose expression is up-regulated in metacyclic trypomastigotes. Acta Trop. 90, 171–179.

Yoshida, N., 2009. Molecular mechanisms of *Trypanosoma cruzi* infection by oral route. Mem. Inst. Oswaldo Cruz 104 (Suppl. 1), 101–107.

Zeledon, R., Bolanos, R., Rojas, M., 1984. Scanning electron microscopy of the final phase of the life cycle of *Trypanosoma cruzi* in the insect vector. Acta Trop. 41, 39–43.

CHAPTER **14**

The Role of Acidocalcisomes in the Stress Response of *Trypanosoma cruzi*

Roberto Docampo, Veronica Jimenez, Sharon King-Keller, Zhu-hong Li, and **Silvia N.J. Moreno**

Contents

Abstract

Acidocalcisomes of *Trypanosoma cruzi* are acidic calcium-containing organelles rich in phosphorus in the form of pyrophosphate (PP_i) and polyphosphate (poly P). Acidification of the organelles is driven by vacuolar proton pumps, one of which, the vacuolar-type proton pyrophosphatase, is absent in mammalian cells. A calcium ATPase is involved in calcium uptake, and an aquaporin is important

Department of Cellular Biology and Center for Tropical and Global Emerging Diseases, University of Georgia, Athens, Georgia, USA

Advances in Parasitology, Volume 75
ISSN 0065-308X, DOI: 10.1016/B978-0-12-385863-4.00014-9

for water transport. Enzymes involved in the synthesis and degradation of PPi and poly P are present within the organelle. Acidocalcisomes function as storage sites for cations and phosphorus, participate in PP_i and poly P metabolism and volume regulation and are essential for virulence. A signalling pathway involving cyclic AMP generation is important for fusion of acidocalcisomes to the contractile vacuole complex, transference of aquaporin and volume regulation. This pathway is an excellent target for chemotherapy as shown by the effects of phosphodiesterase C inhibitors on parasite survival.

ABBREVIATIONS

Ca^{2+}-ATPase	calcium ATPase
cAMP	cyclic AMP
CVC	contractile vacuole complex
PDE	phosphodiesterase
PMCA	plasma membrane type Ca^{2+}-ATPase
poly P	polyphosphate
PPi	pyrophosphate
RVD	regulatory volume decrease
RVI	regulatory volume increase
V-H^+-ATPase	vacuolar-type proton ATPase
V-H^+-PPase	vacuolar-type proton pyrophosphatase
Vtc	vacuolar transporter chaperone

14.1. INTRODUCTION

Acidocalcisomes were first identified in bacteria and named metachromatic granules (Babes, 1895) because they had the property of changing the colour of basic blue dyes. They were also named volutin granules (Meyer, 1904) because of their presence in *Spirillum volutans*. Volutin granules were later found in a number of microorganisms, including trypanosomes (Swellengrebel, 1908). Polyphosphate (poly P), a linear polymer of a few to several hundred orthophosphate residues discovered by Lieberman (Lieberman, 1888), was reported in 1947 as a component of these granules (Wiame, 1947), which then began to be known as poly P granules. More recent work in trypanosomatids and Apicomplexan parasites (Docampo et al., 1995; Moreno and Zhong, 1996; Vercesi et al., 1994) revealed that the poly P granules have proton and calcium pumps, which are responsible for their acidity and calcium content, and were given the name of acidocalcisomes. As these organelles have been found from bacteria (Seufferheld et al., 2003, 2004) to human cells (Ruiz et al.,

2004), it has been suggested that they have been conserved over evolutionary time or have appeared more than one time by convergent evolution (Docampo et al., 2010).

14.2. ACIDOCALCISOMES IN *TRYPANOSOMA CRUZI*

Trypanosoma cruzi acidocalcisomes are electron dense (Fig. 14.1A) and have a vacuolar appearance by conventional electron microscopy (Fig. 14.1B). At the light microscopy level, they can be stained with 4′-6-diamidino-2-phenylindole (DAPI), which labels poly P, and with dyes that accumulate in acidic compartments such as acridine orange (Fig. 14.1C; Docampo et al., 1995) or cycloprodigiosin (Scott and Docampo, 2000). They are spherical with an average diameter of 0.2 μm and randomly distributed in the cells (Fig. 14.1A).

T. cruzi acidocalcisomes are rich in orthophosphate (Pi), pyrophosphate (PPi) and poly P complexed with cations (sodium, potassium, magnesium, calcium, zinc and iron) and basic amino acids (Rohloff

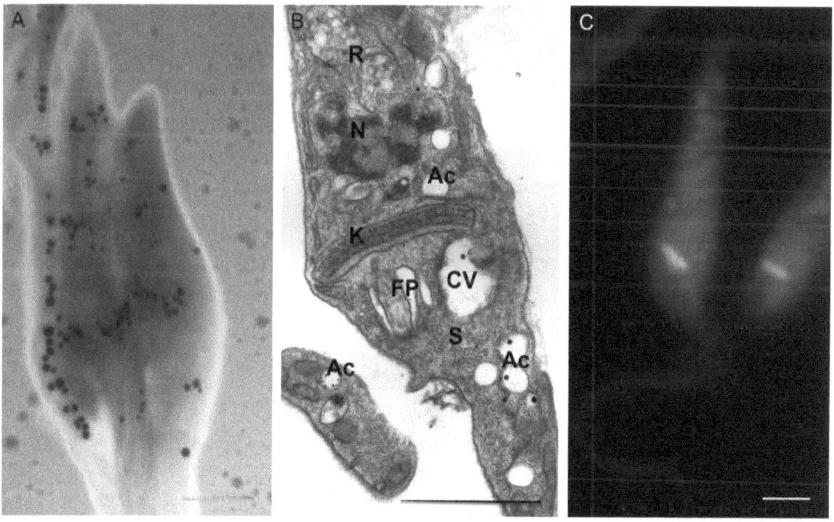

FIGURE 14.1 *Acidocalcisomes in T. cruzi.* (A) Electron micrograph of intact epimastigotes showing the electron-dense acidocalcisomes (black granules) distributed at random; (B) electron micrograph of epimastigote sections showing the acidocalcisomes (Ac) as empty vacuoles containing some electron-dense material (dots and electron-dense material on the membrane of the organelle); the contractile vacuole bladder (CV) and spongiome (S) are also apparent; (C) staining of acidocalcisomes with acridine orange. The acidocalcisomes are shown in orange. Notations are flagellar pocket (FP), acidocalcisomes (Ac), kinetoplast (K), contractile vacuole bladder (CV), tubules forming the spongione (S), reservosomes (R), nucleus (N). Bars, A, B, C = 2.0 μm. (See Color Section.)

et al., 2003; Ruiz et al., 2001a). *T. cruzi* is especially rich in short-chain poly P such as poly P_3, poly P_4 and poly P_5 (Moreno et al., 2000). On the basis of its total concentration (Ruiz et al., 2001a) and the relative volume of acidocalcisomes in the different stages of *T. cruzi* (about 1–2% of the total cell volume; Miranda et al., 2000), it was calculated that the concentration in the organelles would be in the molar range (3–5 M; Docampo et al., 2005). This is congruent with the detection of solid-state condensed phosphates by magic-angle spinning NMR techniques (Moreno et al., 2002) and with the very high electron density of acidocalcisomes (Miranda et al., 2000; Scott et al., 1997). Carbohydrates and lipids could be involved in maintaining these physical characteristics (Salto et al., 2008).

Some enzymatic activities have been detected in acidocalcisomes of *T. cruzi,* such as a poly P kinase and an exopolyphosphatase (Fang et al., 2007b; Ruiz et al., 2001a). Synthesis of poly P in the yeast vacuole (Hothorn et al., 2009) and in acidocalcisomes of trypanosomatids (Fang et al., 2007a) is mediated by the "vacuolar transporter chaperone" (Vtc) complex, which comprises four proteins in yeasts (Vtc 1–4) anchored in the vacuole membrane and probably two (Vtc1 and Vtc4) anchored in the acidocalcisome membrane of trypanosomatids. Vtc4 has the catalytic activity and functions polymerizing and translocating the poly P chain through the vacuole membrane (Hothorn et al., 2009).

A scheme of all the enzymes and transporters identified in acidocalcisomes of *T. cruzi* is depicted in Fig. 14.2. Acidocalcisome membranes possess several pumps and at least one channel. A vanadate-sensitive Ca^{2+}-ATPase was first detected in acidocalcisomes of *T. cruzi* permeabilized with digitonin (Docampo et al., 1995) and later found in the isolated organelles (Scott and Docampo, 2000). A gene encoding the acidocalcisome Ca^{2+}-ATPase was identified and used to complement yeast mutants that were deficient in the vacuolar Ca^{2+}-ATPase gene *PMC1,* giving evidence of its functionality (Lu et al., 1998). This Ca^{2+}-ATPase is closely related to the family of plasma membrane-type Ca^{2+}-ATPases (PMCA), although it does not have a typical calmodulin-binding domain. Two proton pumps have been detected in acidocalcisomes of *T. cruzi.* One is the multisubunit vacuolar-type H^+-ATPase (Docampo et al., 1995) and the other is the vacuolar-type proton pyrophosphatase (V-H^+-PPase; Hill et al., 2000; Scott et al., 1998), which uses PPi instead of ATP as energy source to transport protons. The vacuolar-type proton ATPase (V-H^+-ATPase) was shown, by immunofluorescence and immunoelectron microscopy, to co-localize to acidocalcisomes with the vacuolar-type Ca^{2+}-ATPase (Lu et al., 1998).

The K^+-stimulated V-H^+-PPase of *T. cruzi* was the first example of this type of enzymes found in any organism different from bacteria or plants (Scott et al., 1998). The enzyme was also found in the Golgi apparatus and plasma membrane (Martinez et al., 2002) and in the contractile vacuole

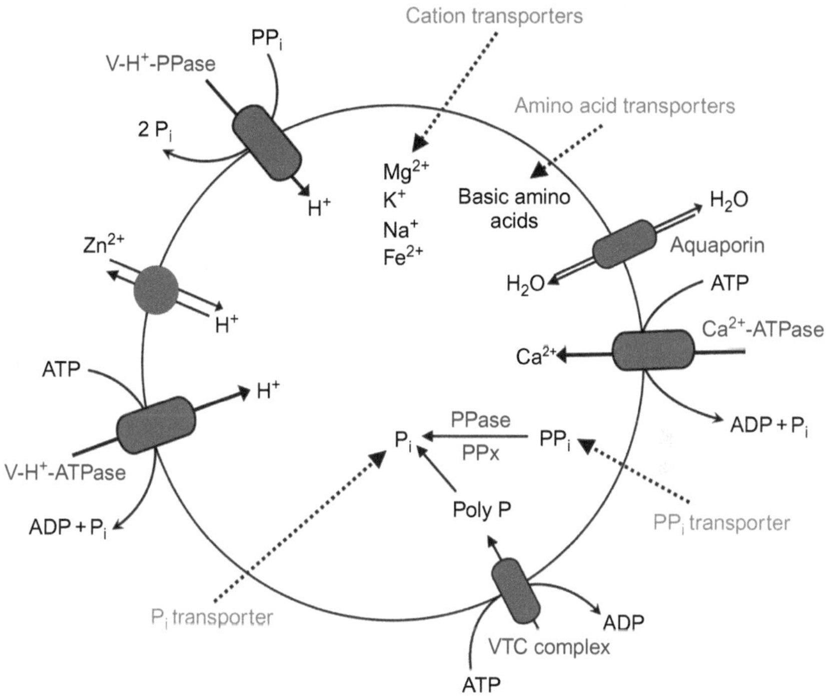

FIGURE 14.2 *Schematic representation of an acidocalcisome.* A H^+ gradient is established by a vacuolar ATPase (V-H^+-ATPase) and a vacuolar pyrophosphatase (V-H^+-PPase). Ca^{2+} transport is driven by a Ca^{2+}-ATPase. Other transporters include a Zn^{2+}/H^+ antiporter, and a water channel or aquaporin. A Vtc complex is involved in synthesis and translocation of poly P. Transporters for basic amino acids, P_i, PP_i and cations are potentially present. The matrix is rich in PP_i and polyphosphate (poly P), and enzymes involved in their metabolism are exopolyphosphatase (PPX) and pyrophosphatase (PPase).

complex (CVC; Rohloff et al., 2004) of *T. cruzi*, although it is predominantly localized in the acidocalcisome and can be used as a marker for this organelle purification (Scott and Docampo, 2000). The gene for the *T. cruzi* V-H^+-PPase could be functionally expressed in yeast (Hill et al., 2000). It was found recently that the N-terminal region of the *T. cruzi* V-H^+-PPase, when fused to other protist enzymes, enhances their functional expression in yeast (Drake et al., 2010). An aquaporin has also been identified in acidocalcisomes of *T. cruzi* (Montalvetti et al., 2004). The protein acts as a water channel and is unable to transport glycerol when expressed in *Xenopus* oocytes (Montalvetti et al., 2004). A zinc-transporter-like protein was also identified by proteomic analysis and by co-localization of the tagged protein with the V-H^+-PPase (Ferella et al., 2008).

14.3. VOLUME REGULATION

Any change in the intracellular and extracellular solute content generates the immediate flow of water into or out of the eukaryotic cell until equilibrium is achieved (Choe and Strange, 2009). This water flow through channels, driven by osmotic pressure gradients, causes swelling or shrinkage of the cells. Cells respond to these volume changes by activating volume-regulatory mechanisms. The processes by which swollen and shrunken cells return to a normal volume are known as *regulatory volume decrease* (RVD) and *regulatory volume increase* (RVI), respectively. Regulation of cell volume in most eukaryotic cells is by the gain or loss of osmotically active solutes that could be inorganic ions such as Na^+, K^+ and Cl^- or small organic molecules known as *organic osmolytes*, such as polyols (e.g. sorbitol, *myo*-inositol), amino acids and their derivatives (e.g. taurine, alanine and proline) and methylamines (e.g. betaine and glycerophosphorylcholine; Choe and Strange, 2009). Some protists, however, rely on a CVC to maintain their water balance both under normal environmental conditions and during dramatic osmotic changes in their environment (Allen et al., 2009). Both mechanisms, the release of ions and osmolytes and the function of the CVC, are important for volume regulation in different stages of *T. cruzi* (Rohloff and Docampo, 2008). It is possible that under normal environmental conditions the CVC is responsible for most water efflux needed to maintain the steady-state volume of the cells.

RVD and RVI are important homeostatic mechanisms needed by all cells under steady-state conditions, and in addition, they are essential for the adaptation of *T. cruzi* to the diverse environmental conditions that the parasite must encounter during its life cycle. For instance, there is a considerable increase in the osmolarity in the lower digestive tract of the insect vector. Osmolarity increases slightly from the faeces to the urine, from 320 to 410 mOsm kg^{-1}, but there is a very strong increase in the yellow rectal content, up to 1000 mOsm kg^{-1} (Kollien et al., 2001). When metacyclic trypomastigotes are introduced into a new host, there is again a dramatic change, back to the normal osmolarity in the tissues and blood (330 mOsm kg^{-1}). Entry of the trypomastigote into a parasitophorous vacuole and its release into the cytosol could potentially involve changes in osmolarity although it is difficult to have a correct estimate of the osmolarity of different regions of a cell. Therefore, the parasite is subjected to both hyperosmotic and hyposmotic stresses during its life cycle and needs mechanisms to adapt to both stress conditions.

Physiological adaptations to hyposmotic stress in different stages of *T. cruzi* have been studied more extensively. The results have indicated that an RVD mechanism is present in all stages, amastigotes, epimastigotes and trypomastigotes (Rohloff et al., 2003). The process is rapid and essentially complete in all *T. cruzi* stages by 5 min. Amino acid efflux accounts for ~50% of the RVD at 150 mOsm in all stages of *T. cruzi* (Rohloff et al., 2003), while the rest depends on K^+ efflux (7%) and the function of the CVC (43%; Rohloff and Docampo, 2008). A number of uncharged or acidic amino acids are mobilized during hyposmotic stress in all three stages, and there is a marked absence of mobilization of cationic amino acids. Glu, Gly, Pro and Ala account for nearly 90% of the total amino acids mobilized (Rohloff et al., 2003). These results suggest that amino acid efflux in *T. cruzi* occurs through anion channels/transporters as proposed in other cells (Lang, 2007; Vieira et al., 1996). Acidocalcisomes contain high concentrations of amino acids, but nearly 90% of them consist of Arg and Lys, minor components of the amino acids released extracellularly during RVD (Rohloff et al., 2003). A rise in intracellular Ca^{2+} occurs upon hyposmotic stress which is completely dependent on extracellular calcium and, although it plays a role in modulating the early phase of amino acid efflux, is not a key determinant of the final outcome of the RVD (Rohloff et al., 2003). Na^+ and phosphate are not released extracellularly. Inositol efflux to the extracellular medium is negligible (Rohloff et al., 2003).

14.4. THE CONTRACTILE VACUOLE COMPLEX

The CVC was first described in *Paramecium* more than 200 years ago (Spallanzani, 1799) and was later found in a wide range of amoeba, photosynthetic and nonphotosynthetic flagellates and ciliates. Clark (1959) was the first to describe the presence of a CVC in *T. cruzi* and reported a pulsation period (time between contractions) in epimastigotes between 1 min and 1 min and 15 s.

The contractile vacuole complex (CVC) of *T. cruzi* has a bipartite structure, consisting of a central vacuole or bladder and a surrounding loose network of tubules and vesicles known as the spongiome (Rohloff et al., 2004; Figs. 14.1B and 14.3). The spongiome and central vacuole form a stable interconnected network that collapses during systole. Functional distinctions between the peripheral and central components of the CVC were evidenced by the localization of different proteins to each compartment. Recent proteomic analysis and fluorescence studies of green fluorescent protein (GFP)-tagged proteins have revealed the presence of the vacuolar H^+-ATPase, Rab11, Rab32, AP180, VAMP1 and a putative phosphate transporter (PT) to the bladder while calmodulin and two SNAREs are localized to the spongiome (Ulrich et al., 2011).

It has been pointed out that because no CV from any organism characterized to date is significantly acidic (e.g. one study (Stock et al., 2002)

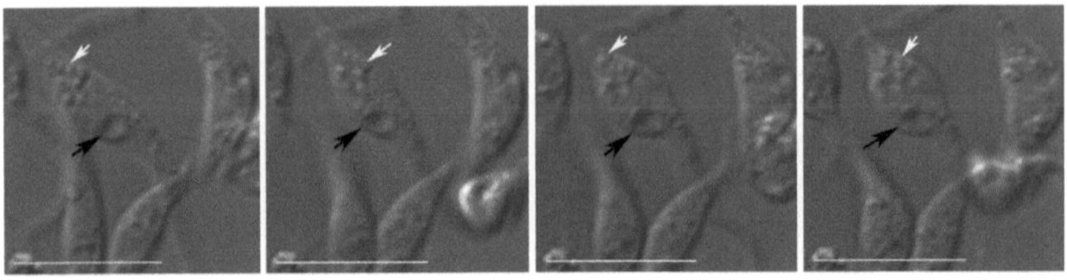

FIGURE 14.3 *Live cell imaging of the contractile vacuole. T. cruzi* epimastigotes were submitted to hyposmotic stress (150 mOsm) to detect swelling of the contractile vacuole bladder (arrows). Note that the cells become rounded after the stress and there is also swelling of smaller vacuoles in the posterior part of the cells. Pictures were taken at 5-s intervals after hyposmotic stress for a total time of 6 min. Initial 20 s of the response are shown in the figure. Bars = 10 μm.

calculated the pH of the CV in *Paramecium multimicronucleatum* to be 6.4), the H^+-ATPases most likely provide instead the primary electrochemical gradient for the movement of other ions (Allen and Naitoh, 2002). Interestingly, the CVC of *T. cruzi* also possesses a vacuolar H^+-pyrophosphatase (Rohloff et al., 2004), which would provide a redundant mechanism for generating an electrochemical potential. The roles of the CVs in protists, though, extend beyond regulation of cell volume to maintenance of Ca^{2+} homeostasis (Malchow et al., 2006; Moniakis et al., 1999; Xie et al., 1996) and transport of proteins to the plasma membrane (Sesaki et al., 1997), although these functions have not been investigated in *T. cruzi*. Recently, Hasne et al. (2010) demonstrated that the CV of *T. cruzi* houses a polyamine transporter that can be transferred to the plasma membrane when the incubation media is deficient in polyamines. The CVC of *T. cruzi* also possesses an aquaporin involved in its periodic filling (Montalvetti et al., 2004; Rohloff et al., 2004).

14.5. ACIDOCALCISOMES AND THE CVC

The acidocalcisome was initially postulated as an osmotically active reservoir linked to the CV function in both *Chlamydomonas reinhardtii* (Ruiz et al., 2001b) and *Dictyostelium discoideum* (Marchesini et al., 2002). Inorganic osmolytes, such as P_i, released from hydrolysed poly P, could be transferred from the acidocalcisome to the CV, setting up a favourable osmotic gradient and facilitating net water flux into the CVC for subsequent water elimination (Marchesini et al., 2002). It was proposed that acidocalcisomes, which usually appear as indistinctive empty vacuoles by electron microscopy (Fig. 14.1B), could correspond to the "vesicles" or "vacuoles" that were identified in free-living protozoa as dynamically fusing with the spongiome portion of the CV. More recent work established that hyposmotic stress conditions result in a significant increase in cyclic AMP (cAMP), swelling of acidocalcisomes and displacement of GFP-labelled aquaporin from the acidocalcisomes to the CVC in a microtubule- and cAMP-dependent fashion (Rohloff et al., 2004). Fusion of acidocalcisomes to the CVC was initially suggested by their apparent continuity in intact cells and subcellular fractions and by electron microscopy observation of similar electron-dense material in both organelles, and was detected by video microscopy (Rohloff et al., 2004). In addition, hyposmotic stress induces a rapid rise in intracellular ammonia, up to 1 mM in whole cell terms, which is rapidly sequestered into acidocalcisomes (Rohloff and Docampo, 2006).

The translocation mechanism of an aquaporin from vesicles to other membranes is similar to that described in mammalian cells; a cAMP-mediated event is involved in fusion of AQP2- (Nielsen et al., 1995) and AQP8- (Garcia et al., 2001) containing vesicles to the plasma membrane. On the other hand, an acetylcholine-induced rise in Ca^{2+} induces fusion of AQP5 vesicles, probably through a protein kinase C-mediated phosphorylation event (Ishikawa et al., 1998).

14.6. SIGNALLING PATHWAYS INVOLVED IN VOLUME REGULATION

The study of the cAMP pathway in *T. cruzi* has been limited. The predicted structure of *T. cruzi* adenylyl cyclases consists of a large presumably extracellular N-terminal domain, followed by a single membrane-spanning helix and an intracellular catalytic domain (Taylor et al., 1999). This is different from the typical 12-transmembrane spanning structure of G-protein-coupled adenylyl cyclases. The structure suggests that these adenylyl cyclases might function as catalytic receptors, ruling out the participation of heterotrimeric G-proteins or other regulatory factors. Further, heterotrimeric G-proteins have not been identified in *T. cruzi* (Parsons and Ruben, 2000). Only one adenylyl cyclase gene of the near 30 genes annotated in the genome of *T. cruzi* (TriTryp.DB) has been studied in detail. The protein product localizes to the flagellum and is activated by calcium (D'Angelo et al., 2002). The increase in cAMP levels after cell swelling might suggest the activation of either a mechanosensitive adenylyl cyclase like the one that occurs in coronary vascular smooth cells (Mills et al., 1990) or of a mechanosensitive channel (Xiao and Xu, 2010) that could lead to the influx of ions, such as Ca^{2+}, and activation of the adenylyl cyclase upon hyposmotic stress. How cAMP exerts its action is unknown. Homologues of a protein kinase A catalytic (Huang et al., 2002) and regulatory (Huang et al., 2006) subunits have been identified in

T. cruzi, but it is still uncertain whether this PKA is stimulated by cAMP. *T. cruzi* AQP1 could be phosphorylated *in vitro* by bovine PKA (Bao et al., 2008), but no experiments were done with the *T. cruzi* enzyme.

cAMP phosphodiesterases (PDEs) are responsible for the termination of cAMP signals by hydrolysing cAMP to 5′-AMP. There are four groups of PDEs in *T. cruzi*: **A** (two genes), **B** (two genes), **C** (one gene) and **D** (two genes). All four PDEs belong to the class I group of PDEs, similar to the large number of class I PDEs found in mammals (Laxman and Beavo, 2007). *T. cruzi* PDEC (TcrPDEC) is a novel and rather unusual PDE that, unlike all other class I PDEs, has its catalytic domain localized in the middle of the polypeptide chain (Alonso et al., 2006; Kunz et al., 2005). In contrast, PDEs have unique N-terminal regulatory domains and the catalytic domain is usually located near their C-terminus. TcrPDEC is the only trypanosome PDE identified to date capable of hydrolysing cyclic guanosine monophosphate (cGMP), although it prefers cAMP as a substrate (cAMP K_m 30 μM and cGMP K_m 80 μM; Kunz et al., 2005). Additionally, TcrPDEC is unusual in that its N-terminal region contains a FYVE-type domain, a functional domain that has not been found in any PDE so far. TcrPDEC was recently found to localize to the CVC (Schoijet et al., 2010). The FYVE domain was shown to be important for the activity of the enzyme and for its localization in the CVC (Schoijet et al., 2010). This is the PDE involved in osmoregulation since the same compounds that inhibit the activity of the recombinant enzyme (Kunz et al., 2005) inhibit CVC swelling that occurs after hyposmotic stress (Rohloff et al., 2004).

Another enzyme potentially involved in volume regulation is the class III phosphatidylinositol 3-kinase (PI3K), related to the yeast vacuolar protein sorting 34, Vps34p, and their homologues from other eukaryotes. These kinases specifically phosphorylate phosphatidylinositol to produce phosphatidylinositol 3-phosphate (PI3P) and are associated with a Vps15p-like protein kinase. *T. cruzi* PI3K was functionally characterized and was able to complement yeast deficient in Vsp34p (Schoijet et al., 2008). Parasites overexpressing TcPI3K showed an enlarged CVC and protection against inhibition of the RVD by the PI3K inhibitors wortmannin and LY294,000 (Schoijet et al., 2008) suggesting a role in volume regulation.

14.7. DRUG TARGETING OF THE VOLUME-REGULATORY PATHWAY

PDEs are validated pharmacological targets for the treatment of several human diseases, such as erectile dysfunction (sildenafil, tadalafil, vardenafil), congestive heart failure (milrinone), platelet aggregation and intermittent claudication (cilostazol) and pulmonary hypertension (sildenafil).

TcrPDEC has sequence similarity to human PDE4. Since many PDE4 inhibitors are currently under development for the treatment of inflammatory diseases, such as asthma, chronic obstructive pulmonary disease, and psoriasis, as well as for treating depression and serving as cognitive enhancers (Houslay et al., 2005), an extensive literature and a number of compounds with potentially little activity against human PDE4s but potentially effective against TcrPDEC are possibly available that could be tested against *T. cruzi*.

A number of compounds originally synthesized as potential PDE4 inhibitors (Zheng et al., 2008) were tested on *T. cruzi* amastigote growth, and several useful hits were obtained (King-Keller et al., 2010). A homology modelling of *T. cruzi* PDEC based on the structure of PDE4B was constructed and other potential inhibitors were obtained through virtual screening (King-Keller et al., 2010). Testing of these compounds on amastigote growth and on the recombinant TcrPDEC activity resulted in several potent inhibitors that caused no toxicity to the host cells (King-Keller et al., 2010). The TcrPDEC was chemically validated as the target for these inhibitors by following the increase in cAMP in the parasites submitted to these inhibitors and the inhibition of their response to hyposmotic stress (King-Keller et al., 2010). The lethal effect of TcrPDEC inhibitors under isosmotic conditions suggests that the cAMP signalling pathway is necessary to overcome dramatic changes in osmolarity that occur not only after hyposmotic stress but also under isosmotic steady-state conditions. Continuous cAMP oscillations, which are known to occur in other cells that have CV mechanisms of water extrusion, such as *D. discoideum* (Monk and Othmer, 1989), could be responsible for the periodic contraction and water expulsion by the CVC that occurs under isosmotic conditions, and explain the absolute essentiality of this mechanism of water regulation in these organisms (King-Keller et al., 2010).

14.8. MODEL FOR VOLUME REGULATION

A model was proposed (Rohloff and Docampo, 2008) in which the stimulus of cell swelling causes a spike in intracellular cAMP through an as yet unidentified adenylyl cyclase, resulting in a microtubule-dependent fusion of acidocalcisomes with the CV and translocation of aquaporin. A simultaneous rise in ammonia (NH_3), and its sequestration in acidocalcisomes as ammonium (NH_4^+), activates an acidocalcisomal exopolyphosphatase, which cleaves poly P, releasing inorganic phosphate residues and also the various poly P-chelated osmolytes, such as basic amino acids and calcium. The resulting osmotic gradient sequesters water through the aid of the aquaporin, which is subsequently ejected into the flagellar pocket. This process is terminated by the action of a PDE (Fig. 14.4).

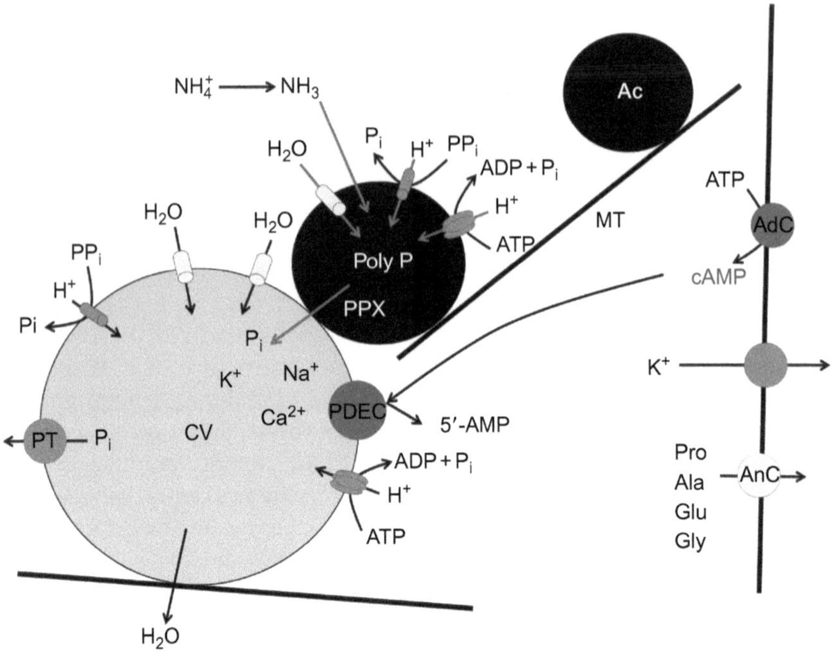

FIGURE 14.4 *Model proposed for regulatory volume decrease in T. cruzi.* Cell swelling causes activation of an adenylyl cyclase (AdC) that results in a spike of intracellular cAMP, resulting in microtubule-dependent movement of acidocalcisomes (Ac) and fusion with the contractile vacuole (CV) with translocation of an aquaporin. A rise in ammonia and its sequestration in acidocalcisomes activates an exopolyphosphatase (PPX) that cleaves poly P, releasing inorganic phosphate residues and also various phosphate-chelated osmolytes, such as calcium and other cations. The resulting osmotic gradient sequesters water, through the aid of the aquaporin, which is subsequently ejected into the flagellar pocket. RVD is completed by the release of amino acids through an anion channel (AnC) and K^+ through a potassium channel both localized in the plasma membrane. Termination of this cycle is by hydrolysis of cAMP through a phosphodiesterase C (PDEC) located in the contractile vacuole (CV). Phosphate is transported back to the cytosol by a phosphate transporter (PT). Proton pumps (V-H^+-ATPase and H^+-PPase) maintain an electrochemical gradient in both the CV and Ac. (See Color Section.)

Since this model was proposed, several supporting results have been reported. For instance, TcrPDEC was shown to localize to the CVC (Schoijet et al., 2010) and inhibitors of this enzyme affect the RVD of *T. cruzi* (King-Keller et al., 2010). This PDE has a FYVE domain, which is a phosphoinositide-binding motif able to bind to PI3P, the product of a PI3K (Alonso et al., 2006; Kunz et al., 2005). Overexpression of TcPI3K was shown to affect the RVD (Schoijet et al., 2008). Several proteins important for vacuolar fusion such as SNAREs and VAMP1 were shown to localize to the CVC and a putative phosphate transporter (PT) was found in the bladder of the CVC (Ulrich et al., 2011). This phosphate transporter (PT) could be involved in recycling of phosphate produced by the hydrolysis of poly P during RVD (Fig. 14.4).

14.9. POLY P, STRESS RESPONSE AND VIRULENCE

Rapid hydrolysis or synthesis of acidocalcisome poly P in *T. cruzi* occurs during hypo- or hyperosmotic stress, respectively (Ruiz et al., 2001a). Overexpression of *T. cruzi* exopolyphosphatase depletes poly P and affects the RVD (Fang et al., 2007b). The use of RNAi to reduce the expression of the acidocalcisomal soluble pyrophosphatase of *T. brucei* (TbVSP1) also resulted in trypanosomes that were deficient in poly P and in their response to hyposmotic stress (Lemercier et al., 2004). Ablation of a vacuolar transporter chaperone 1 (Vtc1) in *T. brucei* by RNAi resulted in abnormal morphology of acidocalcisomes, decrease in their poly P content, and deficient response to hyposmotic stress (Fang et al., 2007a).

In addition to its role in volume regulation, acidocalcisome poly P could have a role in nutritional stress. Knockdown of a TOR-like 1 kinase in *T. brucei* using RNAi leads to growth arrest and accumulation of poly P and PPi inside acidocalcisomes, which increase in size and become heavily stained at the electron microscopy level (de Jesus et al., 2010). It has been suggested that these phenotypic changes would be similar to those occurring during nutritional stress in bacteria (de Jesus et al., 2010). This is known as the "stringent response": amino acid starvation leads to coupled cessation of protein synthesis and stable RNA synthesis. Together with the cessation of nucleic acid synthesis and continued assimilation of Pi from the medium, this results in large accumulations of poly P (Brown and Kornberg, 2004). Knockout of the homologous gene in *Leishmania major* (LmTOR3) resulted in alteration of acidocalcisome morphology, deficient RVD, lower ability to respond to glucose starvation and decreased virulence *in vitro* and *in vivo* (Madeira da Silva and Beverley, 2010). In contrast to the results in *T. brucei* (de Jesus et al., 2010), however, these phenotypic changes were accompanied by an apparent decrease in poly P content of acidocalcisomes although this was not detected by quantitative methods (Madeira da Silva and Beverley, 2010). No studies on this TOR-like kinase 1 (TOR3) have been done on *T. cruzi*. Interestingly, alterations in both acidocalcisomes and poly P content have been associated with reduced *in vivo* virulence in a number of parasites (Besteiro et al., 2008; Lemercier et al., 2004; Luo et al., 2005; Madeira da Silva and Beverley, 2010; Zhang et al., 2005).

14.10. CONCLUSIONS

In *T. cruzi*, acidocalcisomes are rich in short-chain poly P complexed with cations and basic amino acids and possess a number of transporters (Ca^{2+}-ATPase, V-H^{+}-PPase, V-H^{+}-ATPase, zinc transporter) and a channel (aquaporin) involved in the uptake of several ions and water, as well as enzymes involved in poly P metabolism. Acidocalcisomes and their major component, poly P, are essential for the response of *T. cruzi* and other trypanosomatids to different stress conditions. Reduced levels of poly P are associated to decreased ability to respond to osmotic or nutritional stresses and decreased virulence *in vitro* and *in vivo*. A microtubule- and cAMP-dependent signalling pathway is stimulated by hyposmotic stress and results in the transfer of the aquaporin from acidocalcisomes to the CVC. A PI3K is also involved in the response to hyposmotic stress. Acidocalcisomes alkalinize due to ammonia accumulation and also increase their volume in response to hyposmotic stress. A TcrPDEC was localized to the CVC and demonstrated to be essential for volume regulation and survival of the parasite providing a novel target for chemotherapy.

ACKNOWLEDGEMENTS

This work was supported in part by grants AI-077538 (to R. D.) and AI-079625 (to S. N. J. M.) from the U.S. National Institutes of Health. V. J. was supported by a postdoctoral fellowship from the American Heart Association, and S. K.-K. was supported by U.S. NIH training grant AI-060546 to the Center for Tropical and Emerging Global Diseases.

REFERENCES

Allen, R.D., Naitoh, Y., 2002. Osmoregulation and contractile vacuoles of protozoa. Int. Rev. Cytol. 215, 351–394.

Allen, R.D., Tominaga, T., Naitoh, Y., 2009. The contractile vacuole complex and cell volume control in protozoa. In: Evans, D.H. (Ed.), Osmotic and Ionic Regulation. Cells and Animals. CRC Press, Boca Raton.

Alonso, G.D., Schoijet, A.C., Torres, H.N., Flawia, M.M., 2006. TcPDE4, a novel membrane-associated cAMP-specific phosphodiesterase from *Trypanosoma cruzi*. Mol. Biochem. Parasitol. 145, 40–49.

Babes, V., 1895. Beobachtungen über die metachomatischen köperschen, sporenbidung, verzwiegung, kolben- und kapsel-bildung pathogener bakterien. Zentralbl. Bakteriol. Parasitenkd. Infektionskr. Hyg. 20.

Bao, Y., Weiss, L.M., Braunstein, V.L., Huang, H., 2008. Role of protein kinase A in *Trypanosoma cruzi*. Infect. Immun. 76, 4757–4763.

Besteiro, S., Tonn, D., Tetley, L., Coombs, G.H., Mottram, J.C., 2008. The AP3 adaptor is involved in the transport of membrane proteins to acidocalcisomes of *Leishmania*. J. Cell Sci. 121, 561–570.

Brown, M.R., Kornberg, A., 2004. Inorganic polyphosphate in the origin and survival of species. Proc. Natl. Acad. Sci. USA 101, 16085–16087.

Choe, K., Strange, K., 2009. Volume regulation and osmosensing in animal cells. In: Evans, D.H. (Ed.), Osmotic and Ionic Regulation. Cells and Animals. CRC Press, Boca Raton.

Clark, T.B., 1959. Comparative morphology of four genera of trypanosomatidae. J. Protozool. 6, 627–632.

D'Angelo, M.A., Montagna, A.E., Sanguineti, S., Torres, H.N., Flawia, M.M., 2002. A novel calcium-stimulated adenylyl cyclase from *Trypanosoma cruzi*, which interacts with the structural flagellar protein paraflagellar rod. J. Biol. Chem. 277, 35025–35034.

de Jesus, T.C., Tonelli, R.R., Nardelli, S.C., da Silva Augusto, L., Motta, M.C., Girard-Dias, W., et al., 2010. Target of rapamycin (TOR)-like 1 kinase is involved in the control of polyphosphate levels and acidocalcisome maintenance in *Trypanosoma brucei*. J. Biol. Chem. 285, 24131–24140.

Docampo, R., Scott, D.A., Vercesi, A.E., Moreno, S.N., 1995. Intracellular Ca^{2+} storage in acidocalcisomes of *Trypanosoma cruzi*. Biochem. J. 310 (Pt. 3), 1005–1012.

Docampo, R., de Souza, W., Miranda, K., Rohloff, P., Moreno, S.N., 2005. Acidocalcisomes—conserved from bacteria to man. Nat. Rev. Microbiol. 3, 251–261.

Docampo, R., Ulrich, P., Moreno, S.N., 2010. Evolution of acidocalcisomes and their role in polyphosphate storage and osmoregulation in eukaryotic microbes. Philos. Trans. R. Soc. Lond. B Biol. Sci. 365, 775–784.

Drake, R., Serrano, A., Perez-Castineira, J.R., 2010. N-terminal chimaeras with signal sequences enhance the functional expression and alter the subcellular localization of heterologous membrane-bound inorganic pyrophosphatases in yeast. Biochem. J. 426, 147–157.

Fang, J., Rohloff, P., Miranda, K., Docampo, R., 2007a. Ablation of a small transmembrane protein of *Trypanosoma brucei* (TbVTC1) involved in the synthesis of polyphosphate alters acidocalcisome biogenesis and function, and leads to a cytokinesis defect. Biochem. J. 407, 161–170.

Fang, J., Ruiz, F.A., Docampo, M., Luo, S., Rodrigues, J.C., Motta, L.S., et al., 2007b. Over-expression of a Zn^{2+}-sensitive soluble exopolyphosphatase from *Trypanosoma cruzi* depletes polyphosphate and affects osmoregulation. J. Biol. Chem. 282, 32501–32510.

Ferella, M., Nilsson, D., Darban, H., Rodrigues, C., Bontempi, E.J., Docampo, R., et al., 2008. Proteomics in *Trypanosoma cruzi*—localization of novel proteins to various organelles. Proteomics 8, 2735–2749.

Garcia, F., Kierbel, A., Larocca, M.C., Gradilone, S.A., Splinter, P., Larusso, N.F., et al., 2001. The water channel aquaporin-8 is mainly intracellular in rat hepatocytes, and its plasma membrane insertion is stimulated by cyclic AMP. J. Biol. Chem. 276, 12147–12152.

Hasne, M.P., Coppens, I., Soysa, R., Ullman, B., 2010. A high-affinity putrescine–cadaverine transporter from *Trypanosoma cruzi*. Mol. Microbiol. 76, 78–91.

Hill, J.E., Scott, D.A., Luo, S., Docampo, R., 2000. Cloning and functional expression of a gene encoding a vacuolar-type proton-translocating pyrophosphatase from *Trypanosoma cruzi*. Biochem. J. 351, 281–288.

Hothorn, M., Neumann, H., Lenherr, E.D., Wehner, M., Rybin, V., Hassa, P.O., et al., 2009. Catalytic core of a membrane-associated eukaryotic polyphosphate polymerase. Science 324, 513–516.

Houslay, M.D., Schafer, P., Zhang, K.Y., 2005. Keynote review: phosphodiesterase-4 as a therapeutic target. Drug Discov. Today 10, 1503–1519.

Huang, H., Werner, C., Weiss, L.M., Wittner, M., Orr, G.A., 2002. Molecular cloning and expression of the catalytic subunit of protein kinase A from *Trypanosoma cruzi*. Int. J. Parasitol. 32, 1107–1115.

Huang, H., Weiss, L.M., Nagajyothi, F., Tanowitz, H.B., Wittner, M., Orr, G.A., et al., 2006. Molecular cloning and characterization of the protein kinase A regulatory subunit of *Trypanosoma cruzi*. Mol. Biochem. Parasitol. 149, 242–245.

Ishikawa, Y., Eguchi, T., Skowronski, M.T., Ishida, H., 1998. Acetylcholine acts on M3 muscarinic receptors and induces the translocation of aquaporin 5 water channel via cytosolic Ca^{2+} elevation in rat parotid glands. Biochem. Biophys. Res. Commun. 245, 835–840.

King-Keller, S., Li, M., Smith, A., Zheng, S., Kaur, G., Yang, X., et al., 2010. Chemical validation of phosphodiesterase C as a chemotherapeutic target in *Trypanosoma cruzi*, the etiological agent of Chagas' disease. Antimicrob. Agents Chemother. 54, 3738–3745.

Kollien, A.H., Grospietsch, T., Kleffmann, T., Zerbst-Boroffka, I., Schaub, G.A., 2001. Ionic composition of the rectal contents and excreta of the reduviid bug *Triatoma infestans*. J. Insect Physiol. 47, 739–747.

Kunz, S., Oberholzer, M., Seebeck, T., 2005. A FYVE-containing unusual cyclic nucleotide phosphodiesterase from *Trypanosoma cruzi*. FEBS J. 272, 6412–6422.

Lang, F., 2007. Mechanisms and significance of cell volume regulation. J. Am. Coll. Nutr. 26, 613S–623S.

Laxman, S., Beavo, J.A., 2007. Cyclic nucleotide signaling mechanisms in trypanosomes: possible targets for therapeutic agents. Mol. Interv. 7, 203–215.

Lemercier, G., Espiau, B., Ruiz, F.A., Vieira, M., Luo, S., Baltz, T., et al., 2004. A pyrophosphatase regulating polyphosphate metabolism in acidocalcisomes is essential for *Trypanosoma brucei* virulence in mice. J. Biol. Chem. 279, 3420–3425.

Lieberman, L., 1888. Uber das nuclein der hefe und kunstliche darstellung eines nucleus eiweiss und metaphosphatsaure. Ber. Chem-Ges. 21, 598–607.

Lu, H.G., Zhong, L., de Souza, W., Benchimol, M., Moreno, S., Docampo, R., 1998. Ca^{2+} content and expression of an acidocalcisomal calcium pump are elevated in intracellular forms of *Trypanosoma cruzi*. Mol. Cell. Biol. 18, 2309–2323.

Luo, S., Ruiz, F.A., Moreno, S.N., 2005. The acidocalcisome Ca^{2+}-ATPase (TgA1) of *Toxoplasma gondii* is required for polyphosphate storage, intracellular calcium homeostasis and virulence. Mol. Microbiol. 55, 1034–1045.

Madeira da Silva, L., Beverley, S.M., 2010. Expansion of the target of rapamycin (TOR) kinase family and function in *Leishmania* shows that TOR3 is required for acidocalcisome biogenesis and animal infectivity. Proc. Natl. Acad. Sci. USA 107, 11965–11970.

Malchow, D., Lusche, D.F., Schlatterer, C., de Lozanne, A., Muller-Taubenberger, A., 2006. The contractile vacuole in Ca^{2+}-regulation in *Dictyostelium*: its essential function for cAMP-induced Ca^{2+}-influx. BMC Dev. Biol. 6, 31.

Marchesini, N., Ruiz, F.A., Vieira, M., Docampo, R., 2002. Acidocalcisomes are functionally linked to the contractile vacuole of *Dictyostelium discoideum*. J. Biol. Chem. 277, 8146–8153.

Martinez, R., Wang, Y., Benaim, G., Benchimol, M., de Souza, W., Scott, D.A., et al., 2002. A proton pumping pyrophosphatase in the Golgi apparatus and plasma membrane vesicles of *Trypanosoma cruzi*. Mol. Biochem. Parasitol. 120, 205–213.

Meyer, A., 1904. Orientirende untersuchungen über verbreitung, morphologie und chemie des volutins. Bot. Zeitung. 7, 113–152.

Mills, I., Letsou, G., Rabban, J., Sumpio, B., Gewirtz, H., 1990. Mechanosensitive adenylate cyclase activity in coronary vascular smooth muscle cells. Biochem. Biophys. Res. Commun. 171, 143–147.

Miranda, K., Benchimol, M., Docampo, R., de Souza, W., 2000. The fine structure of acidocalcisomes in *Trypanosoma cruzi*. Parasitol. Res. 86, 373–384.

Moniakis, J., Coukell, M.B., Janiec, A., 1999. Involvement of the Ca^{2+}-ATPase PAT1 and the contractile vacuole in calcium regulation in *Dictyostelium discoideum*. J. Cell Sci. 112 (Pt. 3), 405–414.

Monk, P.B., Othmer, H.G., 1989. Cyclic AMP oscillations in suspensions of *Dictyostelium discoideum*. Philos. Trans. R. Soc. Lond. B Biol. Sci. 323, 185–224.

Montalvetti, A., Rohloff, P., Docampo, R., 2004. A functional aquaporin co-localizes with the vacuolar proton pyrophosphatase to acidocalcisomes and the contractile vacuole complex of *Trypanosoma cruzi*. J. Biol. Chem. 279, 38673–38682.

Moreno, S.N., Zhong, L., 1996. Acidocalcisomes in *Toxoplasma gondii* tachyzoites. Biochem. J. 313 (Pt. 2), 655–659.

Moreno, B., Urbina, J.A., Oldfield, E., Bailey, B.N., Rodrigues, C.O., Docampo, R., 2000. ^{31}P NMR spectroscopy of *Trypanosoma brucei*, *Trypanosoma cruzi*, and *Leishmania major*. Evidence for high levels of condensed inorganic phosphates. J. Biol. Chem. 275, 28356–28362.

Moreno, B., Rodrigues, C.O., Bailey, B.N., Urbina, J.A., Moreno, S.N., Docampo, R., et al., 2002. Magic-angle spinning ^{31}P NMR spectroscopy of condensed phosphates in parasitic protozoa: visualizing the invisible. FEBS Lett. 523, 207–212.

Nielsen, S., Chou, C.L., Marples, D., Christensen, E.I., Kishore, B.K., Knepper, M.A., 1995. Vasopressin increases water permeability of kidney collecting duct by inducing translocation of aquaporin-CD water channels to plasma membrane. Proc. Natl. Acad. Sci. USA 92, 1013–1017.

Parsons, M., Ruben, L., 2000. Pathways involved in environmental sensing in trypanosomatids. Parasitol. Today 16, 56–62.

Rohloff, P., Docampo, R., 2006. Ammonium production during hypo-osmotic stress leads to alkalinization of acidocalcisomes and cytosolic acidification in *Trypanosoma cruzi*. Mol. Biochem. Parasitol. 150, 249–255.

Rohloff, P., Docampo, R., 2008. A contractile vacuole complex is involved in osmoregulation in *Trypanosoma cruzi*. Exp. Parasitol. 118, 17–24.

Rohloff, P., Rodrigues, C.O., Docampo, R., 2003. Regulatory volume decrease in *Trypanosoma cruzi* involves amino acid efflux and changes in intracellular calcium. Mol. Biochem. Parasitol. 126, 219–230.

Rohloff, P., Montalvetti, A., Docampo, R., 2004. Acidocalcisomes and the contractile vacuole complex are involved in osmoregulation in *Trypanosoma cruzi*. J. Biol. Chem. 279, 52270–52281.

Ruiz, F.A., Rodrigues, C.O., Docampo, R., 2001a. Rapid changes in polyphosphate content within acidocalcisomes in response to cell growth, differentiation, and environmental stress in *Trypanosoma cruzi*. J. Biol. Chem. 276, 26114–26121.

Ruiz, F.A., Marchesini, N., Seufferheld, M., Govindjee, Docampo, R., 2001b. The polyphosphate bodies of *Chlamydomonas reinhardtii* possess a proton-pumping pyrophosphatase and are similar to acidocalcisomes. J. Biol. Chem. 276, 46196–46203.

Ruiz, F.A., Lea, C.R., Oldfield, E., Docampo, R., 2004. Human platelet dense granules contain polyphosphate and are similar to acidocalcisomes of bacteria and unicellular eukaryotes. J. Biol. Chem. 279, 44250–44257.

Salto, M.L., Kuhlenschmidt, T., Kuhlenschmidt, M., de Lederkremer, R.M., Docampo, R., 2008. Phospholipid and glycolipid composition of acidocalcisomes of *Trypanosoma cruzi*. Mol. Biochem. Parasitol. 158, 120–130.

Schoijet, A.C., Miranda, K., Girard-Dias, W., de Souza, W., Flawia, M.M., Torres, H.N., et al., 2008. A *Trypanosoma cruzi* phosphatidylinositol 3-kinase (TcVps34) is involved in osmoregulation and receptor-mediated endocytosis. J. Biol. Chem. 283, 31541–31550.

Schoijet, A.C., Miranda, K., Medeiros, L.C., de Souza, W., Flawiá, M.M., Torres, H.N., et al., 2010. Defining the role of a FYVE domain in the localization and activity of cAMP phosphodiesterase implicated in osmoregulation in *Trypanosoma cruzi*. Mol. Microbiol. 79 (1), 50–62.

Scott, D.A., Docampo, R., 2000. Characterization of isolated acidocalcisomes of *Trypanosoma cruzi*. J. Biol. Chem. 275, 24215–24221.

Scott, D.A., Docampo, R., Dvorak, J.A., Shi, S., Leapman, R.D., 1997. In situ compositional analysis of acidocalcisomes in *Trypanosoma cruzi*. J. Biol. Chem. 272, 28020–28029.

Scott, D.A., de Souza, W., Benchimol, M., Zhong, L., Lu, H.G., Moreno, S.N., et al., 1998. Presence of a plant-like proton-pumping pyrophosphatase in acidocalcisomes of *Trypanosoma cruzi*. J. Biol. Chem. 273, 22151–22158.

Sesaki, H., Wong, E.F., Siu, C.H., 1997. The cell adhesion molecule DdCAD-1 in *Dictyostelium* is targeted to the cell surface by a nonclassical transport pathway involving contractile vacuoles. J. Cell Biol. 138, 939–951.

Seufferheld, M., Vieira, M.C., Ruiz, F.A., Rodrigues, C.O., Moreno, S.N., Docampo, R., 2003. Identification of organelles in bacteria similar to acidocalcisomes of unicellular eukaryotes. J. Biol. Chem. 278, 29971–29978.

Seufferheld, M., Lea, C.R., Vieira, M., Oldfield, E., Docampo, R., 2004. The H^+-pyrophosphatase of *Rhodospirillum rubrum* is predominantly located in polyphosphate-rich acidocalcisomes. J. Biol. Chem. 279, 51193–51202.

Spallanzani, L., 1799. Tracts on the Nature of Animals and Vegetables. Edinburgh.

Stock, C., Gronlien, H.K., Allen, R.D., 2002. The ionic composition of the contractile vacuole fluid of *Paramecium* mirrors ion transport across the plasma membrane. Eur. J. Cell Biol. 81, 505–515.

Swellengrebel, N.H., 1908. La volutine chez les trypanosomes. C. R. Soc. Biol. Paris 64, 38–43.

Taylor, M.C., Muhia, D.K., Baker, D.A., Mondragon, A., Schaap, P.B., Kelly, J.M., 1999. *Trypanosoma cruzi* adenylyl cyclase is encoded by a complex multigene family. Mol. Biochem. Parasitol. 104, 205–217.

Ulrich, P.N., Jimenez, V., Park, M., Martins, V.P., Atwood, J., III, Moles, K., et al., 2011. Identification of contractile vacuole proteins in *Trypanosoma cruzi*. PLoS One 6, e18013, 1–13.

Vercesi, A.E., Moreno, S.N., Docampo, R., 1994. Ca^{2+}/H^+ exchange in acidic vacuoles of *Trypanosoma brucei*. Biochem. J. 304, 227–233.

Vieira, L.L., Lafuente, E., Gamarro, F., Cabantchik, Z., 1996. An amino acid channel activated by hypotonically induced swelling of *Leishmania major* promastigotes. Biochem. J. 319, 691–697.

Wiame, J.M., 1947. Etude d'une substance polyphosphorée, basophile et métachromatique chez les levures. Biochim. Biophys. Acta 1, 234–255.

Xiao, R., Xu, X.Z., 2010. Mechanosensitive channels: in touch with Piezo. Curr. Biol. 20, R936–R938.

Xie, Y., Coukell, M.B., Gombos, Z., 1996. Antisense RNA inhibition of the putative vacuolar H^+-ATPase proteolipid of *Dictyostelium* reduces intracellular Ca^{2+} transport and cell viability. J. Cell Sci. 109 (Pt. 2), 489–497.

Zhang, K., Hsu, F.F., Scott, D.A., Docampo, R., Turk, J., Beverley, S.M., 2005. *Leishmania* salvage and remodelling of host sphingolipids in amastigote survival and acidocalcisome biogenesis. Mol. Microbiol. 55, 1566–1578.

Zheng, S., Kaur, G., Wang, H., Li, M., Macnaughtan, M., Yang, X., et al., 2008. Design, synthesis, and structure–activity relationship, molecular modeling, and NMR studies of a series of phenyl alkyl ketones as highly potent and selective phosphodiesterase-4 inhibitors. J. Med. Chem. 51, 7673–7688.

CHAPTER 15

Signal Transduction in *Trypanosoma cruzi*

Huan Huang

Contents

Abstract

Signal transduction plays a key role in regulating important functions in both multicellular and unicellular organisms and largely controls the manner in which cells respond to stimuli. Signal transduction pathways coordinate the functions in different type of cells in animals and control the growth and differentiation in unicellular organisms. Intracellular signal transduction pathways are largely activated by second messenger molecules. *Trypanosoma cruzi* has a complex life cycle involving four morphogenetic stages with various second messenger systems able to regulate its growth and differentiation. Signal transduction often alters the status of phosphorylation in target proteins and thus alters the

Department of Pathology, Albert Einstein College of Medicine, Bronx, New York, USA

Advances in Parasitology, Volume 75
ISSN 0065-308X, DOI: 10.1016/B978-0-12-385863-4.00015-0

activities of these proteins. In this review, two major signal transduction pathways, cyclic AMP-dependent pathway and mitogen-activated protein kinase pathway, are discussed. Protein phosphatases are also discussed due to their importance in dephosphorylating target proteins and terminating signal transduction. Understanding of the unique pathways in this pathogen may lead to the development of novel therapeutic agents.

15.1. INTRODUCTION

Signal transduction pathways convert extracellular stimuli into specific cellular responses (Campbell and Reece, 2004). Typically, signal transduction begins with a signal to a receptor and ends with a change in cell function. Sometimes, there is a cascade of signals within the cell. With each step of the cascade, the signal can be amplified, so a small signal can result in a large response (Campbell and Reece, 2004). Eventually, the signal creates a change in the cell, either in the expression of the DNA in the nucleus or in the activity of enzymes in the cytoplasm. Most signal transduction involves the binding of extracellular signalling molecules (and ligands) to cell-surface receptors. Intracellular signal transduction is largely carried out by second messenger molecules such as cyclic-AMP (cAMP) and -GMP (cGMP), calcium (Ca^{2+}), nitric oxide and lipophilic second messenger molecules (diacylglycerol, ceramide and the eicosanoids). In multicellular organisms, numerous signal transduction processes are required for coordinating the behaviour of individual cells to support the function of the organism as a whole (Campbell and Reece, 2004). Many disease processes, such as diabetes, heart disease, autoimmunity and cancer, arise from defects in signal transduction pathways, further highlighting the critical importance of signal transduction to biology, as well as the development of medicine (Huang et al., 2010). Unicellular organisms may also respond to environmental stimuli through activation of signal transduction pathways. For example, slime moulds secrete cAMP upon starvation, which stimulates individual cells in the immediate environment to aggregate (Hanna et al., 1984). Yeast employs mating factors to determine the mating types of other yeast and to participate in sexual reproduction (Sprague, 1991).

Trypanosoma cruzi has a complex life cycle involving four morphogenetic stages (Tanowitz et al., 1992). The epimastigote and metacyclic trypomastigote are insect-specific stages, whereas the blood form trypomastigote and the amastigote are mammalian host-specific, extra- and intracellular stages, respectively. Each developmental stage can be distinguished morphologically and displays stage-specific differences in surface antigens and intracellular components (Andrews et al., 1998;

Contreras et al., 1985). This parasite can adapt to hostile environments such as starvation and host responses by differentiation to a specific life form to survive.

Surface and soluble molecules in *T. cruzi* are important in triggering Ca^{2+} signalling both in the parasite and in the target host cells to achieve invasion (Burleigh and Andrews, 1995; Caler et al., 1998; Yoshida and Cortez, 2008). *T. cruzi* possesses a large and unique organelle called acidocalcisome which can be used for Ca^{2+} storage (Moreno and Docampo, 2009). The details of invasion and acidocalcisome-related Ca^{2+} signalling are discussed in other reviews in this issue of *Advances in Parasitology*. In addition, molecular signalling using eicosanoids was recently discovered in *T. cruzi* (Ashton et al., 2007), and this topic is also covered in this issue.

In this review, two major signal transduction pathways, cAMP-dependent pathway and mitogen-activated protein kinase (MAPK) pathway, will be discussed. Both pathways are highly relevant to modulation of differentiation and proliferation in *T. cruzi* by phosphorylating a set of specific substrate proteins. Reversible protein phosphorylation is one of the most important biological mechanisms for the regulation of adaptive responses to intra- and extracellular signals in many organisms (Cohen, 1989; Kutuzov and Andreeva, 2008; Luan, 2003). Therefore, protein phosphatases are also discussed in this review.

15.2. cAMP-DEPENDENT PATHWAY IN *TRYPANOSOMA CRUZI*

15.2.1. Background

cAMP is a common second messenger with important roles in cell differentiation, growth, hormone regulation, sensory signal transduction and various diseases (Kasai et al., 2010). In the majority of eukaryotes, cAMP homeostasis is regulated by a set of enzymes. It is synthesized by adenylyl cyclases (ACs) using ATP as a substrate (Diel et al., 2008). AC is activated by a range of signalling molecules through the activation of AC stimulatory (G_s) coupled heptahelical receptors and inhibited by agonists of AC inhibitory (G_i) coupled receptors (Pavan et al., 2009). The cyclic nucleotide phosphodiesterases (PDEs) degrade the phosphodiester bond in cAMP to 5′-AMP (Dorsey et al., 2010), abrogating signal transduction. Typical effector proteins of cAMP are protein kinase A (PKA) (Pidoux and Taskén, 2010), exchange proteins directly activated by cAMP (EPACs) and ion channels (Gloerich and Bos, 2010). These pathways have proven to be important clinically, and numerous drugs target receptors coupled to ACs or PDEs. The components of the cAMP pathways in *T. cruzi* are significantly different from their mammalian counterparts; therefore, the cAMP pathways in this parasite should provide an attractive target for the development of new therapeutic agents.

15.2.2. Adenylyl cyclases

With completion of the *T. cruzi* genome, 20 orthologs of ACs have been annotated; five of these ACs are presumably pseudogenes (http://tritrypdb.org/tritrypdb/); and the reminders are orthologs of receptor-type ACs. AC activity was described in purified plasma membrane fractions from epimastigote several decades ago (Zingales et al., 1979). Taylor et al. was the first to describe and characterize the multigene family of ACs in *T. cruzi.* Two complete genes and one pseudogene have been sequenced. D'Angelo et al. also characterized a novel Ca^{2+}-stimulated AC which interacts with the structural flagellar protein paraflagellar rod. Recombinant catalytic domains of all these proteins display AC activity *in vitro*, which was enhanced by divalent cations in a dose-dependent manner (D'Angelo et al., 2002; Taylor et al., 1999). This finding suggests that Ca^{2+} signalling may activate these ACs and increase cAMP concentration in *T. cruzi.* This is interesting for both cAMP and Ca^{2+} second messengers have been described to be the main signals involved in the differentiation process of these parasites (Lammel et al., 1996).

The significant differences between *T. cruzi* ACs (*Tc*ACs) and their mammalian counterparts are striking. *T. cruzi* ACs lack a binding region for heterotrimeric G proteins and do not require G proteins for biochemical activity (D'Angelo et al., 2002; Taylor et al., 1999). Consistent with this, no ortholog of heterotrimeric G protein has been annotated in the *T. cruzi* genome. All trypanosome cyclases have long, diverse extracellular regions and a single transmembrane domain, which is followed by a single, well-conserved intracellular catalytic region. The extracellular domain may serve as a receptor or environmental sensor similar to the guanylyl cyclase receptors of the olfactory epithelium (Yu et al., 1997). The intracellular catalytic region likely generates cAMP upon the activation signals relayed from the sensor (the extracellular domain). *Tc*ACs may require dimerization for activity, based on the biochemical and structural studies of *Trypanosoma brucei* ACs which are similar to *Tc*ACs. Functionally, the dimerization of *Tc*ACs has been verified *in vitro* (D'Angelo et al., 2002). The mechanism(s) involved in regulation of *Tc*ACs remain unknown. It is likely that extracellular stimulation or environmental stresses trigger the activation of these ACs. To this end, it has been reported that a peptide produced by proteolysis of α^{d}-globin in the hindgut of *Triatoma infestans* vector can stimulate AC activity and induce differentiation of epimastigotes to metacyclic trypomastigotes (Fraidenraich et al., 1993; Garcia et al., 1995). These observations are particularly intriguing because they suggest that initial AC activation and subsequent trypanosome differentiation may be triggered by factors synthesized within the host, but not by the parasite itself, indicating parasite–host interaction plays a key role in differentiation. However, extensive studies in this field by independent laboratories are necessary to verify this concept.

15.2.3. Cyclic nucleotide PDEs

PDEs comprise a group of enzymes that degrade the phosphodiester bond in the second messenger molecules cAMP and cGMP. They regulate the localization, duration and amplitude of cyclic nucleotide signalling within subcellular domains. PDEs are therefore important regulators of signal transduction mediated by these second messenger molecules. The PDE superfamily of enzymes is classified into 11 families in mammals, namely PDE1–PDE11 (Keravis and Lugnier, 2010). The classification is based on amino acid sequence, substrate specificity, regulatory properties, pharmacological properties and tissue distribution. PDEs have a great deal of clinical significance as inhibitors of PDE can prolong or enhance the effects of physiological processes mediated by cAMP or cGMP by inhibition of their degradation. For example, Sildenafil, an inhibitor of cGMP-specific PDE type 5, enhances the vasodilatory effects of cGMP and is used to treat erectile dysfunction (Dorsey et al., 2010). Other PDE inhibitors have been identified as new potential therapeutics in variety of other diseases (Galie et al., 2010; Ghofrani et al., 2006; Jaski et al., 1985; Movsesian and Alharethi, 2002).

Several groups have studied PDEs in *T. cruzi*. Three decades ago, Goncalves et al. reported that epimastigote forms of *T. cruzi* contain a soluble cAMP PDE. The *T. cruzi* genome database provides additional information about PDEs in this parasite, with four well-conserved families being defined. A unified nomenclature for these enzymes has been proposed (Kunz et al., 2006), with all four *T. cruzi* PDEs belonging to the Class I group of PDEs, and all being similar to the large number of Class I PDEs found in mammals (Keravis and Lugnier, 2010). Much of our current molecular, biochemical and pharmacological understanding of PDEs in *T. cruzi* comes from the cloning and characterization of *T. cruzi* PDEs identified by several investigations. Alonso et al. reported the identification and characterization of an ortholog of PDEA, a singular PDE of *T. cruzi* (Alonso et al., 2007). In addition, orthologs of the PDEB family in *T. cruzi* have been identified and characterized by two independent groups (D'Angelo et al., 2004; Diaz-Benjumea et al., 2006). Another PDE family in *T. cruzi*, the FYVE-domain containing PDEC family, was identified and characterized (Kunz et al., 2005). Interestingly, this PDEC is a dual-specificity PDE that accepts both cAMP and cGMP as its substrates. Mammalian PDE inhibitors, such as methylxanthines (including 3-isobutyl-1-methylxanthine, caffeine or theophylline), are poor inhibitors of *T. cruzi* PDEs either in intact parasites (Goncalves et al., 1980) or of the recombinant enzymes (Alonso et al., 2007, D'Angelo et al., 2004; Diaz-Benjumea et al., 2006). Thus, experiments in different *T. cruzi* life forms using mammalian PDE inhibitors should be carefully interpreted, for these inhibitors have not been shown to be effective to *T. cruzi* PDEs.

All of the studies of PDEs in *T. cruzi* indicate that the parasitic enzymes are insensitive to mammalian PDE inhibitors. This suggests that the active sites in the parasitic PDEs are substantially different than that of the mammalian counterparts. Therefore, it should be possible to design inhibitors that are selective for the parasitic PDEs without causing side effects due to simultaneous inhibition of the mammalian counterparts. Since the majority of *T. cruzi* recombinant proteins were expressed in PDE null yeasts but purified recombinant proteins or crystal structures are not yet available for any *T. cruzi* PDE, the molecular differences between mammalian and parasitic PDEs active sites remain to be defined. Screening chemical libraries using the partial purified recombinant proteins would be a feasible approach for drug discovery.

15.2.4. Protein kinase A

The PKA, or cAMP-dependent protein kinase family of enzymes, is a collection of serine/threonine kinases whose activity is dependent on the level of cAMP in the cell. Each PKA is a holoenzyme that consists of two regulatory and two catalytic subunits. Under low levels of cAMP, the holoenzyme remains intact and is catalytically inactive. When the concentration of cAMP rises (e.g. activation of ACs by G protein-coupled receptors coupled to G_s or inhibition of PDEs that degrade cAMP), cAMP binds to the two binding sites on the regulatory subunits resulting in release of the catalytic subunits. The free catalytic subunits then mediate the transfer of ATP terminal phosphates to protein substrates at serine or threonine residues. This phosphorylation usually results in a change in activity of the substrate. Since PKAs are present in a variety of cells and act on different substrates, PKA and cAMP regulation are involved in many different pathways. In animals, the two regulatory subunits of PKA are important for localizing the kinase inside the cell in conjunction with A-kinase anchor protein (AKAP). AKAP binds both to the regulatory subunits and to either a component of the cytoskeleton or a membrane of an organelle, anchoring the enzyme complex to a particular subcellular compartment.

cAMP–PKA regulates fundamental functions in many organisms. It has been extensively studied and is one of the best-known members of the PK family (Suzuki et al., 1990; Thevelein and de Winde, 1999). In *Saccharomyces cerevisiae*, PKA regulates cell growth by conveying signals from the small GTP-binding Ras proteins (Broach, 1991; Herman, 2002; Taylor et al., 1990). The two Ras proteins, Ras1 and Ras2, increase AC activity and stimulate the production of cAMP (Field et al., 1990; Taylor et al., 2004). This stimulation results in elevated PKA activity and the increased phosphorylation of substrates that are important for cell growth and proliferation (Toda et al., 1987).

In response to starvation, *Dictyostelium discoideum* becomes a multicellular organism. cAMP acts as both an extracellular messenger, which is secreted by cells in response to starvation, and an intracellular activator of PKA in *Dictyostelium*. Components of the cAMP pathway, including PKA, are essential for differentiation of the cellular components of the fruiting body (Loomis, 1998). In African trypanosomes, cAMP induces the cell cycle arrest that occurs in the differentiation of bloodstream trypanosomes to procyclic forms (Vassella et al., 1997). In *Plasmodium* species that cause malaria, cAMP and levels of PKA have been implicated in gametocyte differentiation (Read and Mikkelsen, 1991).

Since cAMP signalling was found to mediate *T. cruzi* differentiation (Flawia et al., 1997) and PKAs are the major effectors in most eukaryotic cells, the identification of PKA in *T. cruzi* has been pursued by several laboratories. The presence of a PKA activity was suggested by Ulloa in *T. cruzi* (Ulloa et al., 1988), and a catalytic kinase subunit was purified by Ochatt (Ochatt et al., 1993). The molecular weight of the reconstituted holoenzyme suggested a tetrameric structure for the *T. cruzi* PKA. In recent years, Huang et al. cloned and characterized both catalytic (TcPKAc) and regulatory (TcPKAr) subunits (Huang et al., 2002, 2006). Generation of specific mAbs to both subunits indicated that the two gene products were developmentally regulated in different life forms. Co-immunoprecipitation indicated that the two subunits are associated *in vivo*. The complex showed TcPKAc activity and was inhibited by the PKA-specific inhibitor PKA inhibitor (PKI) (Huang et al., 2006). This was the first clear demonstration of a TcPKAr and TcPKAc complex that is activated by cAMP in *T. cruzi*, an important breakthrough in the field. Both TcPKAc and TcPKAr localized to the plasma membrane and the flagellar region (Bao et al., 2010; Huang et al., 2006) in trypomastigote form. TcPKAr was found to interact with several P-type ATPases which suggests that these P-type ATPases may play a role in anchoring PKA to the plasma membrane (Bao et al., 2009).

The functional importance of the TcPKAc has been examined in *T. cruzi*. A gene encoding a PKI containing a specific PKA pseudosubstrate, R-R-N-A, was subcloned into a pTREX vector and introduced into epimastigotes by electroporation. Expression of PKI has a lethal effect in this parasite. Similarly, a pharmacological inhibitor, H89, killed epimastigotes at a concentration of 10 μM. Thus, PKA enzymatic activity is essential for the survival of the parasites (Bao et al., 2008). To understand the biology of PKA, identification of the particular substrates of this enzyme was carried out. Using a yeast two-hybrid system, 38 candidates interacting with TcPKAc were identified. Eighteen of these were hypothetical proteins with unknown functions, while the others had putative or known functions. Eight genes were presumably important in regulating *T. cruzi* growth, adaptation and differentiation, including a type III PI3 kinase (Vps34), a putative PI3 kinase, a MAPK, a cAMP-specific phosphodiesterase (PDEC2), a hexokinase, a putative ATPase, a DNA excision repair protein and an aquaporin. PKA phosphorylated the recombinant proteins of these genes. These findings support the importance of cAMP–PKA signalling in this organism (Bao et al., 2008).

Research also suggests that TcPKAc may mediate protein trafficking of members of the *trans*-sialidase super family which enable the parasite to adhere and invade host cells (Bao et al., 2010). Using a yeast two-hybrid system, several members of the *trans*-sialidase super family were found to interact with TcPKAc. Bidirectional immunoprecipitation using *T. cruzi* lysate confirmed the interactions. An *in vitro* phosphorylation assay demonstrated that PKA phosphorylated the recombinant protein of an active *trans*-sialidase. In addition, a phospho-(Ser/Thr) PKA substrate antibody detected bands on immunoblot analysis of *trans*-sialidase antibody precipitated proteins from parasite lysate and the media of L_6E_9 myoblasts infected with trypomastigotes as well as from a SA85-1.1 antibody precipitated proteins from parasite lysate. The identified *trans*-sialidases have PKA consensus phosphorylation sites located near the endoplasmic reticulum retention motif in the N-terminal (Bao et al., 2010). The correlation that exists between the increased cAMP level, elevated PKA activity and *trans*-sialidase expression in late stage epimastigotes before they differentiate into invasive trypomastigotes is interesting, suggesting that TcPKAc activity may be important for *T. cruzi* differentiation and invasion.

With the completion of the *T. cruzi* genome, two isoforms of TcPKAc were annotated (PKA catalytic subunit isoform-1 [Tc00.1047053508461.310] and isoform-2 [Tc00.1047053508461.280]). So far, only one typical TcPKAr gene has been annotated in the genome, and this has been characterized (Huang et al., 2006). Phosphoproteome analysis of different life stages of *T. cruzi* and bioinformatic analysis of *T. cruzi* genome should help identify additional TcPKAc substrates and the involved pathways. Other known cAMP effector pathways such as EPACs have not been found, and there are no orthologs of EPAC in *T. cruzi* genome. Ion channels that can respond to cAMP or cAMP–PKA pathways in *T. cruzi* plasma membrane have also not been found.

15.3. MAPK PATHWAYS IN *TRYPANOSOMA CRUZI*

MAPKs are well-known mediators of signal transduction of higher eukaryotes regulating important processes like proliferation, differentiation, stress response and apoptosis. They display a high level of evolutionary conservation and are essential for many cellular functions in response to extracellular stimuli. In mammalian cells, four mammalian MAPK cascades are currently recognized, including extracellular signal-regulated kinase (ERK), c-Jun NH_2-terminal kinase/stress-activated protein kinase (JNK/SAPK), p38 and big mitogen-activated protein kinase-1/ERK5 (BMK-1/ERK5) pathways (Avruch, 2007; Camps et al., 2000; Ramos, 2008). These MAPKs are activated by phosphorylation that occurs at specific threonine and tyrosine residues localized within the activation loop motif TxY (T, threonine; x, any amino acids; Y, tyrosine) of kinase subdomain VIII. A prototypical three-component cascade is involved in this activation. MAPKs are activated by a range of diverse stimuli. Activation of MAPKs in cells occurs by several modes, including receptor tyrosine kinase, G protein-coupled receptors and PKC. MAPK pathways may crosstalk with other signal transduction pathways to regulate cellular responses. The PKA pathway and MAPK cascades modulate common processes in the cell, and multiple levels of crosstalk between these signalling pathways have been described. PKA can phosphorylate MAPK signalling components leading to activation or inhibition of MAPKs (Gerits et al., 2008). PKA can inhibit protein phosphatases, by phosphorylating its kinase interaction motif, resulting in the dissociation of MAPKs and protein phosphatases. ERK can inhibit cAMP-specific PDEs, which in turn increases the activity of PKA.

Studies of MAPKs in pathogenic protozoa have revealed the importance of this kinase family in the development of many organisms. Identification of novel MAPKs, TgMAPK1 and TgMAPK2, in *Toxoplasma gondii* has been reported (Lacey et al., 2007). TgMAPK1 and TgMAPK2 are evolutionarily very distant from other MAPK family members. In malaria parasites, *Plasmodium berghei* and *Plasmodium falciparum*, MAPK-2 is required for male gamete formation (Dorin et al., 2005; Rangarajan et al., 2005; Tewari et al., 2005). An atypical activator of MAPK was reported in *P. falciparum* (Dorin et al., 2005; Low et al., 2007; Lye et al., 2006), and the typical three-component signalling cascade does not exist in malaria parasites, suggesting that mechanisms for the activation of MAPKs in malaria are different than their mammalian host. *Giardia lamblia*, an intestinal protozoan parasite, possesses homologues of ERK1 and ERK2, which are involved in encystation (Ellis et al., 2003). In *T. brucei*, deletion of MAP kinase homologue, TbMAPK5, resulted in lower parasitemia and premature differentiation (Domenicali et al., 2006). Deletion of TbMAPK2 affected the differentiation of the parasite (Müller et al., 2002). TbMAPK4 was reported to confer resistance to temperature stress (Güttinger et al., 2007). In *Leishmania* parasites, 15 putative MAPKs have been described (Bengs et al., 2005; Erdmann et al., 2006; Kuhn and Wiese, 2005; Wiese, 1998, 2007; Wiese et al., 2003). Three-component kinase signal transduction pathways are present; however, typical surface activators such as cell-surface receptors are missing, indicating that alternative mechanisms for MAPKs activation exist in these parasites. Members of MAPKs in *Leishmania* parasites have been found to play important roles in flagellar length as well as parasite survival in the infected host (Bengs et al., 2005; Erdmann et al., 2006; Kuhn and Wiese, 2005; Wiese, 2007).

Recently, a *T. cruzi* homologue of ERK2 (TcMAPK2) was cloned and characterized (Bao et al., 2010). TcMAPK2 has high homology with lower eukaryotic ERK2 but has significant differences from mammalian ERK2. Enzymatic assays of both recombinant TcMAPK2 and native protein of TcMAPK2 were catalytically active. The subcellular localization of TcMAPK2 is mainly cytoplasmic in epimastigotes, along the flagella in trypomastigotes and on the plasma membrane of intracellular amastigotes. Phosphorylated TcMAPK2 (active form) was highest in trypomastigotes and lowest in amastigotes. TcMAPK2 was found to interact with TcPKAc- and cAMP-specific phosphodiesterase (TcPDEC)2, suggesting that crosstalk between these signalling pathways may exist in this parasite. Recombinant TcMAPK2 was able to phosphorylate recombinant TcPDEC2, suggesting that TcMAPK2 may participate in regulating cAMP homeostasis in *T. cruzi*. Over-expression of TcMAPK2 in epimastigotes inhibited growth and development leading to death. All these data indicate that TcMAPK2 may have an important role in the stress response of the parasite and may be important in regulating proliferation and differentiation.

With the availability of *T. cruzi* genome, the identification of MAPKs with limited or no homology to mammalian counterparts is becoming feasible. The identification of such TcMAPKs should allow the development of highly parasite-specific therapeutic tools to interdict the pathways. Thirteen TcMAPKs could be identified using the amino acid pattern (TxYxxxRxYRxPE) in a motif search of the *T. cruzi* genome. We analyzed protein sequences of all these TcMAPKs by BLAST and found that five of them are significantly different from mammalian MAPKs (Table 15.1). TcMAPK1, 2, 3, 4 and 9 showed high homology with lower eukaryotes and plant MAPKs but very little homology with mammalian MAPKs. These MAPKs may be good candidates for new drug development. Examination of their role in *T. cruzi* biology should advance our understanding of signalling in this organism. In addition, the identification of substrates for a particular MAPK will also provide understanding of its signalling pathway. The typical consensus for MAP kinases is ΨX [ST] P in which Ψ represents a proline or an aliphatic amino acid (Gonzalez et al., 1991); therefore, MAP kinases can have many substrates. For example, mammalian ERK is a promiscuous kinase which can phosphorylate more than 100 different substrates. TriTrypDB (http://tritrypdb.org) has become a very useful tool in the identification of putative substrates of TcMAPKs. Using ΨX[ST]P as the TcMAPKs consensus

TABLE 15.1 Identification of MAPKs in CL *T. cruzi* genome

Candidates	Motif and position	Copy	Gene ID
Tc MAPK1	TEYVVTRWYRPPE (189–201)	1	Tc00.1047053511299.70
TcMAPK2	TDYIMTRWYRPPE (173–185)	2	Tc00.1047053506007.40 Tc00.1047053510295.50
TcMAPK3	TDYVITRWYRPPE (192–204)	1	Tc00.1047053509553.60
TcMAPK4	TDYVVTRWYRPPE (206–218)	1	Tc00.1047053509065.20 Tc00.1047053506943.10
TcMAPK5	TDYVATRWYRAPE (157–169)	1	Tc00.1047053511025.30
TcMAPK6	TEYVSTRWYRAPE (162–174)	2	Tc00.1047053506211.180 Tc00.1047053511289.50
TcMAPK7	THYVTHRWYRAPE (189–201)	2	Tc00.1047053506229.10 Tc00.10470535511573.40
TcMAPK8	TDYVIMRWYRAPE (182–194)	2	Tc00.1047053511837.70 Tc00.1047053510123.20
TcMAPK9	THYVVTRWYRPPE (270–282)	1	Tc00.1047053511491.80
TcMAPK10	TEYISTRWYRAPE (159–171)	1	Tc00.1047053506885.120
TcMAPK11	TDYVSTRWYRAPE (174–186)	1	Tc00.1047053509719,50
TcMAPK12	TFYVCTRYYRPPE (242–254)	1	Tc00.1047053509105.120
TcMAPK13	TGYLATRWYRAPE (172–184)	1	Tc00.1047053504167.30

Using the amino acid pattern (TxYxxxRxYRxPE) to search homologues of MAPKs in TriTryDB(http:/tritrypdb.org). This motif contains two typical feature of MAPKs, the dual-phosphorylation motif TxY and the (P + 1)-specificity pocket determining the site-directed substrate phosphorylation at serine/threonine followed by proline. 13 MAPKs homologues were identified. Five candidates have two copies in the genome. The five unique TcMAPKs are underlined.

([IVLAPM]x[ST]P) to screen possible substrates of TcMAPKs, we can identify a large number of candidate substrates many of which are hypothetical proteins. Among these proteins are some very interesting MAPK candidate substrates such as dual-specificity phosphatases (DSPs), RNA-editing proteins, cell cycle proteins and PI3 kinases. These proteins contain multiple ΨX[ST]P sites. Some of these proteins are unique to trypanosomatid such as RNA-editing proteins (Table 15.2). Biochemical approaches can now be applied to evaluate if these interesting proteins identified by this bioinformatic approach meet the criteria for being true

TABLE 15.2 Putative substrates of TcMAPKs identified by a bioinformatics approach using ΨX[ST]P

Candidates	Gene ID
RNA-editing complex protein MP81, putative	Tc00.1047053503515.20
RNA-editing complex protein MP81, putative	Tc00.1047053508741.270
RNA-editing complex protein MP61, putative	Tc00.1047053506679.210
Dual specificity protein phosphatase, putative	Tc00.104753508385.40
Dual specificity protein phosphatase, putative	Tc00.1047053504075.6
Dual specificity protein phosphatase, putative	Tc00.1047053506933.98
Tyrosine phosphatase, putative	Tc00.1047053511127.340
Phosphatidylinositol 3-kinase, putative	Tc00.1047053511903.160
Phosphatidylinositol 3-kinase 2, putative	Tc00.104753508859.90
Cell division cycle protein, putative	Tc00.1047053511907.260

These proteins contain at least three ΨX[ST]P sites.

MAPK substrates (e.g. forming complex *in vivo*, *in vitro* phosphorylated by a particular *T. cruzi* MAPK and phosphorylation at ΨX[ST]P site in lysates by phosphoproteomic analysis).

15.4. PROTEIN PHOSPHATASES IN *TRYPANOSOMA CRUZI*

Protein phosphatases dephosphorylate substrates of protein kinases, including PKA and MAPKs, and regulate kinase activity of the MAPKs. Dephosphorylation of either the threonine or the tyrosine residue within the MAPK activation loop T*x*Y motif alone can result in their enzymatic inactivation. Protein phosphorylation is one of the major tools to regulate cellular responses. The immense importance of the phosphorylation networks in eukaryotic biology is underscored by the estimated one-third of cellular proteins that are phosphorylated, with the vast majority of the modifications occurring on serines and threonines. To manage this complex, signalling network requires over 400 serine/threonine kinases encoded in the human genome (Virshup and Shenolikar, 2009). To provide the tight reversible and adjustable control in the robust signalling networks, there exists a similar complexity in the number of serine/threonine phosphatases. However, for phosphatases, unlike kinases, this complexity does not lie in the number of genes encoding phosphatase catalytic subunits. The two most abundant serine/threonine phosphatases, PP1 and PP2A, are encoded by only five catalytic subunit genes in mammals. These serine/threonine phosphatases are obligate multimeric enzymes, assembled from only a small number of catalytic subunits combining with many hundreds of regulatory subunits. The combinatorial and regulatory complexity of protein phosphatases creates specifically targeting enzymes that decode environmental cues and coordinate and control highly regulated biochemical events (Virshup and Shenolikar, 2009).

In mammals, there are four major classes of mammalian serine/threonine phosphatases defined by substrate specificity, divalent cation requirements and specificity of activators/inhibitors: PP1, PP2A and PP2B and PP2C. The first three, PP1, PP2A and PP2B, together form the PPP superfamily of protein phosphatases. PP2C, classified as a PPM, for Mg^{2+}-dependent protein phosphatase, is structurally and mechanistically unrelated (Barford, 1996; Burns et al., 1993). The original classification into type 1 and type 2 phosphatases was based on the observation that type 1 enzymes are inhibited by two heat stable protein inhibitors, protein phosphatase inhibitor-1 (PPI-1) and inhibitor-2 (PPI-2), whereas type 2 enzymes are not inhibited by PP1-1 and PP1-2. PPP classification now takes into account sequence data and other inhibitor profiles.

In *T. cruzi*, the PP1 and PP2A inhibitors, okadaic acid (OA), tautomycin (TA) and calyculin A (CA), were found to trigger differentiation from trypomastigote to extracellular amastigotes (Grellier et al., 1999). Trypomastigotes treated with low concentrations (1 nM) of CA underwent differentiation, forming a rounded amastigote form, and expressing all the markers of amastigotes after the normal differentiation process. Two PP1 isoforms, *Tc*PP1α (Tc00.1047053506201.70) and *Tc*PP1β (Tc00.1047053507671.39), were identified in *T. cruzi*, and the mRNAs were detected in both epimastigote and metacyclic parasites (Orr et al., 2000). CA, but not OA, had profound effects on the *in vitro* replication and morphology of *T. cruzi* epimastigotes. Low concentrations of CA (1–10 nM) caused growth arrest. CA-treated epimastigotes underwent flagellar duplication and both kinetoplast and nuclear divisions but were incapable of successfully completing cytokinesis. These cells also lost their characteristic elongated, epimastigote phenotype and adopted a more rounded morphology, suggesting these PP1 phosphatases are important for the completion of cell division and the maintenance of cell shape in *T. cruzi*. González et al. (2003) characterized *Tc*PP2A (Tc00.1047053511021.10) and found a critical role of PP2As in the transformation of trypomastigotes into amastigotes. In transformation assays at pH 5.0, even low concentrations (0.1 μM) of OA profoundly blocked the transformation of trypomastigotes to extracellular amastigotes. With the completion of *T. cruzi* genome, *T. cruzi* phosphatase catalytic domains were identified by an ontology-based scan of the genome (Brenchley et al., 2007). As compared to other eukaryotic genomes, *T. cruzi* has a low proportion of tyrosine phosphatases and expansion of serine/threonine phosphatases. Additionally, *T. cruzi* has a large number of atypical protein phosphatases, representing more than one-third of the total phosphatases. Most of the atypical phosphatases belong to the DSPs family and show considerable divergence from classic DSPs in both the domain organization and the sequence features (Brenchley et al., 2007).

15.5. PROTEIN KINASES AND PROTEIN PHOSPHATASES AS DRUG TARGET IN *TRYPANOSOMA CRUZI*

There is a very limited arsenal of drugs for *T. cruzi*, and they are highly toxic. Protein kinases are important regulators of many different cellular processes such as transcriptional control, cell cycle progression and differentiation, and have drawn much attention as potential drug targets to treat a wide range of diseases and syndromes, such as cancer, cardiovascular disease and Alzheimer's disease. In recent years, pharmaceutical companies have invested heavily in the development of new compounds directed against specific protein kinase targets, and there are wide ranges of protein kinase inhibitors that have entered clinical trials. Two tyrosine kinase inhibitors, Gleevec and Iressa, are approved to treat chronic myeloid leukaemia and gastrointestinal stromal tumours/ non-small-cell lung cancer, respectively (Naula et al., 2005). Gleevec targets the BCR–ABL tyrosine kinase, and Iressa targets the tyrosine kinase domain of the epidermal growth factor receptor.

Protein kinase inhibitors fall into four main groups: substrate-specific inhibitors, ATP-competitive inhibitors, activation inhibitors and irreversible inhibitors. The ideal protein kinase inhibitor prevents activation rather than competing with the ATP cofactor or the substrate. An example of such an inhibitor is Gleevec, which upon binding induces a conformational change that mimics substrate binding and therefore prevents activation by upstream kinases. However, most inhibitors currently in clinical trials fall into the ATP-competitive inhibitor class. The ATP-binding pocket is well suited to bind specifically designed inhibitors and, despite the relatively high degree of conservation of the ATP-binding pocket, specific inhibitors have been developed. My laboratory group has reported that TcPKAc activity is essential in *T. cruzi* (Bao et al., 2010; Huang et al., 2006). In addition, some TcPKAc substrates identified by yeast two-hybrid screens suggest that TcPKAc may have unique pathways in this organism. Five unique MAPKs were identified all of which are significantly different from their mammalian counterparts. Once their biological role in this organism is defined, they may be useful drug targets.

Protein phosphatases have become "hot" targets in drug discovery in recent years (Cohen, 2002; Guergnon et al., 2006). Specific inhibitors of PPP phosphatases have been widely used to infer the involvement of these enzymes in cellular physiology of parasitic protozoa. Blockade of *Tc*PP1s by inhibitor resulted in failure of cytokinesis in this organism. Inhibition of TcPP2As blocked transformation of trypomastigotes to amastigotes. If a key parasitic protein phosphatase which is crucial in regulating important biological processes in *T. cruzi* but significantly different to mammalian counterpart is well characterized, an inhibitor specific to that parasitic protein phosphatase may be developed. Therefore, parasites will be killed without harming the host. With the availability of the *T. cruzi* genome, detailed analysis of protein phosphatases will improve our understanding of their biochemical features, from which unique targets can be used to develop new therapeutic agents.

15.6. CONCLUDING REMARKS

It is almost three decades since some studies indicated the importance of signal transduction in *T. cruzi* for its proliferation and differentiation. To this end, our knowledge has been steadily improved by the efforts of many scientists. With the availability of the *T. cruzi* genome, many pathways can be evaluated by the presence or the absence of the key components of certain pathways in this organism. Genetic, biochemical and bioinformatic approaches are important in defining the biological significance of these pathways in *T. cruzi*. Cyclic AMP-PKA and MAPK signalling as well as protein phosphatases are significantly different in this pathogen as compared to mammal; therefore, they should be able to be exploited for drug development.

ACKNOWLEDGEMENTS

This work was supported by National Institutes of Health Grants AI 058893 (H. H.) and AI 076248.

REFERENCES

Alonso, G.D., Schoijet, A.C., Torres, H.N., Flawiá, M.M., 2007. TcrPDEA1, a cAMP-specific phosphodiesterase with atypical pharmacological properties from *Trypanosoma cruzi*. Mol. Biochem. Parasitol. 152, 72–79.

Andrews, N.W., Hong, K.S., Robbins, E.S., Nussenweig, V., 1998. Stage-specific surface antigen expressed during the morphogenesis of the vertebrate forms of *Trypanosoma cruzi*. Exp. Parasitol. 64, 474–484.

Ashton, A.W., Mukherjee, S., Nagajyothi, F., Huang, H., Braunstein, V.L., Desruisseaux, M.S., et al., 2007. Thromboxane A2 is a key regulator of pathogenesis during *Trypanosoma cruzi* infection. J. Exp. Med. 204, 929–940.

Avruch, J., 2007. MAPP kinase pathways: the first twenty years. Biochim. Biophys. Acta 1773, 1150–1160.

Bao, Y., Weiss, L.M., Braunstein, V.L., Huang, H., 2008. The role of protein kinase A in *Trypanosoma cruzi*. Infect. Immun. 76, 4757–4763.
Bao, Y., Weiss, L.M., Hashimoto, M., Nara, T., Huang, H., 2009. Protein kinase A regulatory subunit interacts with P-type ATPases in *Trypanosoma cruzi*. Am. J. Trop. Med. Hyg. 80, 941–943.
Bao, Y., Weiss, L.M., Ma, Y.F., Kahn, S., Huang, H., 2010. Protein kinase A catalytic subunit interacts and phosphorylates members of trans-sialidase super-family in *Trypanosoma cruzi*. Microbes Infect. 202, 1104–1113.
Barford, D., 1996. Molecular mechanisms of protein serine/threonine phosphatases. Trends Biochem. Sci. 21, 407–412.
Bengs, F., Scholz, A., Kuhn, D., Wiese, M., 2005. LmxMPK9, a mitogen-activated protein kinase homologue affects flagellar length in Leishmania mexicana. Mol. Microbiol. 55, 1606–1615.
Brenchley, R., Tariq, H., McElhinney, H., Szöor, B., Huxley-Jones, J., Stevens, R., et al., 2007. The TriTryp phosphatome: analysis of the protein phosphatase catalytic domains. BMC Genomics 26 (8), 434.
Broach, J.R., 1991. RAS genes in *Saccharomyces cerevisiae*: signal transduction in search of a pathway. Trends Genet. 7, 28–33.
Burleigh, B.A., Andrews, N.W., 1995. A 120-kDa alkaline peptidase from *Trypanosoma cruzi* is involved in the generation of a novel Ca (2+)-signaling factor for mammalian cells. J. Biol. Chem. 270, 5172–5180.
Burns, J.M., Parsons, M., Rosman, D.E., Reed, S.G., 1993. Molecular cloning and characterization of a 42 kDa protein phosphatase of *Leishmania chagasi*. J. Biol. Chem. 268, 17155–17161.
Caler, E.V., Vaena de Avalos, S., Haynes, P.A., Andrews, N.W., Burleigh, B.A., 1998. Oligopeptidase B-dependent signaling mediates host cell invasion by *Trypanosoma cruzi*. EMBO J. 17, 4975–4986.
Campbell, N.A., Reece, J.B., 2004. Hormones and the endocrine system. In: Biology. Benjamin Cummings, San Francisco, pp. 943–959 (Unit 7).
Camps, M., Nichols, A., Arkinstall, S.J., 2000. Dual specificity phosphatases: a gene family for control of MAP kinase function. FASEB J. 14, 6–16.
Cohen, P., 1989. The structure and regulation of protein phosphatases. Annu. Rev. Biochem. 58, 453–508.
Cohen, P., 2002. Protein kinases—the major drug targets of the twenty-first century? Nat. Rev. Drug Discov. 1, 309–315.
Contreras, V.T., Morel, C.M., Goldenberg, S., 1985. Stage specific expression precedes morphological change during *Trypanosoma cruzi* metacyclogenesis. Mol. Biochem. Parasitol. 14, 83–96.
D'Angelo, M.A., Montagna, A.E., Sanguineti, S., Torres, H.N., Flawia, M.M., 2002. A novel calcium-stimulated adenylyl cyclase from *Trypanosoma cruzi*, which interacts with the structural flagellar protein paraflagellar rod. J. Biol. Chem. 277, 35025–35034.
D'Angelo, M.A., Sanguineti, S., Reece, J.M., Birnbaumer, L., Torres, H.N., Flawia, M.M., 2004. Identification, characterization and subcellular localization of TcPDE1, a novel cAMP-specific phosphodiesterase from *Trypanosoma cruzi*. Biochem. J. 378, 63–72.
Diaz-Benjumea, R., Laxman, S., Hinds, T.R., Beavo, J.A., Rascon, A., 2006. Characterization of a novel cAMP-binding, cAMP-specific cyclic nucleotide phosphodiesterase (TcrPDEB1) from *Trypanosoma cruzi*. Biochem. J. 399, 305–314.
Diel, S., Beyermann, M., Navarro-LLorens, J.M., Wittig, B., Kleuss, C., 2008. Two interaction sites on mammalian adenylyl cyclase type I and II: modulation by calmodulin and Gbg. Biochem. J. 411, 449–456.
Domenicali, P.D., Burkard, G., Morand, S., Renggli, C.K., Roditi, I., Vassella, E., 2006. A mitogen-activated protein kinase controls differentiation of bloodstream forms of *trypanosoma brucei*. Eukaryot. Cell 5, 1126–1135.

Dorin, D., Semblat, J.P., Poullet, P., Alano, P., Goldring, J.P., Whittle, C., et al., 2005. PfPK7, an atypical MEK-related protein kinase, reflects the absence of classical three-component MAPK pathways in the human malaria parasite *plasmodium falciparum*. Mol. Microbiol. 55, 184–196.

Dorsey, P., Keel, C., Klavens, M., Hellstrom, W.J., 2010. Phosphodiesterase type 5 (PDE5) inhibitors for the treatment of erectile dysfunction. Expert Opin. Pharmacother. 11, 1109–1122.

Ellis, J.G., 4th, Davila, M., Chakrabarti, R., 2003. Potential involvement of extracellular signal-regulated kinase 1 and 2 in encystations of a primitive eukaryote, *Giardia lamblia*. J. Biol. Chem. 278, 1936–1945.

Erdmann, M., Scholz, A., Melzer, I.M., Schmetz, C., Wiese, M., 2006. Interacting protein kinase involved in the regulation of flagellar length. Mol. Biol. Cell 17, 2035–2045.

Field, J., Xu, H.P., Michaeli, T., Ballester, R., Sass, P., Wigler, M., et al., 1990. Mutations of the adenylyl cyclase gene that block RAS. Science 247, 464–467.

Flawia, M.M., Tellez-Inon, M.T., Torres, H.N., 1997. Signal transduction mechanisms in *Trypanosoma cruzi*. Parasitol. Today 13, 30–33.

Fraidenraich, D., Peña, C., Isola, E.L., Lammel, E.M., Coso, O., Añel, A.D., et al., 1993. Stimulation of *Trypanosoma cruzi* adenylyl cyclase by an alpha D-globin fragment from Triatoma hindgut: effect on differentiation of epimastigote to trypomastigote forms. Proc. Natl. Acad. Sci. USA 90, 10140–10144.

Galie, N., Rubin, L.J., Simonneau, G., 2010. Phosphodiesterase inhibitors for pulmonary hypertension. N. Engl. J. Med. 362, 559–560.

Garcia, E.S., Gonzalez, M.S., de Azambuja, P., Baralle, F.E., Fraidenraich, D., Torres, H.N., et al., 1995. Induction of *Trypanosoma cruzi* metacyclogenesis in the gut of the hematophagous insect vector, *Rhodnius prolixus*, by hemoglobin and peptides carrying alpha D-globin sequences. Exp. Parasitol. 81, 255–261.

Gerits, N., Kostenko, S., Shiryaev, A., Johannessen, M., Moens, U., 2008. Relations between the mitogen-activated protein kinase and the cAMP-dependent protein pathways: comradeship and hostility. Cell. Signal. 20, 1592–1607.

Ghofrani, H.A., Osterloh, I.H., Grimminger, F., 2006. Sildenafil: from angina to erectile dysfunction to pulmonary hypertension and beyond. Nat. Rev. Drug Discov. 5, 689–702.

Gloerich, M., Bos, J.L., 2010. Epac: defining a new mechanism for cAMP action. Annu. Rev. Pharmacol. Toxicol. 50, 355–375.

Goncalves, M.F., Zingales, B., Colli, W., 1980. cAMP phosphodiesterase and activator protein of mammalian cAMP phosphodiesterase from *Trypanosoma cruzi*. Mol. Biochem. Parasitol. 1, 107–118.

Gonzalez, F.A., Raden, D.L., Davis, R.J., 1991. Identification of substrate recognition determinants for human ERK1 and ERK2 protein kinases. J. Biol. Chem. 266, 22159–22163.

González, J., Cornejo, A., Santos, M.R., Cordero, E.M., Gutiérrez, B., Porcile, P., et al., 2003. A novel protein phosphatase 2A (PP2A) is involved in the transformation of human protozoan parasite *Trypanosoma cruzi*. Biochem. J. 374, 647–656.

Grellier, P., Blum, J., Santana, J., Bylen, E., Mouray, E., Sinou, V., et al., 1999. Involvement of calyculin A-sensitive phosphatase(s) in the differentiation of *Trypanosoma cruzi* trypomastigotes to amastigotes. Mol. Biochem. Parasitol. 98, 239–252.

Guergnon, J., Dessauge, F., Dominguez, V., Viallet, J., Bonnefoy, S., Yuste, V.J., et al., 2006. Use of penetrating peptides interacting with PP1/PP2A proteins as a general approach for a drug phosphatase technology. Mol. Pharmacol. 69, 1115–1124.

Güttinger, A., Schwab, C., Morand, S., Roditi, I., Vassella, E., 2007. A mitogen-activated protein kinase of *Trypanosoma brucei* confers resistance to temperature stress. Mol. Biochem. Parasitol. 153, 203–206.

Hanna, M.H., Nowicki, J.J., Fatone, M.A., 1984. Extracellular cyclic AMP (cAMP) during development of the cellular slime mold *Polysphondylium violaceum*: comparison of accumulation in the wild type and an aggregation-defective mutant. J. Bacteriol. 157, 345–349.

Herman, P.K., 2002. Stationary phase in yeast. Curr. Opin. Microbiol. 5, 602–607.

Huang, H., Werner, C., Weiss, L.M., Wittner, M., Orr, G.A., 2002. Molecular cloning and expression of the catalytic subunit of protein kinase A from *Trypanosoma cruzi*. Int. J. Parasitol. 32, 1107–1115.

Huang, H., Weiss, L.M., Nagajyothi, F., Tanowitz, H.B., Wittner, M., Orr, G.A., et al., 2006. Molecular cloning and characterization of the protein kinase A regulatory subunit of *Trypanosoma cruzi*. Mol. Biochem. Parasitol. 149, 242–245.

Huang, R., Martinez-Ferrando, I., Cole, P.A., 2010. Enhanced interrogation: emerging strategies for cell signaling inhibition. Nat. Struct. Mol. Biol. 17, 646–649.

Jaski, B.E., Fifer, M.A., Wright, R.F., Braunwald, E., Colucci, W.S., 1985. Positive inotropic and vasodilator actions of milrinone in patients with severe congestive heart failure. Dose–response relationships and comparison to nitroprusside. J. Clin. Invest. 75, 643–649.

Kasai, H., Hatakeyama, H., Ohno, M., Takahashi, N., 2010. Exocytosis in islet beta-cells. Adv. Exp. Med. Biol. 654, 305–338.

Keravis, T., Lugnier, C., 2010. Cyclic nucleotide phosphodiesterases (PDE) and peptide motifs. Curr. Pharm. Des. 16, 1114–1125.

Kuhn, D., Wiese, M., 2005. LmxPK4, a mitogen-activated protein kinase kinase homologue of *Leishmania mexicana* with a potential role in parasite differentiation. Mol. Microbiol. 56, 1169–1182.

Kunz, S., Oberholzer, M., Seebeck, T., 2005. A FYVE-containing unusual cyclic nucleotide phosphodiesterase from *Trypanosoma cruzi*. FEBS J. 272, 6412–6422.

Kunz, S., Beavo, J.A., D'Angelo, M.A., Flawia, M.M., Francis, S.H., Johner, A., et al., 2006. Cyclic nucleotide specific phosphodiesterases of the kinetoplastida: a unified nomenclature. Mol. Biochem. Parasitol. 45, 133–135.

Kutuzov, M.A., Andreeva, A.V., 2008. Protein Ser/Thr phosphatases of parasitic protozoa. Mol. Biochem. Parasitol. 161, 81–90.

Lacey, M.R., Brumlik, M.J., Yenni, R.E., Burow, M.E., Curiel, T.J., 2007. *Toxoplasma gondii* expresses two mitogen-activated protein kinase genes that represent distinct protozoan subfamilies. J. Mol. Evol. 64, 4–14.

Lammel, E.M., Barbieri, M.A., Wilkowsky, S.E., Bertini, F., Isola, E.L., 1996. *Trypanosoma cruzi*: involvement of intracellular calcium in multiplication and differentiation. Exp. Parasitol. 83, 240–249.

Loomis, W.F., 1998. Role of PKA in the timing of developmental events in *Dictyostelium* cells. Microbiol. Mol. Biol. Rev. 62, 684–694.

Low, H., Lye, Y.M., Sim, T.S., 2007. Pfnek3 functions as an atypical MAPKK in *Plasmodium falciparum*. Biochem. Biophys. Res. Commun. 361, 439–444.

Luan, S., 2003. Protein phosphatases in plants. Annu. Rev. Plant Biol. 54, 63–92.

Lye, Y.M., Chan, M., Sim, T.S., 2006. Pfnek3: an atypical activator of a MAP kinase in *Plasmodium falciparum*. FEBS Lett. 580, 6083–6092.

Moreno, S.N., Docampo, R., 2009. The role of acidocalcisomes in parasitic protists. J. Eukaryot. Microbiol. 56, 208–213.

Movsesian, M.A., Alharethi, R., 2002. Inhibitors of cyclic nucleotide phosphodiesterase PDE3 as adjunct therapy for dilated cardiomyopathy. Expert Opin. Invest. Drugs 11, 1529–1536.

Müller, I.B., Domenicali-Pfister, D., Roditi, I., Vassella, E., 2002. Stage-specific requirement of a mitogen-activated protein kinase by *Trypanosoma brucei*. Mol. Biol. Cell 13, 3787–3799.

Naula, C., Parsons, M., Mottram, J.C., 2005. Protein kinases as drug targets in trypanosomes and Leishmania. Biochim. Biophys. Acta 1754, 151–159.

Ochatt, C.M., Ulloa, R.M., Torres, H.N., Tellez-Inon, M.T., 1993. Characterization of the catalytic subunit of *Trypanosoma cruzi* cyclic AMP-dependent protein kinase. Mol. Biochem. Parasitol. 57, 73–81.

Orr, G.A., Werner, C., Xu, J., Bennett, M., Weiss, L.M., Takvorkan, P., et al., 2000. Identification of novel serine/threonine protein phosphatases in *Trypanosoma cruzi*: a potential role in control of cytokinesis and morphology. Infect. Immun. 68, 1350–1358.

Pavan, B., Biondi, C., Dalpiaz, A., 2009. Adenylyl cyclases as innovative therapeutic goals. Drug Discov. Today 14, 982–991.

Pidoux, G., Taskén, K., 2010. Specificity and spatial dynamics of protein kinase A signaling organized by A-kinase-anchoring proteins. J. Mol. Endocrinol. 44, 271–284.

Ramos, J.W., 2008. The regulation of extracellular signal-regulated kinase (ERK) in mammalian cells. Int. J. Biochem. Cell Biol. 40, 2707–2719.

Rangarajan, R., Bei, A.K., Jethwaney, D., Maldonado, P., Dorin, D., Sultan, A.A., et al., 2005. A mitogen-activated protein kinase regulates male gametogenesis and transmission of the malaria parasite *Plasmodium berghei*. EMBO Rep. 6, 464–469.

Read, L.K., Mikkelsen, R.B., 1991. Comparison of adenylate cyclase and cAMP-dependent protein kinase in gametocytogenic and nongametocytogenic clones of *Plasmodium falciparum*. J. Parasitol. 77, 346–352.

Sprague, G.F., Jr., 1991. Signal transduction in yeast mating: receptors, transcription factors, and the kinase connection. Trends Genet. 7, 393–398.

Suzuki, N.H.R., Choe, Y., Nishida, Y., Yamawaki-Kataoka, S., Ohnishi, T., Kataoka, T., 1990. Leucine-rich repeats and carboxyl terminus are required for interaction of yeast adenylate cyclase with RAS proteins. Proc. Natl. Acad. Sci. USA 87, 8711–8715.

Tanowitz, H.B., Kirchhoff, L.V., Simon, D., Morris, S.A., Weiss, L.M., Wittner, M., 1992. Chagas' disease. Clin. Microbiol. Rev. 5, 409–419.

Taylor, S.S., Buechler, J.A., Yonemoto, W., 1990. cAMP-dependent protein kinase: framework for a diverse family of regulatory enzymes. Annu. Rev. Biochem. 5, 971–1005.

Taylor, M.C., Muhia, D.K., Baker, D.A., Mondragon, A., Schaap, P.B., Kelly, J.M., 1999. *Trypanosoma cruzi* adenylyl cyclase is encoded by a complex multigene family. Mol. Biochem. Parasitol. 104, 205–217.

Taylor, S.S., Yang, J., Wu, J., Haste, N.M., Radzio-Andzelm, E., Anand, G., 2004. PKA: a portrait of protein kinase dynamics. Biochim. Biophys. Acta 1697, 259–269.

Tewari, R., Dorin, D., Moon, R., Doerig, C., Billker, O., 2005. An atypical mitogen-activated protein kinase controls cytokinesis and flagellar motility during male gamete formation in a malaria parasite. Mol. Microbiol. 58, 1253–1263.

Thevelein, J.M., de Winde, J.H., 1999. Novel sensing mechanisms and targets for the cAMP-protein kinase A pathway in the yeast *Saccharomyces cerevisiae*. Mol. Microbiol. 33, 904–918.

Toda, T., Cameron, S., Sass, P., Zoller, M., Wigler, M., 1987. Three different genes in *S. cerevisiae* encode the catalytic subunits of the cAMP-dependent protein kinase. Cell 50, 277–287.

Ulloa, R.M., Mesri, E., Esteva, M., Torres, H.N., Tellez–Inon, M.T., 1988. Cyclic AMP-dependent protein kinase activity in *Trypanosoma cruzi*. Biochem. J. 255, 319–326.

Vassella, E., Reuner, B., Yutzy, B., Boshart, M., 1997. Differentiation of African trypanosoma is controlled by a density sensing mechanism which signals cell cycle arrest via the cAMP pathway. J. Cell Sci. 110, 2661–2671.

Virshup, D.M., Shenolikar, S., 2009. From promiscuity to precision: protein phosphatases get a makeover. Mol. Cell 33, 537–545.

Wiese, M., 1998. A mitogen-activated protein (MAP) kinase homologue of *Leishmania mexicana* is essential for parasite survival in the infected host. EMBO J. 17, 2619–2628.

Wiese, M., 2007. Leishmania MAP kinases—familiar proteins in an unusual context. Int. J. Parasitol. 37, 1053–1062.

Wiese, M., Kuhn, D., Grünfelder, C.G., 2003. Protein kinase involved in flagellar-length control. Eukaryot. Cell 2, 769–777.

Yoshida, N., Cortez, M., 2008. *Trypanosoma cruzi:* parasite and host cell signaling during the invasion process. Subcell. Biochem. 47, 82–91.

Yu, S., Avery, L., Baude, E., Garbers, D.L., 1997. Guanylyl cyclase expression in specific sensory neurons: a new family of chemosensory receptors. Proc. Natl. Acad. Sci. USA 94, 3384–3387.

Zingales, B., Carniol, C., Abramhamsohn, P.A., Colli, W., 1979. Purification of an adenylyl cyclase-containing plasma membrane fraction from *Trypanosoma cruzi*. Biochem. Biophys. Res. Commun. 550, 722–733.

INDEX

CONTENTS OF VOLUMES IN THIS SERIES

Volume 45

Volume 46

Volume 47

Volume 48

Volume 59

Volume 60

Volume 61

Volume 66

Volume 67

Volume 68

Volume 69

Volume 70

Volume 71

Volume 72

Volume 73

Volume 74

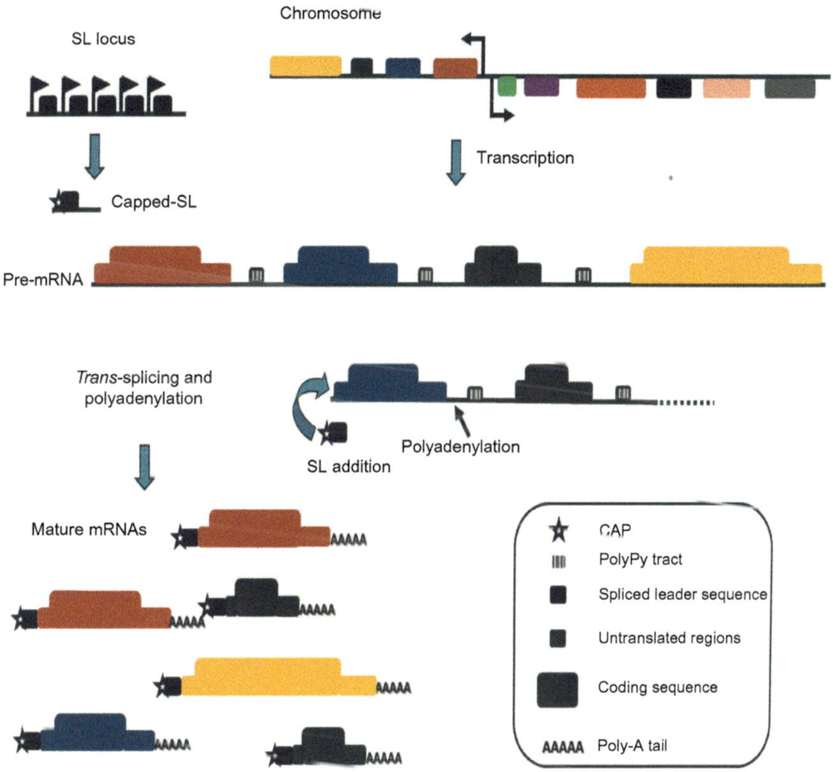

chapter 10, Figure 10.2 **(See page 213 of this volume.)**

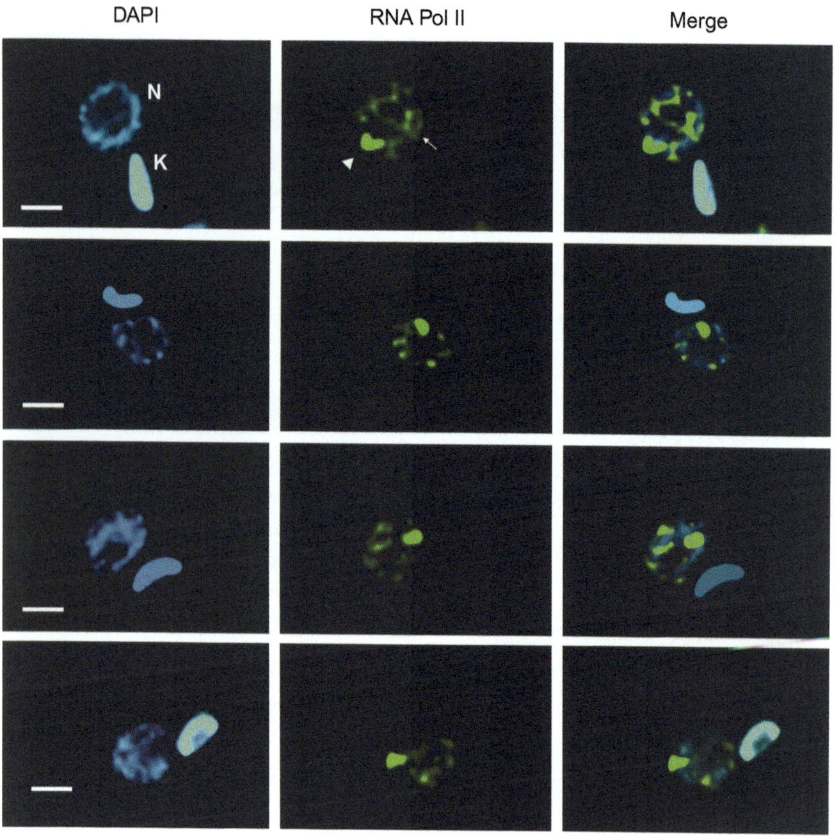

chapter 12, Figure 12.2 (See page 272 of this volume.)

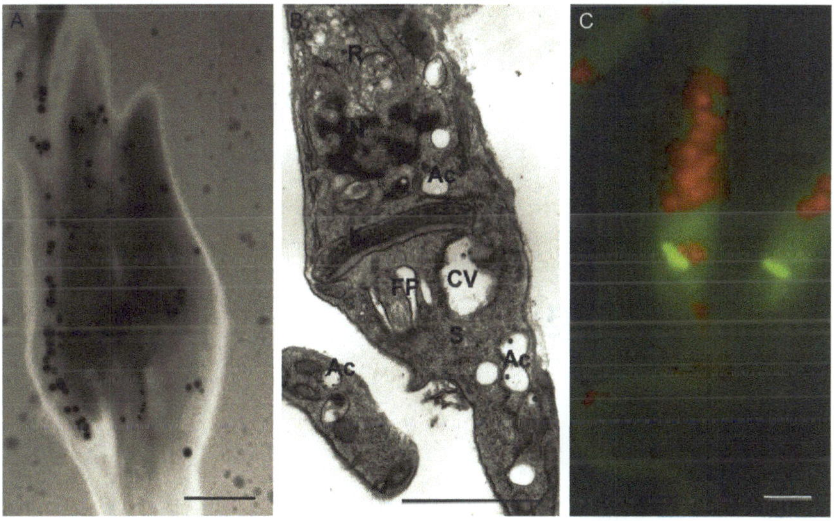

chapter 14, Figure 14.1 (See page 309 of this volume.)

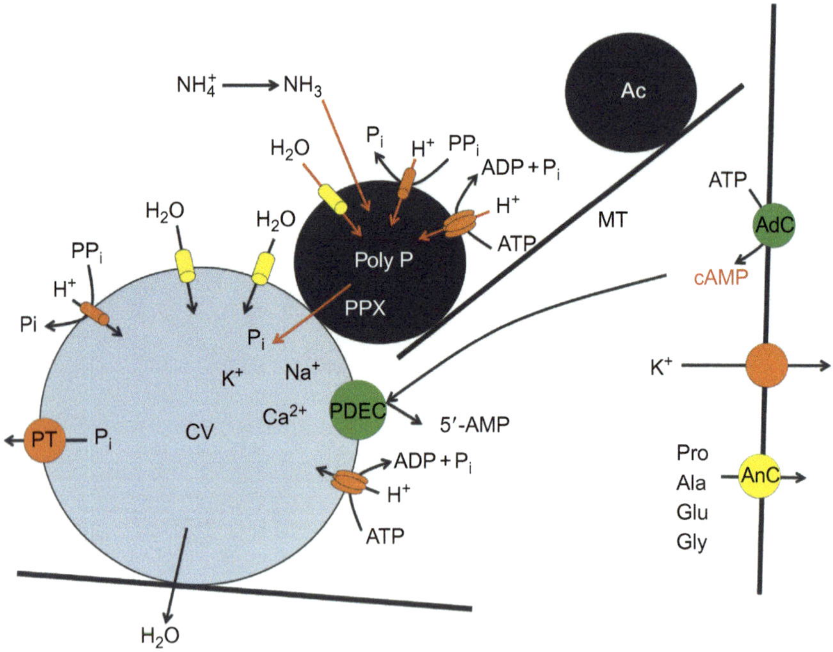

chapter 14, Figure 14.4 (See page 318 of this volume.)

FSC
www.fsc.org
MIX
Papier | Fördert gute Waldnutzung
FSC® C083411

Kolibri 360 GmbH
Ferdinand-Jühlke-Straße 7
99095 Erfurt, Deutschland
produktsicherheit@kolibri360.de